Carolyn Hilarski, PhD
Editor

Addiction, Ass
and Treatr
with Adolescents Adults,
and Families

Addiction, Assessmer
Adults, and Families
as *Journal of Evidence*
bers 1/2 2005.

Pre-publication
REVIEWS,
COMMENTARIES,
EVALUATIONS . . .

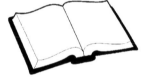

The Haworth Social Work Practice Press
An Imprint of The Haworth Press, Inc.

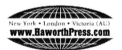

New York • London • Victoria (AU)
www.HaworthPress.com

Addiction, Assessment, and Treatment with Adolescents, Adults, and Families

Addiction, Assessment, and Treatment with Adolescents, Adults, and Families has been co-published simultaneously as *Journal of Evidence-Based Social Work*, Volume 2, Numbers 1/2 2005.

Monographic Separates from the *Journal of Evidence-Based Social Work*™

For additional information on these and other Haworth Press titles, including descriptions, tables of contents, reviews, and prices, use the QuickSearch catalog at http://www.HaworthPress.com.

Addiction, Assessment, and Treatment with Adolescents, Adults, and Families, edited by Carolyn Hilarski, PhD (Vol. 2, No. 1/2, 2005). *An overview of current theory and practice concerning addiction treatment and assessment issues for all populations.*

Kids and Violence: The Invisible School Experience, edited by Catherine N. Dulmus, PhD, and Karen M. Sowers, PhD (Vol. 1, No. 2/3, 2004). *"Important . . . . will benefit school adminstrators, counselors, teachers, and personnel as they come to identify, understand, and act on violence in school settings." (Peter A. Newcombe, PhD, BEd, BA (Hons), Acting Program Director, Behavioural Studies, School of Social Work and Applied Human Sciences, The University of Queensland, Australia)*

Addiction, Assessment, and Treatment with Adolescents, Adults, and Families

Carolyn Hilarski, PhD
Editor

Addiction, Assessment, and Treatment with Adolescents, Adults, and Families has been co-published simultaneously as *Journal of Evidence-Based Social Work*, Volume 2, Numbers 1/2 2005.

The Haworth Social Work Practice Press
An Imprint of The Haworth Press, Inc.

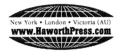

New York • London • Victoria (AU)
www.HaworthPress.com

Published by

The Haworth Social Work Practice Press, 10 Alice Street, Binghamton, NY 13904-1580 USA

The Haworth Social Work Practice Press is an imprint of The Haworth Press, Inc., 10 Alice Street, Binghamton, NY 13904-1580 USA.

Addiction, Assessment, and Treatment with Adolescents, Adults, and Families has been co-published simultaneously as *Journal of Evidence-Based Social Work*, Volume 2, Numbers 1/2 2005.

The development, preparation, and publication of this work has been undertaken with great care. However, the publisher, employees, editors, and agents of The Haworth Press and all imprints of The Haworth Press, Inc., including The Haworth Medical Press® and The Pharmaceutical Products Press®, are not responsible for any errors contained herein or for consequences that may ensue from use of materials or information contained in this work. Opinions expressed by the author(s) are not necessarily those of The Haworth Press, Inc. With regard to case studies, identities and circumstances of individuals discussed herein have been changed to protect confidentiality. Any resemblance to actual persons, living or dead, is entirely coincidental.

Cover design by Kerry E. Mack.

Library of Congress Cataloging-in-Publication Data

Addiction, assessment, and treatment with adolescents, adults, and families/Carolyn Hilarski, editor.
     p. cm.
    "Co-published simultaneously as Journal of evidence-based social work, Volume 2, Numbers 1/2 2005."
    Includes bibliographical references and index.
    ISBN-13: 978-0-7890-2886-0 (hc.: alk. paper)
    ISBN-10: 0-7890-2886-7 (hc.: alk. paper)
    ISBN-13: 978-0-7890-2887-7 (pbk.: alk. paper)
    ISBN-10: 0-7890-2887-5 (pbk.: alk. paper)
    1. Social work with teenagers. 2. Teenagers-Counseling of. 3. Teenagers-Substance use. 4. Teenagers-Alcohol use. 5. Teenagers-Family relationships. 6. Substance abuse-Prevention. 7. Alcoholism-Prevention. I. Hilarski, Carolyn. II. Journal of evidence-based social work.
    HV1421.A33 2005
    362.29'1532–dc22
                                           2004030050

Indexing, Abstracting & Website/Internet Coverage

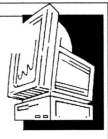

This section provides you with a list of major indexing & abstracting services and other tools for bibliographic access. That is to say, each service began covering this periodical during the year noted in the right column. Most Websites which are listed below have indicated that they will either post, disseminate, compile, archive, cite or alert their own Website users with research-based content from this work. (This list is as current as the copyright date of this publication.)

Abstracting, Website/Indexing Coverage . . . . Year When Coverage Began

- *CareData: the database supporting social care management and practice <http://www.elsc.org.uk/caredata/caredata.htm>* 2004
- *DH-Data (available via DataStar and in the HMIC [Health Management Information Consortium] CD ROM* 2005
- *EBSCOhost Electronic Journals Service (EJS) <http://ejournals.ebsco.com>* 2004
- *Family & Society Studies Worldwide <http://www.nisc.com>* 2003
- *Family Index Database <http://www.familyscholar.com>* 2004
- *Google <http://www.google.com>* 2004
- *Google Scholar <http://scholar.google.com>* 2004
- *Haworth Document Delivery Center <http://www.HaworthPress.com/journal/dds.asp>* 2004
- *National Center for Chronic Disease Prevention & Health Promotion (NCCDPHP) <http://chid.nih.gov>* 2004
- *National Clearinghouse on Child Abuse & Neglect Information Documents Database <http://nccanch.acf.hhs.gov>* 2004
- *Sage Family Studies Abstracts (SFSA)* 2004
- *Social Services Abstracts <http://www.csa.com* 2004
- *Sociedad Iberoamericana de Información Científica (SIIC) <http://www.siicsalud.com>* 2004
- *Women, Girls & Criminal Justice Newsletter. Civic Research Institute, 4490 Rte 27 Box 585, Kingston, NJ 08528* 2004

(continued)

*Special Bibliographic Notes related to special journal issues
(separates) and indexing/abstracting:*

- indexing/abstracting services in this list will also cover material in any "separate" that is co-published simultaneously with Haworth's special thematic journal issue or DocuSerial. Indexing/abstracting usually covers material at the article/chapter level.
- monographic co-editions are intended for either non-subscribers or libraries which intend to purchase a second copy for their circulating collections.
- monographic co-editions are reported to all jobbers/wholesalers/approval plans. The source journal is listed as the "series" to assist the prevention of duplicate purchasing in the same manner utilized for books-in-series.
- to facilitate user/access services all indexing/abstracting services are encouraged to utilize the co-indexing entry note indicated at the bottom of the first page of each article/chapter/contribution.
- this is intended to assist a library user of any reference tool (whether print, electronic, online, or CD-ROM) to locate the monographic version if the library has purchased this version but not a subscription to the source journal.
- individual articles/chapters in any Haworth publication are also available through the Haworth Document Delivery Service (HDDS).

Addiction, Assessment, and Treatment with Adolescents, Adults, and Families

CONTENTS

ABOUT THE EDITOR

Carolyn Hilarski, PhD, is currently Assistant Professor, Rochester Institute of Technology, Rochester, NY. She earned her MSW and PhD from SUNY Buffalo, and holds a clinical social work license in the state of New York. Dr. Hilarski's research interests and publications concern trauma and abusive behavior-such as substance abuse. She serves on the editorial boards of *Stress, Trauma, and Crisis: An International Journal* and the *Journal of Evidence-Based Social Work: Advances in Practice, Programming, Research, and Policy.* She also serves as Research Consultant and Co-Investigator for several grants concerning youth substance abuse and trauma.

Beliefs About Confrontation Among Substance Abuse Counselors: Are They Consistent with the Evidence?

Thomas Dale Davis, PhD

SUMMARY. Substance abuse researchers have recommended that substance abuse counselors and helping professionals use a non-confrontational counseling approach when addressing client denial. Yet little is known about substance abuse counselor beliefs about the use of confrontation. The purpose of this study was to use the Theory of Reasoned Action to qualitatively capture, quantitatively evaluate, and theoretically interpret beliefs about confrontation among 124 substance abuse counselors in residential and outpatient treatment facilities. Counselor beliefs accounted for nearly one-third of the variance in counselor intention to use a confrontational counseling approach. Counselors who engaged in professional development activities held more favorable beliefs toward a non-confrontational counseling approach than counselors who had not engaged in such activities. Based on the findings in this study, counselor beliefs hold promise as critical components in developing an

Thomas Dale Davis is Assistant Professor, Department of Social Work, California State University, San Bernardino 5500 University Parkway, San Bernardino, CA 92407-2397 (E-mail: mtomdavis@csusb.edu).

[Haworth co-indexing entry note]: "Beliefs About Confrontation Among Substance Abuse Counselors: Are They Consistent with the Evidence?" Davis, Thomas Dale. Co-published simultaneously in *Journal of Evidence-Based Social Work* (The Haworth Social Work Practice Press, an imprint of The Haworth Press, Inc.) Vol. 2, No. 1/2, 2005, pp. 1-17; and: *Addiction, Assessment, and Treatment with Adolescents, Adults, and Families* (ed: Carolyn Hilarski) The Haworth Social Work Practice Press, an imprint of The Haworth Press, Inc., 2005, pp. 1-17. Single or multiple copies of this article are available for a fee from The Haworth Document Delivery Service [1-800-HAWORTH, 9:00 a.m. - 5:00 p.m. (EST). E-mail address: docdelivery@haworthpress.com].

http://www.haworthpress.com/web/JEBSW
Digital Object Identifier: 10.1300/J394v02n01_01

1

empirical and theoretical understanding of the gap between research and practice in substance abuse counseling. *[Article copies available for a fee from The Haworth Document Delivery Service: 1-800-HAWORTH. E-mail address: <docdelivery@haworthpress.com> Website: <http://www.HaworthPress.com> ©2005 by The Haworth Press, Inc. All rights reserved.]*

KEYWORDS. Beliefs, confrontation, counselor, evidence-based practice, technology transfer, theory of reasoned action

INTRODUCTION

As evidence-based treatments emerge for addictions (Volpicelli, Pettinati, McLellan, & O'Brien, 2001), substance abuse researchers have recommended that substance abuse counselors and helping professionals use a non-confrontational counseling approach when addressing client denial (Miller & Rollnick, 2002). The use of confrontation has long been associated with substance abuse treatment (Fisher & Harrison, 1997). The traditional view has been that individuals with substance abuse disorders are manipulative and in denial. As a consequence, confrontation was viewed as necessary in order to break down patterns of conduct and psychological defenses. Addictions treatment research in the last ten years, however, has forced the field to reevaluate client motivation, stages of change, and the effectiveness of a confrontational counseling approach to address client denial. Miller and Rollnick (2002) have identified a range of studies suggesting that a supportive, reflective, and non-confrontational style of counseling is more effective in lowering client resistance than a confrontational style. Reducing client resistance is an important part of any treatment procedure. Resistant clients experience less benefit and are more prone to prematurely terminate from treatment than those who are cooperative (Beutler, Moleiro, & Talebi, 2002).

Increasingly, contrasts are drawn between a confrontational and a non-confrontational counseling approach to address client denial in substance abuse treatment (Connors, Donovan, & DiClemente, 2001; Miller & Rollnick, 2002; Velasquez, Maurer, Crouch, & DiClemente, 2001). Broadly, these contrasts include differences between collaborative and confrontational styles of counseling. A collaborative style involves a partnership that honors the client's expertise and perspective, while a confrontational style involves replacing client expertise with imposed counselor directives. Additional contrasts include differences between evocation and education in the treatment process, where evocation presumes that motivation for change resides within the client, and education presumes that the client lacks key knowledge and is in need of counselor enlightenment.

Despite researcher-led efforts to promulgate a non-confrontational counseling approach among substance abuse counselors, little is known about substance abuse counselor beliefs about the use of confrontation. Identifying substance abuse counselor beliefs holds promise as an essential first step in understanding the gap (Lamb, Greenlick, & Mc-Carty, 1998) between a science-based recommendation and its reception among counselors in communities of clinical practice. In the field of decision-making in clinical medicine, for example, studies have found that physician beliefs are factors that influence clinician decision making when it comes to adhering to science-based recommendations in clinical practice (Fang, Mittman, & Weingarten, 1996; Flores, 2000; Langley, Faulkner, Watkins, Gray, & Harvey, 1998). Support for beliefs as determinants of subsequent behavior has been summarized in a meta-analysis (Armitage & Conner, 2000) and in a review of the literature (Ajzen, 2001; Sutton, 1998).

Theory of Reasoned Action

This study used Ajzen and Fishbein's (1980) Theory of Reasoned Action (TRA) to qualitatively capture, quantitatively evaluate, and theoretically interpret beliefs about confrontation among substance abuse counselors. The TRA posits that antecedent, belief-based constructs offer explanatory power for subsequent intention and behavior. In the TRA, these constructs include intention, attitude, norms, and beliefs.

According to the TRA, and as applied to this study, a counselor's intention to perform a behavior is the best predictor of subsequent behavior. In deciding whether or not to perform a behavior, the counselor as decision-maker is influenced both by his or her own attitude and by the social norms the counselor perceives. A counselor's attitude is, in turn, based on the counselor's beliefs about the expected outcomes, or consequences, of the behavior, as well as his or her beliefs about the likelihood of those outcomes occurring. The counselor's perceived social norms are based on his or her expectations about how people important to the counselor feel about the counselor performing the behavior, as well as the counselor's motivation to comply with these referents. In deciding whether or not to use a confrontational counseling approach to address client denial, then, and according to the TRA, the counselor as decision-maker is influenced by his or her own attitude, social norms, intentions, and beliefs about the use of confrontation to address client denial.

METHOD

Study Overview

In summary, the purpose of this study was to use the Theory of Reasoned Action to qualitatively capture, quantitatively evaluate, and theoretically interpret beliefs about confrontation among 124 substance abuse counselors in residential and outpatient treatment facilities. This study also examined the influence of counselor characteristics on specific beliefs and normative referents. These counselor characteristics included research experience, conference attendance, gender, journal subscriptions, and membership in a professional organization.

Counselors were recruited from outpatient and residential treatment facilities in four urban counties surrounding a Pacific Northwest metropolitan city. Of 18 treatment facilities contacted, 10 (56%) agreed to participate in the study. Study fliers were given to prospective respondents, with dates and times for the administration of a survey. Counselors were informed that they would be paid $13 for completing the survey. Surveys were administered during clinical staff meetings. The 11-page survey took an average of 20 minutes to complete.

Respondent Characteristics

Respondents were all certified substance abuse counselors who worked full-time in outpatient (36%) and residential (64%) chemical addiction treatment facilities in a Pacific Northwestern state. The sample was predominantly female (65%), had a mean age of 45 (SD = 11.3), and was predominantly Caucasian (83%). Number of years respondents had worked in the addictions treatment field ranged from 2- to 23-years, with an average of nine years (SD = 8.4). Most of the respondents had not participated in a research project (62%), did not subscribe to a professional journal (71%), were not members of a professional organization (56%), and had not attended a professional conference in the last year (70%). Educational background of counselors included some college with no degree (21%), AA degree (26%), BA (30%), Masters degree (20%), and Doctorate (3%). Counselor characteristics were consistent with a Pacific Northwest treatment workforce survey of substance abuse counselors (Gallon, Gabriel, & Knudsen, 2003).

PROCEDURES

Clinical Terminology

Four certified substance abuse counselors, each with ten to fifteen years of substance abuse counseling experience, were consulted regarding the phrase "a confrontational counseling approach." Believing the phrase would create reactivity in a survey of substance abuse counselors, all four counselors independently recommended using a more neutral sounding phrase. Following the work of Atkinson (1995) on the importance of clinical practice discourse in communities of practice, the counselors were asked by the researcher to devise three alternative phrases for "a confrontational approach."

Counselors offered the following alternative phrases: (1) "a counselor-directive approach," (2) "a strategic-challenge approach," and (3) "a direct approach." Counselors were asked to independently classify each phrase as having low acceptability, medium acceptability, or high acceptability for use in a survey. Interrater reliability was 100 percent, with high acceptability for the phrase " a direct approach."

With consultation from the same counselors, the researcher constructed formal definitions for the new phrase and related terms. Counselors were asked to independently classify each definition as having low acceptability, medium acceptability, or high acceptability. Interater reliability was 100 percent, with high acceptability for the following definitions. A "direct counseling approach" to client denial is when the "counselor builds on good client rapport and tells the client directly that he or she is in denial." An "indirect counseling approach" to client denial is when the "counselor sustains empathic accepting responses toward the client, but does not focus on the client's denial." "Client denial" is present when the "client does not acknowledge or does not recognize the facts, implications, feelings, or need for change regarding their problem use with drugs or alcohol." Counselor consultants did not participate in the subsequent TRA survey.

Belief-Elicitation Interviews

To capture salient beliefs about the use of "a direct approach" to address client denial, and using TRA recommendations, the researcher conducted belief-elicitation interviews with a sample of substance abuse counselors similar to the larger sample of counselors to be surveyed (Ajzen & Fishbein, 1980). Eligible counselors for elicitation interviews were required to be certified substance abuse counselors with at least five to ten years of counseling experience. Counselors were recruited from two inpatient treatment facilities for one-on-one elicitation interviews. Residential treatment facilities were selected based on the high number of certified substance abuse counselors in each facility and the high number of years of counseling experience.

Counselors were given a written description of the study, with a sign-up sheet if they wanted to participate in an elicitation interview. Out of a total of 34 counselors who were offered participation in an elicitation interview, 19 counselors (56%) completed a one-on-one interview. Six males and thirteen females were interviewed by the same researcher. Each interview lasted an average of 30 to 40 minutes. Subjects were paid $13 for completing an interview.

In each belief-elicitation interview, the counselor was offered a short list with definitions used in the study. Each counselor was asked the following three belief-based questions: (1) "from your perspective, what are some positive outcomes associated with using a direct approach to address client denial?" (2) "what are some negative outcomes associated with using a direct approach to address client denial?" and (3) "which individuals or groups would have strong opinions about whether or not the average substance abuse counselor used a direct approach to address client denial?" Counselor responses were captured in notes taken by the researcher.

Following Lofland and Lofland (1995) on qualitative data analysis, beliefs and normative referents were coded by theme and were culled to reflect modal responses. The three modal beliefs identified for question one were: "Creating an honest dialogue about substance abuse"; "showing that clients can't play games about their use"; and "showing clients that you care about them even if they use." The three modal beliefs for question two were: "Making clients feel less bonded with counselor"; "making clients angry in treatment"; and "becoming judgmental about clients." The six modal normative referents for question three were "12-step programs"; "clients"; "client's spouses or partners"; "courts"; "substance abuse researchers"; and "substance abuse continuing education courses." These modal beliefs and normative referents were then embedded in the TRA survey questionnaire. Counselors who participated in the elicitation interviews did not participate in the subsequent TRA survey.

Measures

Variables measured included all of the belief-based variables suggested by Ajzen and Fishbein (1980): intention to use a direct approach to address client denial, overall attitude toward the use of a direct approach, overall social norm about the use of a direct approach, perceived likelihood and evaluation of salient outcomes of using a direct approach, and perceived norms of salient referents and motivation to comply with those referents with regard to using a direct approach to address client denial.

Parametric tests were chosen after a visual inspection of detrended normal plots revealed reasonably normal distributions. The parametric tests and semantic scales used in this study are delineated by TRA founders Ajzen and Fishbein (1980), examined by Eagly and Chaiken (1993) for the measurement of complex constructs like attitudes, norms, beliefs, and intentions, and are used in a range of TRA studies. A draft of the initial questionnaire was pretested in a residential treatment facility for clarity and readability, and revised before beginning data collection. The wording and anchors of the items are listed below. Included in the survey were definitions of key terms.

Intentions. "How likely is it that you will use a direct counseling approach?" The response scale anchors were *very unlikely* [0] and *very likely* [6], with a midpoint labeled *50/50 chance* [3]. Higher scores indicate greater likelihood.

Attitudes. "Using a direct approach to address client denial would be . . ." Three semantic differential response scales were used. Anchors for the three scales were: *bad/good, pleasant/unpleasant,* and *harmful/helpful.* Two questions were reverse coded, and higher scores were assigned to the positive anchor. The average of the three items was used as the respondents' overall attitude toward using a direct counseling approach. For this multiple-item scale, a Cronbach alpha of .68 was recorded.

Perceived social norms. Perceived social norm was measured with one item: "What do most people and organizations that are important to you think about you using a direct counseling approach to address client denial?" This question was used with a response scale anchored with *think I definitely should not* [1] use a direct counseling approach to *think I definitely should* [5] use a direct approach. Higher scores indicate more positive perceived norms.

Outcome beliefs. Six beliefs about the effects of using a direct approach were measured. These beliefs were: "creating an honest dialogue about substance abuse problems"; "making clients angry in treatment"; "showing that clients can't play games with you about their substance use"; "becoming judgmental about my clients"; "showing clients that you care about them even if they use"; and "making clients feel less bonded with you in treatment." Two items were constructed for each belief. The first was the individual's estimate of the likelihood of the outcome (*very unlikely* [0] to *very likely* [4]); the second was the individual's evaluation of that outcome (*very negative* [−2] to *very positive* [+2]), with a midpoint of *neither positive or negative* [0]. The computed value of each belief item is the product of the likelihood and evaluation ratings. These product terms are then summed to form the overall value of the outcome beliefs.

Normative beliefs. Norms of six referents were measured, under the general question, "How might other individuals and organizations view your use of a direct counseling approach to address client denial?" The referents were: "12-step programs"; "clients"; "client's spouses or partners"; "courts"; "substance abuse researchers"; and "substance abuse continuing education courses." Two items were constructed for each referent. The first was the respondent's perception of each referent's expectational norm: "[Referent] thinks that you . . ." Response anchors were *definitely should not* [−2] use a direct counseling approach to *definitely should* [+2] use a direct approach, with a midpoint of *don't care one way or another* [0] about using a direct counseling approach. The second item required the respondent to rate the statement, "Generally speaking, how much do you want to do what [referent] think(s) you should do?" Response anchors were *very little* [1] to *very much* [5]. The computed value for each normative belief is the product of the perceived referent norm and motivation to comply with the referent. These product terms are then summed to form the value of the normative referent beliefs. Mean scores for intention, overall attitude and norms, and outcome and normative beliefs, are reported in Table 1.

TABLE 1. Mean Scores on Intention, Overall Attitude and Norm, and Outcome and Normative Beliefs (N = 124)

Variable	Mean	SD
Intention	4.17	1.81
Overall Attitude	3.46	.57
Overall Norm	3.83	.80
Outcomes Beliefs		
Create Dialogue	1.54	.64
Anger Client	−.18	.86
Prevent Games	.53	1.13
Be Judgmental	−1.67	.58
Show Care	1.37	.77
Reduce Bonding	−.71	.93
Outcomes Likelihood		
Create Dialogue	2.72	.85
Anger Client	2.28	.72
Prevent Games	2.38	.99
Be Judgmental	.83	.92
Show Care	2.59	1.05
Reduce Bonding	1.65	.76
Norms		
Expectations		
12-Step	1.17	.90
Client	.26	1.01
Spouse/Partner	.83	.92
Courts	1.32	.76
Researchers	.33	.89
Continuing Education	.48	.86
Motivation		
12-Step	3.79	1.03
Client	2.22	.90
Spouse/Partner	1.83	.82
Courts	3.09	.99
Researchers	3.21	1.02
Continuing Education	3.50	.92

ANALYSIS STRATEGY

There were three steps in the analysis. First, correlations between the sum of the outcome belief cross-products and overall attitude were computed, as were correlations between the sum of the normative belief cross-products and overall perceived social norm. These correlations assess the adequacy of the sets of counselor beliefs to predict overall attitude or norm. Second, correlations between overall attitude and each outcome belief, and between overall perceived social norm and each normative belief, were also computed. These correlations assess the relationship of each specific belief or referent to overall attitude or social norm. Third, intention was regressed onto overall attitude and norm.

RESULTS

Outcome beliefs and attitude. All six of the outcome beliefs were significantly correlated with overall attitude, as was the sum of the outcome beliefs. Correlations ranged from .26 to .51, as shown in Table 2.

Perceived social norm and normative beliefs. Four of the six normative referents were significantly correlated with overall norm, as was the sum of these normative referents. Correlations ranged from .19 to .31, as shown in Table 3.

Regression of intention to use a direct counseling approach onto attitude and norm yielded a significant R of .574, $F(2, 122) = 30.25$, $p < .001$. Using a hierarchical regression analysis, the independent variable of attitude was entered first followed by the variable norm. This strategy was based on the theoretical reasoning in TRA and its posited relationships among variables. In this study, an adjusted R^2 of .32 was used. Use of an adjusted R^2 offers a truer, though smaller, estimate of the degree to which attitude and norm account for variance in counselor intention to use a direct counseling approach when addressing client denial. Subse-

TABLE 2. Correlations of Outcome Belief Product Terms with Overall Attitude

Outcome Belief	Correlation with overall attitude toward using a direct approach *r*
Creating an honest dialogue about substance abuse	.51**
Becoming judgmental about clients	.41**
Making clients angry in treatment	.33**
Showing that clients can't "play games" about their use	.32**
Making clients feel less bonded with counselor	.31**
Show clients that you care about them even if they use	.26**
r, attitude with the sum of outcomes	.59**
n	124

**$p < .001$, two-tailed

quent stepwise regression techniques did not detect additional associations. Regression results are displayed in Table 4.

Independent-sample t-tests were conducted to determine influence of counselor characteristics on specific beliefs. Counselors who had not attended a professional conference in the last year (M = 3.54, SD = .05) held on average a more favorable belief that substance abuse researchers wanted counselors to use a direct counseling approach when addressing client denial, as opposed to counselors who had attended a professional conference in the last year (M = 3.18, SD = .84), t(122) =

TABLE 3. Correlations of Normative Belief Product Terms with Overall Norm

Normative Belief	Correlation with overall perceived social norm toward using a direct approach
	r
Substance abuse researchers	.31**
Continuing education courses	.31**
12-step program	.27**
Clients	.19*
Partners	.15(NS)
Courts	.10(NS)
r, social norm with the sum of normative	.39**
n	124

*p < .01, two-tailed. **p < .001, two-tailed.

TABLE 4. Regression Analysis Summary for Overall Attitude and Subjective Norm Predicting Intention to Use a Direct Counseling Approach to Address Client Denial

Variable	B	SEB	β
Overall Attitude	1.28	.30	.41**
Overall Norm	.51	.21	.23*

Note. Adjusted R-squared = .32 (N = 122, p < .001)
**p < .001, *p < .05.

−2.20, p = .02. Male counselors (M = 4.70, SD = .47) on average held a more favorable belief that using a direct approach would create an honest dialogue about substance abuse, as opposed to female counselors (M = 4.45, SD = .71), t(122) = 2.34, p = .02. Counselors with no research experience (M = 2.86, SD = .74) also held on average a more favorable belief that a direct approach would create an honest dialogue, as opposed to counselors with research experience (M = 2.46, SD, .93), t(122) = 2.44, p = .04. Counselors who did not subscribe to a professional journal (M = 2.70, SD = 1.05) held on average a more favorable belief that a direct approach would show clients that they care about them even if they use, as opposed to counselors who did subscribe to a professional journal (M = 2.30, SD = 1.0), t(122) = −2.00, p = 0.4. Counselors who were a member of a professional organization (M = 2.43, SD = .63) held on average a more favorable belief that using a direct approach would make clients angry in treatment, as opposed to counselors who were not a member of a professional organization (M = 2.15, SD = .79), t(122) = 2.06, p = .04. Differential effects based on ethnic identity, education, or treatment setting were not detected.

DISCUSSION

The purpose of this study was to use the Theory of Reasoned Action to qualitatively capture, quantitatively evaluate, and theoretically interpret beliefs about confrontation among 124 substance abuse counselors in residential and outpatient treatment facilities. Also examined was the influence of counselor characteristics on specific beliefs about the use of a direct approach.

This study found that all six of the outcome beliefs were associated with overall attitude. That counselors believed that a direct approach to client denial might also create a judgmental attitude about clients, make clients angry, and make clients feel less bonded with the counselor, may suggest that these counselors are more aware of the risks that accompany the use of a direct counseling approach than the science-based literature seems to imply (Schneider, Casey, & Kohn, 2000). Due to an absence of ecological validity (Brunswik, 1943), research studies commonly underestimate (Garb & Boyle, 2003) the extent to which everyday counseling strategies among counselors are already congruent with best-practice recommendations. Additionally, these counselor beliefs about confrontation corroborate research on the effects of ruptures in counselor-client bonds (Horvath & Symonds, 1991) and therapeutic alliances (Safran & Muran, 2000).

That counselors believed that a direct approach would create an honest dialogue about substance abuse, show that clients can't play games about their use, and show clients that counselors care about them even if they use, suggests the possibility that these counselors, in their everyday practices, have discovered a proactive utility in the use of a direct approach. These particular beliefs seem to run contrary to research on the deleterious effects of a direct counseling approach to address client denial. Yet it is possible to interpret these same beliefs as the kind of tacit and *in situ* expertise that are often eclipsed from research studies in clinical reasoning (Downie & Macnaughton, 2000).

The study also found four of the six normative beliefs were associated with overall norm. That counselors identified substance abuse researchers, continuing education courses, 12-step programs, and clients as holding strong beliefs about the use of a direct counseling approach, corroborates counseling texts on the importance of these specific groups in disseminating and offering feedback on counseling strategies among addictions treatment counselors (Perkinson, 2002).

Counselor attitude and norm predicted counselor intention to use a direct approach. Given research on the influence of attitudes (Petty, Wegener, & Fabrigar, 1997) and norms (Wood, 2000) on subsequent behavior, these two belief-based factors may hold explanatory power for understanding counselor utilization of science-based recommendations. Science-based recommendations in clinical medicine, for example, have had a limited effect on clinician behavior and often do not affect clinical practice (Davis & Taylor-Vaisey, 1997). As a result, studies have turned to, and have identified, clinician-beliefs as factors that influence clinician adoption of science-based interventions (Flores, 2000; Langley et al., 1998). Such clinician-centric studies hold promise for a deeper understanding of the gap (Lamb et al., 1998; Marinelli-Casey, Domier, & Rawson, 2002) between research and practice in substance abuse treatment counseling.

Yet in contrast to types of treatment and client characteristics, substance abuse counselors have been little studied in the substance abuse field (Ball et al., 2002; Najavits, 2002; Najavits, Crits-Christoph, & Dierberger, 2000; Najavits & Weiss, 1994; Siqueland et al., 2000). Wampold (2001) and Hubble, Duncan, and Miller (1999) have examined a broad range of empirical evidence in the counseling and psychotherapy literature, concluding that counselor effects account for greater variance in treatment outcome than adherence to treatment protocol in manuals or particular treatment modality.

In this study, norm appears less important than attitude in predicting intention to use a direct approach to address client denial. Counselors across a range of clinical disciplines and settings hold eclectic orientations to counseling strategies (Jensen, Bergin, & Greaves, 1990). Counselors in this study may feel that attempts to instantiate science-based prescriptions around a direct counseling approach are incompatible with the kind of eclectic counseling frameworks developed in communities of local practice.

Counselors who engaged in the professional development activities of subscribing to a journal, being a member of a professional organization, and attending a professional conference in the last year, were more likely to hold accurate beliefs about what current researchers believe about the use of a direct, or confrontational, approach to address client denial. Counselors who did not engage in such professional development activities believed, erroneously, that substance abuse researchers wanted counselors to use a direct approach to address client denial. Also, clinicians with research experience held a less favorable belief that a direct approach would lead to an authentic dialogue about substance abuse problems, as opposed to clinicians without research experience. It may be that professional development and research experience, as socialization processes, keep counselors current on what the research community holds about substance abuse counseling strategies. While no published studies have addressed the influence of professional development on substance abuse counselors, there is evidence that substance abuse counselors desire increased professional development (Nall, Amodeo, Shaffer, & Bilt, 2000). Of additional interest, males held a more favorable belief that a direct approach created an honest dialogue with the client about substance abuse, as opposed to females. Studies have indicated that counselor gender can be an important component in treatment outcomes (Najavits & Weiss, 1994). A potential implication is that gender may moderate the way counselors view certain evidence-based counseling strategies.

Limitations of Study

This study and its findings are limited in a number of ways. First, a majority of counselors in the study were drawn from residential facilities, making generalization to outpatient facilities limited. Second, the majority of counselors were Caucasian. Counselor beliefs about a direct approach may vary based on ethnic identity. Third, surveys about beliefs are vulnerable to errors in self-report recall (Fineberg, 1985; Manfredo & Shelby, 1988). Fourth, exchanging the phrase "a confrontational approach" for "a direct approach" was based on a consensus among experienced substance abuse counselors. It is likely that such a consensus, while necessary, is not a sufficient condition to determine clinical phrase equivalency. Fifth, while the use of multiplicative composites for outcome beliefs has been criticized on the grounds that it makes assumptions of ratio level measurements that are questionable (Evans & Sullivan, 2001; Hankins, French, & Horne, 2000; van den Putte & Hoogstraten, 1997), there is no consensus about a better way to operationalize beliefs. In addition, because multiplicative composites are the standard in the TRA literature, using another method would undermine comparisons between the analyses in this study and others. Also, because beliefs in TRA instruments are often limited to one question per belief construct, criticisms about the absence of reliability analysis in TRA instruments are a concern but not a focus in this study.

Based on the findings in this study, counselor beliefs hold promise as critical components in developing an empirical and theoretical understanding of the gap between research and practice in substance abuse counseling.

REFERENCES

Ajzen, I. (2001). Nature and operation of attitudes. *Annual Review of Psychology, 52,* 27-58.

Ajzen, I., & Fishbein, M. (1980). *Understanding attitudes and predicting social behavior.* New Jersey: Prentice-Hall.

Armitage, C. J., & Conner, M. (2000). Efficacy of the theory of planned behavior: A meta-analytic review. *British Journal of Social Psychology,* 40(4), 471-499 (2001).

Atkinson, P. A. (1995). *Medical talk and medical work.* London: Sage.

Ball, S., Bachrach, K., DeCarlo, J., Farentinos, C., Keen, M., McSherry, T., Polcin, D., Snead, N., Sockriter, R., Wrigley, P., Zammarelli, L., & Carroll, K. (2002). Characteristics, beliefs, and practices of community clinicians trained to provide manual-guided therapy for substance abusers. *Journal of Substance Abuse Treatment,* 23(4), 309-318.

Beutler, L. E., Moleiro, C. M., & Talebi, H. (2002). Resistance. In J. C. Norcross (Ed.), *Psychotherapy relationships that work: Therapist contributions and responsiveness to patients* (pp. 129-143). New York: Oxford University Press.

Brunswik, E. (1943). Organismic achievement and environmental probability. *The psychological review, 50,* 255-272.

Connors, G. J., Donovan, D. M., & DiClemente, C. C. (2001). *Substance abuse treatment and the stages of change: Selecting and planning interventions.* New York: The Guilford Press.

Davis, D. A., & Taylor-Vaisey, A. (1997). Translating guidelines into practice: A systematic review of theoretic concepts, practical experience, and research evidence in the adoption of clinical practice guidelines. *Canadian Medical Association Journal, 157*(4), 408-416.

Downie, R. S., & Macnaughton, J. (2000). *Clinical judgment: Evidence in practice.* New York: Oxford University Press.

Eagley, A. H., and Chaiken, S. (1993). *The psychology of attitudes.* Belmont, CA: Thompson and Wadsworth.

Evans, K., & Sullivan, J. M. (2001). *Dual diagnosis: Counseling the mentally ill substance abuser* (2nd ed.). New York: The Guilford Press.

Fang, E., Mittman, B. S., & Weingarten, S. (1996). Use of clinical practice guidelines in managed care physician groups. *Archives of Family Medicine, 5*, 528-531.

Fineberg, S. (1985). Cognitive aspects of health survey. *Milbank Memorial Fund Quarterly, 63*(3), 547-564.

Fisher, G. L., & Harrison, T. C. (1997). *Substance abuse: Information for school counselors, social workers, and therapists.* Boston: Allyn and Bacon.

Flores, G. (2000). Pediatricians' attitudes, beliefs, and practices regarding clinical practice guidelines: A national study. *Pediatrics, 105*(3), 496-501.

Gallon, S. L., Gabriel, R. M., & Knudsen, J. R. (2003). The toughest job you'll ever love: A Pacific Northwest treatment workforce survey. *Journal of Substance Abuse Treatment, 24*, 183-196.

Garb, H. N., & Boyle, P. A. (2003). Understanding why some clinicians use pseudoscientific methods: Findings from research on clinical judgment. In S. O. Lilienfeld, S. J. Lynn, & J. M. Lohr (Eds.), *Science and pseudoscience in clinical psychology* (pp. 17-38). New York: The Guilford Press.

Hankins, M., French, D., & Horne, R. (2000). Statistical guidelines for studies of the theory of reasoned action and the theory of planned behavior. *Psychology and Health, 15*, 151-296.

Horvath, A. O., & Symonds, B. D. (1991). Relation between working alliance and outcome in psychotherapy: A Meta-Analysis. *Journal of Counseling Psychology, 38*, 139-149.

Hubble, M. A., Duncan, B. L., & Miller, S. D. (1999). Introduction. In M. A. Hubble, B. L. Duncan, & S. D. Miller (Eds.), *The heart and soul of change: What works in therapy* (pp. 1-19). Washington, DC: American Psychological Association.

Jensen, J. P., Bergin, A. E., & Greaves, D. W. (1990). The meaning of eclecticism: New survey and analysis of components. *Professional Psychology: Research and Practice, 21*, 124-130.

Lamb, S., Greenlick, M. R., & McCarty, D. (Eds.). (1998). *Bridging the gap between practice and research: Forging partnerships with community-based drug and alcohol treatment.* Washington DC: National Academy Press.

Langley, C., Faulkner, A., Watkins, C., Gray, S., & Harvey, I. (1998). Use of guidelines in primary care: Practitioners' perspectives. *Family Practice, 15*(2), 105-111.

Lofland, J., & Lofland, L. H. (1995). *Analyzing social settings* (3rd ed.). Boston: Wadsworth.

Manfredo, M. J., & Shelby, B. (1988). The effect of using self-report measures in tests of attitude-behavior relationships. *The Journal of Social Psychology, 128*(6), 731-743.

Marinelli-Casey, P., Domier, C. P., & Rawson, R. A. (2002). The gap between research and practice in substance abuse treatment. *Psychiatric Services, 53*(8), 984-987.

Miller, W. R., & Rollnick, S. (2002). *Motivational interviewing: Preparing people for change* (2nd. ed.). New York: THe Guilford Press.

Najavits, L. M. (2002). Clinicians' views on treating posttraumatic stress disorder and substance use disorder. *Journal of Substance Abuse Treatment, 22*, 79-85.

Najavits, L. M., Crits-Christoph, P., & Dierberger, A. (2000). Clinicians' impact on the quality of substance use disorder treatment. *Substance Use and Misuse, 35*(12-14), 2161-2190.

Najavits, L. M., & Weiss, R. D. (1994). Variations in therapist effectiveness in the treatment of patients with substance use disorders: An empirical review. *Addiction, 89*(6), 679-688.

Nall, M. N., Amodeo, M., Shaffer, H. J., & Bilt, J. V. (2000). Social workers employed in substance abuse treatment agencies: Training needs assessment. *Social Work, 45*(2), 141-154.

Perkinson, R. R. (2002). *Chemical dependency counseling: A practical guide.* Thousand Oaks: Sage.

Petty, R. E., Wegener, D. T., & Fabrigar, L. R. (1997). Attitudes and attitude change. *Annual Review of Psychology, 48*, 609-647.

Safran, J. D., & Muran, J. C. (2000). *Negotiating the therapeutic alliance: A relational treatment guide.* New York: The Guilford Press.

Schneider, R. J., Casey, J., & Kohn, R. (2000). Motivational versus confrontational interviewing: A comparison of substance abuse assessment practices at employee assistance programs. *The Journal of Behavioral Health Services & Research, 27*(1), 60-74.

Siqueland, L., Crits-Christoph, P., Barber, J. P., Butler, S. F., Thase, M., Najavits, L., & Onken, L. S. (2000). The role of therapist characteristics in training effects in cognitive, support-expressive, and drug counseling therapies for cocaine dependence. *Journal of Psychotherapy Practice & Research, 9*, 123-130.

Sutton, S. (1998). Predicting and explaining intentions and behavior: How well are we doing? *Journal of Applied Social Psychology, 28*, 1317-1338.

van den Putte, B., & Hoogstraten, J. (1997). Applying structural equation modeling in the context of the theory of reasoned action: Some problems and solutions. *Structural Equation Modeling, 4*, 320-337.

Velasquez, M. M., Maurer, G. G., Crouch, C., & DiClemente, C. C. (2001). *Group treatment for substance abuse: a stages-of-change therapy manual.* New York: The Guilford Press.

Volpicelli, J. R., Pettinati, H. M., McLellan, A. T., & O'Brien, C. P. (2001). *Combining medication and psychosocial treatments for addictions.* New York: The Guildford Press.

Wampold, B. E. (2001). *The great psychotherapy debate: Models, methods, and findings.* New Jersey: Lawrence Erlbaum.

Wood, W. (2000). Attitude change: Persuasion and social influence. *Annual Review of Psychology, 51*, 539-570.

Twelve-Step Programs and Faith-Based Recovery: Research Controversies, Provider Perspectives, and Practice Implications

Kathleen M. Tangenberg, PhD

SUMMARY. This paper draws upon empirical research literature and faith-related provider perspectives on addiction and recovery to address practice and research challenges posed by 12-step and other spiritually oriented treatment approaches. The paper is organized to provide clarification of relevant terminology, review research literature and controversies surrounding the effectiveness of 12-step recovery approaches and other treatment models, present faith-related provider narratives, and discuss the implications of existing research and faith-related treatment ideologies for evidence-based practice. *[Article copies available for a fee from The Haworth Document Delivery Service: 1-800-HAWORTH. E-mail address: <docdelivery@haworthpress.com> Website: <http://www.HaworthPress.com> © 2005 by The Haworth Press, Inc. All rights reserved.]*

Kathleen M. Tangenberg is affiliated with the School of Social Work, University of Iowa.

[Haworth co-indexing entry note]: "Twelve-Step Programs and Faith-Based Recovery: Research Controversies, Provider Perspectives, and Practice Implications." Tangenberg, Kathleen M. Co-published simultaneously in *Journal of Evidence-Based Social Work* (The Haworth Social Work Practice Press, an imprint of The Haworth Press, Inc.) Vol. 2, No. 1/2, 2005, pp. 19-40; and: *Addiction, Assessment, and Treatment with Adolescents, Adults, and Families* (ed: Carolyn Hilarski) The Haworth Social Work Practice Press, an imprint of The Haworth Press, Inc., 2005, pp. 19-40. Single or multiple copies of this article are available for a fee from The Haworth Document Delivery Service [1-800-HAWORTH, 9:00 a.m. - 5:00 p.m. (EST). E-mail address: docdelivery@haworthpress.com].

http://www.haworthpress.com/web/JEBSW
© 2005 by The Haworth Press, Inc. All rights reserved.
Digital Object Identifier: 10.1300/J394v02n01_02

KEYWORDS. Substance abuse treatment, addiction, 12-step, spiritually oriented treatment

Recovery from chemical dependency may be considered a cognitive, spiritual, physical, social, and emotional process influenced by multiple individual and environmental circumstances. The term *recovery* is often associated with Alcoholics Anonymous (AA) and other twelve-step programs encouraging complete sobriety and reliance on a higher power to change patterns of behavioral dependency and self-understanding. Religious and spiritual dimensions of recovery have received considerable scholarly attention (Gregoire, 1995; Hooks, 1993; Miller, 1998; Tangenberg, 2001), though the perspectives on addiction and recovery expressed by service providers in faith-based service agencies are rarely included in professional literature. Many social work clients are likely to receive assistance from faith-related providers, especially if they utilize shelters, food banks, or any other forms of emergency services often provided through faith communities. Faith-based shelters, drop-in centers, and other organizations frequently offer 12-step programs and other chemical dependency programs consistent with spiritual and religious values. Research indicates that between 40 and 57% of homeless adults experience alcoholism, and between 10 and 20% have other chemical dependencies (Liberty et al., 1998). To better assist individuals likely to access faith-related agencies and treatment programs, it is important for social workers to understand diverse philosophies of addiction and recovery. Greater awareness of treatment approaches and evaluations of their effectiveness may assist evidence- based assessments of treatment needs, as well as inform possible collaborations between secular and faith-related providers. The following article draws on interviews with providers in faith-related shelter settings to provide greater understanding of organizational and personal ideologies guiding treatment programs and related clinical and ethical issues. The goals of this article are to: (1) provide conceptualizations of recovery, spirituality, and religion relevant to practice involving 12-step programs; (2) review research literature and controversies regarding 12-step program effectiveness; (3) present perspectives on addiction and recovery expressed by faith-related service providers in shelter settings; and (4) discuss implications of existing research and faith-related treatment perspectives for evidence-based social work. Although the 12-step approach of Alcoholics Anonymous has been applied to a number of addictive behaviors, the paper will focus mostly on alcoholism due to its dominance in recovery literature and high rates of alcoholism documented among individuals who rely on faith-related shelter organizations (Liberty et al., 1998).

SPIRITUAL AND RELIGIOUS ASPECTS OF RECOVERY AND 12-STEP PROGRAMS

In social work practice focused on addictions, the term recovery typically refers to following the principles and twelve steps of Alcoholics Anonymous, and agreement with the program philosophy of the Minnesota Model, currently considered the most widely practiced addiction treatment model in the United States (Winters, Stinchfield, Opland, Weller, & Latimer, 2000). The Minnesota model is predicated upon four key elements: (1) Changing addictive beliefs, attitudes, and behaviors is possible; (2) General agreement with the disease concept suggesting that some individuals are physically vulnerable to developing alcoholism and drug addiction; (3) Beliefs that total abstinence from all mood altering chemicals and lifestyle changes are necessary for treatment success; and (4) Adherence to the principles of Alcoholics Anonymous and Narcotics Anonymous as summarized in the 12-steps (Cook, 1988). These steps include admitting powerlessness over addiction, coming to believe in a higher power and turning one's will over to this higher power, taking a moral inventory, admitting wrongdoing, asking for forgiveness, making amends with others, seeking to improve conscious contact with a higher power through prayer and meditation, and using one's spiritual awakening to carry this message to others who are addicted (Hazelden, 1996). Recovery has been described as an "ongoing, life-long program for living" in which "an alcoholic's best, if not only, hope for sobriety is through recognizing, appealing to, accepting help from an directing his or here life toward a transcendent higher power, referred to as God" (Miller, 1998, p. 982). Miller's (1998) association of the higher power with God is common in recovery narratives (Fitzgerald, 1996; O'Reilly, 1997), though program literature suggests that interpretation of the higher power is highly subjective, and participants are free to draw inspiration from any theological or non-theological entity.

Questions of how to define and discuss spiritual aspects of twelve step programs have generated controversy since the inception of Alcoholics Anonymous. Bill Wilson, founder of AA, was closely associated with the Oxford Group, a religious reform movement that attempted to emulate early Christian practices of spiritual awakening and fellowship.

When writing *Alcoholics Anonymous* (the Big Book), Wilson (1939) deliberately avoided exclusive affiliation with Christianity, preferring theistic yet non-doctrinal allusions to a higher power. Beliefs guiding the twelve steps drew heavily from the work of William James and Carl Jung. In his book titled *The Varieties of Religious Experience*, William James (1902) asserted the scientific validity of conversion experiences, and described their spiritual and psychological aspects. Having experienced his own religious conversion in a treatment setting, Wilson was especially interested in the conversion experiences of others and the potential of spiritual interventions to end addictions. Carl Jung's writings about the spiritual dimensions of alcoholism also influenced Wilson's belief that spiritual transformation was necessary for true sobriety. Wilson's work has consistently been regarded as more religious than scientific (Raphael, 2000), although it has been closely integrated in recovery programs adhering to medical and scientific treatment models.

Attributions of disease associated with early proponents of the 12-steps focused on the spiritual, existential nature of alcoholism rather than somatic, biological forms of illness. Although Wilson had once been comforted by a physician's assertion that his alcoholism was attributable to physical factors, subsequent relapses convinced him that scientific and self-knowledge were inadequate to end addiction. Wilson strongly criticized exclusively medical models of addiction because he believed they could result in abdication of personal responsibility for alcoholic behavior and create expectations for relapse.

As addiction treatment was increasingly professionalized in the latter part of the 20th century, holistic models emerged that integrated the spiritual and self-help traditions of Alcoholics Anonymous with recognition of physiological and cultural addiction processes. Research conducted by Madsen (1974) concluded that alcoholism resulted from a complex set of individual and cultural dynamics. Asserting that alcoholism was probably both inherited *and* learned, Madsen asserted that American cultural anxiety and social pressures contributed to alcoholism and required holistic intervention approaches. Gregory Bateson (1971) also explored the contributions of cultural values and pressures to individual alcoholism in a study describing the experiences of AA members. Bateson drew upon member narratives to develop a theory of alcoholism addressing various social systems and cognitions contributing to excessive alcohol use. Nearly all participants in Bateson's study described painful feelings of separation from others that could be remedied by alcohol. Rather than viewing these beliefs in separateness as cognitive distortions, Bateson argued that they were reinforced by American cultural beliefs in individual autonomy and control. Participants in Bateson's study stated that identification with individualistic values and beliefs generated errors of "alcoholic thinking" or "alcoholic epistemology" (Wilcox, 1998, p. 120) that were positively transformed by 12-step program participation and adherence to spiritual beliefs in a higher power and willingness to surrender control. In an ethnographic study of over six hundred 12-step groups, Wilcox (1998) similarly found that many members had rejected religious beliefs in favor of individualistic rationalist paradigms prior to program participation. Awareness of their addictions and feelings of powerlessness led many to reconsider the existence of God. According to Wilcox (1998), "Members claimed that in the beginning, they did not want to accept that God was real, but they decided that they needed the help so badly, they were willing to try to believe" (p. 80). Participants in Wilcox's study typically avoided discussions of how or why the steps worked, but instead described experiences of "a mysterious healing power that they could call anything they wanted, but which most chose to call God" (p. 81).

Definitions of *spirituality* found in recovery literature tend to describe transcendent, transpersonal aspects of individual connections to God or other forms of a higher power, whereas *religion* is associated with social practices, beliefs, rituals, and forms of governance (Miller, 1998). Spiritual dimensions of 12-step programs have generally been less controversial than formal religious affiliations. In social work and feminist literature, the cultural appropriateness and gender sensitivity of 12-step programs and the Minnesota model have been challenged, often in light of historical referents to the Oxford Group and continued associations of 12-step meetings with Christian churches and ideologies (Saulnier, 1996; Tallen, 1990). Adaptations of 12-step principles and practices to fit different cultural groups and faith traditions have been well documented in professional literature (Brandes, 2002; Krestan, 2000), yet serious concerns remain. Allegations of anti-Semitism, racism, classism, sexism, heterosexism, and cultism in the recovery movement have contributed to professional distance from recovery programs and challenged their credibility (Bufe, 1998).

Arguing for a socio-spiritual approach to recovery, Morell (1996) described tensions between professional social work and 12-step recovery philosophies linking spirituality and religion. Identified concerns included: "The understanding that specific religious beliefs exclude many who need help, a sense that 'otherworldliness' precludes necessary politicization of this life, and fear of the power of right-wing religious ideology" (Morell, 1996, p. 309). To address these concerns, Morell encouraged social workers to draw upon the spiritually based social justice traditions of many marginalized groups, and to appreciate the potential for political empowerment in the recovery movement. Using the 4-step approach to recovery adopted by Glide Memorial Church in San Francisco (Williams, 1992), Morell (1996) encouraged modifications of the original 12-steps to provide emphasis on: "(1) recognition (not powerlessness); (2) self-definition (not society's definition); (3) re-birth (facing the pain and telling the truth); and (4) community (moving further into relationship with people of all colors)" (p. 310). Qualitative research conducted by Kurtz and Fisher (2003) explored the relationship between 12-step program participation and community service, and found that group members frequently viewed community empowerment activities as integral to the recovery process. Activities pursued by members included the organization of neighborhood groups, participation in community task forces, and political advocacy. Although links between spirituality, religion, 12-step program involvement, and political action have not been extensively studied, social worker awareness of historical traditions of self-help and collective spiritual strength in many marginalized communities may enhance recognition of the complex, multidimensional nature of recovery efforts.

RESEARCH EVIDENCE AND CONTROVERSIES

Hazelden and other treatment facilities currently utilizing the Minnesota Model have integrated the 12-step program philosophy of Alcoholics Anonymous with additional therapeutic strategies recognizing physical, psychological, social, and spiritual aspects of addiction. Researchers describing characteristics and outcomes of Hazelden inpatient treatment programs stated, "The primary agent of change is group affiliation, and practicing behaviors consistent with the Twelve-Step Program of Alcoholics Anonymous" (Stinchfield & Owen, 1998). According to client self-report data submitted by 767 participants at a 12-month follow-up, 405 (52.8%) stated they had not used alcohol or drugs since discharge and 267 (34.8%) stated that had not used as much. Over half of the respondents reported attending 12-step meetings at least once a week. Results from the Hazelden study are consistent with findings from other studies examining the effectiveness of the Minnesota model (Cook, 1988). Research based on the 8-year, $27 million Project MATCH study of the effectiveness of different treatment modalities for different types of alcoholics indicated that 12-step facilitation therapy was comparable to motivational enhancement therapy and cognitive behavioral therapy in treating alcoholism, though researchers cautioned that findings were predicated upon on individual counseling technique promoting active participation in the traditional AA activities (Project MATCH Research Group, 1998). This technique guided participants through the first five steps of Alcoholics Anonymous and actively encouraged AA affiliation. More definitive information regarding 12-step program effectiveness was anticipated from the Project MATCH study, and the research has been criticized for lack of a non-treatment control group and failure to explore the experiences of involuntary program participants, the effects of the therapeutic relationship on treatment outcomes, and factors likely to facilitate sustained recovery (Bower, 1997).

The lack of research examining ways therapist education and treatment orientation may influence treatment success is of specific concern to social workers since the one of the profession's core values promotes the central importance of human relationships. In the Project MATCH study, no therapist attributes, including gender, experience, and beliefs about alcoholism or recovery status, were consistently related to outcomes across treatment conditions (Carroll, 2001). Though not outcome related, research exploring the attitudes of treatment providers toward different treatment approaches has indicated correlations between treatment preferences and provider roles and educational levels. In a study of 317 treatment staff members associated with the Delaware Valley Clinical Trials Network, participants with doctoral degrees expressed the lowest degree of endorsement for 12-step and other spiritual approaches, although staff members with other credentials indicated very positive support for 12-step oriented approaches (82%) and greater attention to spirituality in general (84%) (Forman, Bovasso, & Woody, 2001). Physicians and psychiatrists were more likely to support pharmacologic interventions than other staff members, and staff members were divided in their opinions of confrontation. Based on these findings, researchers argued for closer bridging of the practice-research gap, and suggested that spiritually based approaches warranted careful, systematic study (Forman, Bovasso, & Woody, 2001).

Evaluations of research examining the effectiveness of 12-step programs have identified numerous methodological weaknesses, including reliance on client self-report, lack of long-term follow-up, poor instrument quality, and biases related to professional affiliations between researchers and treatment centers. Disparities in the implementation of 12-step program models, lack of formal records regarding program participation, emphasis on self-help, and beliefs in mystical forms of spiritual transformation have also complicated empirical research efforts to understand 12-step program effectiveness.

Critics of 12-step programs suggest that the experiences of individuals who have become sober without any form of treatment or group participation have been ignored due to unquestioned acceptance of claims made by treatment professionals (Sobell, Ellingstad, & Sobell, 2000). Trimpey (1996), founder of the Rational Recovery approach to alcoholism and other addictions, has been especially critical of treatment success outcomes claimed by many organizations relying on the Minnesota Model. Rational Recovery asserts that "there is no treatment for addiction any more than there would be a treatment for dancing" (Trimpey, 1996, p. 72), and argues that no credible scientific evidence exists supporting the disease model or the need for treatment participation to end addiction. Although substantial evidence exists that large number of people have been able to end addictions independently, further research is needed to clarify environmental factors and demographic characteristics contributing to success, the effectiveness of natural recovery in addressing different forms of addiction, pre-recovery problem severity, and other factors associated with self-change processes (Fiorentine & Hillhouse, 2001; Sobell, Ellingstad, & Sobell, 2000).

Harm reduction approaches to alcohol use challenge the abstinence-only, spiritual directives of Alcoholics Anonymous by focusing on reducing alcohol use to avoid harmful consequences. Alan Marlatt, a leading proponent of harm reduction, has argued that abstinence goals are unrealistic for many people, and instead supports the use of cognitive-behavioral and pharmacological treatments to encourage reduced alcohol consumption (Marlatt & Witkiewitz, 2002). Citing evidence of natural, unassisted recovery and moderate alcohol use among a large number of former alcoholics, Marlatt and Witkiewitz (2002) suggested that 12-step program participation may intensify addiction-related stigmas by forcing self-identification as an addict and requiring disclosure of addiction narratives. Research exploring the effectiveness of harm reduction strategies has indicated a reduction of excessive alcohol consumption among college-age adults, though interventions with adults requiring more intensive treatment have failed to determine whether harm reduction is more effective in limiting drinking than 12-step program involvement and other strategies associated with the Minnesota Model (Marlatt & Witkiewitz, 2002).

The absence of strong research evidence to support any particular treatment approach poses significant challenges to social workers interested in evidence-based practice. Evidence-based practice principles encourage communication with clients about the likely outcomes of intervention participation, and suggest that empirical research findings can assist decision-making regarding intervention appropriateness and likely effectiveness (Gambrill, 2003). Recovery principles frequently challenge evidence-based practice as they rely on spiritual paradigms for which empirical evidence is rarely available. In 1987, the National Association of Social Workers (NASW) formally expressed agreement with the disease concept of addiction, and many social workers are currently employed by treatment centers using the Minnesota model, although the dominance of this model has been attributed "a fluke of history and professional neglect rather than on scientific support" (van Wormer, 1995, p. 73).

Questions regarding the relevance and appropriateness of 12-step involvement for members of disenfranchised groups have been especially challenging for social workers (Morell, 1996). Findings from Project MATCH and other quantitative studies comparing treatment effectiveness among different cultural groups have been inconclusive (Tonigan, Connors & Miller, 1998). Although ethnographic and qualitative studies have suggested the benefits of program participation for individuals experiencing multiple social stigmas (Allahyari, 2000; Kurtz & Fisher, 2003; Tangenberg, 2001; Washington & Moxley, 2003), further studies of cultural and psychosocial dimensions of recovery are needed.

Research exploring 12-step programs and other treatment activities in faith-related service settings is also important for the social work profession since many clients access emergency services offered through faith communities that also provide opportunities for 12-step program participation. In 2001, worldwide membership in Alcoholics Anonymous was estimated to include 2 million individuals participating in nearly 100,800 groups meeting in 150 different countries (Alcoholics Anonymous World Services, 2001). Findings from a national study of congregationally based social services indicated that 28.3% of the congregations surveyed housed AA programs. Discussing this finding, Cnaan (2001) stated, "The association between twelve-step programs and congregations has become so well known that it is not unusual to find it depicted in movies, novels, and even songs" (p. 73). Recovery groups organized through religious congregations are likely to lack professional guidance, and the self-help orientation of meetings refutes any presumptions of expertise beyond personal experience. Staff members of organizations such as the Salvation Army are unlikely to have professional degrees, yet often describe personal experiences of addiction and 12-step recovery that shape their service orientations (Allahyari, 2000).

Although social workers may navigate research literature to address possible benefits and risks of 12-step program involvement, work with clients already possessing strong religious and spiritual orientations, or already involved with 12-step recovery, may present beliefs that challenge evidence-based paradigms. Greater knowledge of how faith-related providers understand and respond to addictive behavior may enhance practitioner understanding of different treatment philosophies and belief systems encountered by clients, and assist facilitation of possible collaborations or other treatment plans.

PROVIDER PERSPECTIVES ON ADDICTION AND RECOVERY

The following interview excerpts were obtained in a research project exploring the values, beliefs, and practices guiding faith-based service programs and organizations. Twenty-two providers of faith-based social services in northwestern and Midwestern regions of the U.S. participated in semi-structured interviews asking: (1) how the program's spiritual base was integrated in activities and interpersonal relationships; (2) what characterized this spiritual base (values, religion, practices such as prayer, attendance of services); (3) the distinction between a spiritually-based service *community* and social service *program*; and (4) the distinction between a social service *ministry* and social *work* (Tangenberg, 2002). In interviews focused on work in shelter and hospice settings where clients often experienced alcoholism and other addictions, providers were also asked to discuss their perspectives on addiction and recovery. Twelve providers worked at organizations offering treatment services, and all of these services integrated 12-step recovery groups. Certified chemical dependency counselors were responsible for individual treatment planning and private counseling sessions, and self-help recovery groups provided ongoing support, often several times a day. Qualitative analysis of interview transcripts was conducted using constructivist methods derived from grounded theory (Strauss, 1998; Denzin, 1987). Themes that emerged in analysis of provider statements describing their perspectives on addiction and recovery included: (1) unanimous agreement that authentic spiritual awareness is an integral part of the recovery process; (2) understanding addiction as a condition of bondage that could easily be transferred to other behaviors, people, or other entities, including faith itself; (3) expressions of belief that a higher power will often have different intentions for a recovering addict than that person will have for themselves; and, (4) descriptions of how provider experiences of recovery influenced current activities and beliefs in the twelve steps.

Providers concurred that spiritual awareness was integral to the recovery process. None of the providers interviewed described the need for conversion experiences, though some closely integrated Christian beliefs in their recovery programs:

> I don't think there's any doubt that faith plays a major part in recovery. People can have faith in different things that can look different to different people, but when we go back to our faith-based kinds of programs I think that recognizing that there's nothing that we can do on our own, like the first step acknowledges that we're powerless, that's basically what we do in our faith. We acknowledge that on our own we're not worthy or we can't do what we can do with God's help, with the help of Christ, with the help of whatever it is that we believe in. So people who are in recovery that already have that kind of a faith have something to start with, something to lean on, something to depend on.

> And I think faith can, you know, if it is real faith, it can overcome the addictions. Just because I believe God is real and I believe that He can do anything and that's what the Bible says, so all things are possible through Christ and his ministry, it says in the Philippians, and I truly believe that.

> The only way out for an alcoholic, in terms of the AA program, it's the only way out, is to find a higher power and to stay in conscious spiritual contact. And that is the answer to being powerless over alcohol, is to find a power greater than yourself and avail yourself of that assistance. People are able to stay sober without that. I've been told that; I don't know anyone, but I'm sure there are many people who can. But we say for the true alcoholic-which I don't know what that means, but-the answer's a spiritual one, which is fascinating. And it seems to be true for addicts as well, that the answer is spiritual. That's very interesting to me and always has been.

> It's the twelve-step spiritual journey. It's the same as AA except we know who our higher power is. It's not a group conscience; it's not a doorknob or a sponsor. Our higher power is the Lord. They

are taught how to approach the Lord. We have what's called the twelve-step spiritual journey that I teach, and we go through all the steps.

When asked their perspectives of addiction, several providers expressed beliefs that addiction created a condition of bondage or attachment that could easily be transferred to other behaviors, people, or ideologies. Perspectives on ending addiction typically reflected the program's religious beliefs and 12-step orientation.

Addiction is, you end up giving your world over to a substance or a thing, whether it's gambling or . . . I had a lady that, she had a fishing business, she had a home, and she lost it all to bingo. Yes. Addiction is, you don't have a choice anymore; you've given it up that will to that substance or that urge. When you have faith, you have the Lord to turn to and let it go. You get the baggage off your back; you get the baggage out of your system. You get the needs taken care of. You learn the right way to do things so you can become the best that you can be.

When a person has been delivered from something, they've been totally set free by God, and God does deliver us. Christ, you see some of the works he did in the Bible where He set people free from all sorts of bondages, that work is still happening today. When He delivered me, I was free. I don't classify myself as an alcoholic anymore or a cigarette smoker in recovery anymore or anything like that. I've been set free from those, you know. I think that, to me, is the thing that makes the difference in people that participate in programs outside the faith and get free, that's great. I believe like this. I know a lot of people would not agree with this, but I do believe it. I believe God is always operating, even in programs that we don't think are, quote, "Christian." I believe God operates through circumstances and situations and He will step into a person's life at whatever point they allow Him, even if they're in a secular place. And I believe He moves in secular places. He's a secular guy. He wants to reach the world. He doesn't just move in the church. So there are some people that would argue that, but I guess I've just seen too much to say any different.

People wouldn't make it if they didn't have some connection with spirituality. They won't. You'll find another form of addiction, whether it be women, food, cigarettes, running, shopping. Those are all addictions and you just substitute something else. Or bingo, I mean that's the big one in Indian country, because when you're drinking you get that high. That's the same way when you go to bingo or when you're gambling, it's like, "Oh, I'm almost on!" You know, you get that same high again and it is the same high, but it's just a temporary thing. But if you're spiritually connected that high just stays there.

If they have faith and that faith is real, then they recognize that it may only be that one that they believe in that hasn't let them down and won't let them down. That there's a strength there that they have to have to get through this, there is such a tremendous pull in chemical dependency that it's a minute-by-minute struggle for a lot of individuals. And there isn't any social worker, there isn't any counselor, there isn't any addiction treatment person that be with you every minute of every day. But that one that you believe in can be there and it's at those times when you're most vulnerable that may be the only thing that you've got that can pull you through and help you stay strong.

One provider described how addictions to the idea of faith and faith-related activities could develop following different forms of addiction:

I think, you know, a lot of addiction can be overcome by faith, but I also think it's possible to be addicted to faith. And I don't know if that makes sense or not to you, but some people replace their chemical . . . or some people have relationship addictions. Like they're addicted to unhealthy relationships, or they're addicted to sex, or they're addicted to alcohol, but it's very easy to replace that kind of addiction with "faith," "faith" in quotes, okay, because it's not real faith it's just a replacement. How do you describe that? If you don't internalize what the Bible teaches or what, you know, what your faith entails, if you're just going through the motions you can get really caught up in going through the motions and doing the faith thing which is like praying out loud but you're not really praying in your room. Does this make sense? Because, you know, you can look really good on the outside and you can replace . . . you know, going to church a lot, or going, you know, or being involved in Bible study, but it's not really faith unless you do it in private and you really truly believe.

Beliefs in divine intervention, and the intercession of God to provide experiences the individual may not have chosen, were described by a number of providers. Such beliefs challenge many empirically derived treatment models emphasizing individual control and autonomy to achieve desired outcomes.

As the Bible says: "All things are possible for those who love the Lord." Now, you've got to remember, you know, as the Bible says: "Ask and ye shall have; seek and ye shall find." Well, it's got to be in the Lord's will. Just because I want a new car or I want a new roof or something on my house, doesn't mean it's gonna actually just happen just because I want it. And it's gotta be in the Lord's will. If you wait upon Him, things will turn around. It may not be to your liking, but things will turn around.

I think that if you have faith, and that you truly believe that God is in control and knows what's best for you, and even if He doesn't give you the answer that you want or are expecting, He still will honor what you do for him . . . I've seen a lot of people overcome homelessness and poverty. I mean they don't become wealthy and they don't live in a castle but they can get their lives back on track if they know and believe God and trust him that He's got their best interest in mind. And that doesn't mean it always happens. That doesn't mean that every bad situation will turn out okay because it doesn't obviously.

Several providers also described how their own experiences of addiction and recovery influenced their current work activities and commitment to 12-step programs:

Well, I've been addicted to alcohol and cigarettes. I haven't walked a deep addiction like some people, so . . . From my experience, though, I can tell you that I understood that there are people, and from working with this program and working with people who have been through our drug treatment program; they have said, and I have experienced the same thing, that there are people who go through programs that are non-faith-based or whatever, and they say, "I'm an alcoholic, still, in recovery." They could be clean for ten, fifteen, twenty years, but they would still classify them-selves as an alcoholic. When I was delivered from alcohol, and to be delivered means to be totally set free from the bondage of it, God totally delivered me from it, and I feel no inkling of any type of urge to want to touch a drop of alcohol again. Or a cigarette-same thing. So I don't know what people that are outside of faith-based solutions experience in their bodies, but I know what I did before I came to Christ, and there were many times I tried to quit drinking or smoking and I couldn't. I would go for a few months or whatever and the urge would just take over my body and I had to do it. When God came in and gave me direction on how to get free and I fol-lowed those instructions, it has been fifteen years now, and I have not even had the slightest urge to even want to consider a drink or anything like that because I've been set free. So I think there's a dif-ference, I think.

Twelve-step spiritual healing. And God is our higher power. I'm in recovery. I've been sober for thirty-six years.

A lot of the answers I gave you are answers that have been relevant in my life. And I think in order to be effective in a faith-based min-istry, you know, it's good to have some experience in life where faith has lifted you up. And it has lifted me up, you know, obvi-ously, I was homeless for two years, and you know, among a lot other things, and so I can step into this role and they can look at me and say "how did you do that", and say "you did it. I want to do it too", you know, and I can say that you can come out of it. You know, I won't tell all when I'm with the residents, you know, they don't know everything about me. They know a lot about me be-cause I've shared some of my experiences. I don't share them all the time, but if I'm talking to somebody and it's relevant then I do because it gives them hope and gives them something to look at and say "you were just like me and look where you're at now" and it's cool, this one girl there . . . she's homeless, she was in the hos-pital, she's lost custody of her kids . . . She's very intelligent and nobody's ever told her. Now since she's been there it's so awe-some because, you know, she's writing stories, and she's just re-ally looking forward to going back to school and finishing her degree, she's had a year-and- a-half of college, and she wants to go back and finish and she really believes that she can do it. So it's awesome to watch.

Social worker fears identified by Morell (1996) regarding the promotion of right-wing religious ideology and an over-emphasis on other-worldliness were not substantiated in the interviews, as most of the providers has a strong sense of social justice, engaged in advocacy efforts for homeless individuals and families, and were acutely aware of practical, real-world needs for employment, housing, food, and other material assistance. Concerns regarding possibly exclusionary aspects of 12-step program participation were substantiated in the Christian programs integrating religious and recovery ideologies. Although the religious orientations of these programs were evident in their names, informational materials, icons, and treatment consent agreements, and no discriminatory policies existed regarding potential participants, it is likely that individuals who did not ascribe to Christian beliefs would feel isolated and possibly stigmatized.

None of the providers interviewed stated beliefs that addiction was linked to evil, sin, weakness, or wrongdoing. Likely because of their own personal histories of addiction and 12-step recovery experiences, some providers suggested that addictive behaviors developed as attempts to find security and love. One provider stated:

> I think, in some respects, that chemical . . . the use of chemicals to alter consciousness is what it's really about, and I think people do that because they're looking for something that they can't find, and there's a hollowness inside that is terrifying and cannot be tolerated. People who are fortunate enough from day one to be shown how to fill that through prayer, right living, right action, who are well-loved and so it's not so terrifying to find that hole, tend to do okay, and perhaps some don't wind up getting addicted. Other people whose lives are intolerable, who may on the outside look fine but inside their psychic and spiritual life is intolerable for whatever reason, turn to drugs and alcohol.

Only one provider described alcoholism and drug addiction as "physiological" issues, and there were no references to medical treatment models or the disease concept of addiction. In general, providers maintained very positive expectations that individuals committed to recovery and following the twelve steps could end their addictions permanently.

PRACTICE IMPLICATIONS OF EXISTING RESEARCH AND PROVIDER PERSPECTIVES

Research controversies surrounding the effectiveness of different treatment approaches and the dominance of the 12-step program philosophy create both challenges and opportunities for evidence-based social work. Although the Minnesota Model and 12-step programs are strongly abstinence focused, research has consistently indicated that approximately half of the participants in programs utilizing the Minnesota Model have maintained sobriety a year following treatment (Cook, 1988; Stinchfield & Owen, 1998). Such findings suggest the correctness of Marlatt's (2002) opinion that abstinence goals are unrealistic for many people, although harm reduction models have not proven more effective for long-term drinkers than abstinence approaches. The proliferation of 12-step programs since the 1940s and their value to group members and professional treatment providers suggest their positive effects despite less than dramatic research conclusions.

According to Gambrill (2003), "Given the many burdens social work clients confront, we could argue that accurate brokering of knowledge and ignorance is especially important in our field" (p. 19). Evidence-based practice principles encourage practitioners to be transparent in sharing information about the evidentiary status of treatment interventions, and to consider client values, culture, individual circumstances, and expectations in decision-making. Such considerations are especially important when working with clients involved in 12-step programs or contemplating future involvement. Evidence-based practice supports the development of critical appraisal skills among both workers and clients to assess intervention appropriateness. In work with individuals who are actively addicted, the physical effects of alcohol use and other chemical dependencies may compromise such cognitive abilities. Research literature and anecdotal evidence describing the process of recovery have suggested that rational thinking becomes nearly impossible at certain stages of addiction, and the individual's best hope is to let go of trying to manage their life and surrender to a higher power. For people likely to positively respond to the recovery philosophy of AA, meeting attendance may facilitate validation, social support, and helpful spiritual practices. For others, the AA philosophy of surrender may seem defeating, irrational, and stigmatizing. Attention to context and personal values and beliefs is a crucial element of evidence-based practice. As revealed in the provider narratives, faith-related ideologies of addiction and recovery are seldom scientific, yet their effects are often profound. It is important for social workers to challenge the Minnesota Model and recovery based on 12-step program participation in a way that supports transformative spiritual experiences and faith-related treatment strategies valued by clients, yet also recognizes the possible cultural, spiritual, and religious influences on client outcomes.

Views of addiction and recovery conveyed by faith-related providers emphasize a spiritual process that opens the individual to possibilities and relationships they may not have before considered. Acceptance of mystery and the relinquishment of control are central to a number of faith traditions, many of which may already be familiar to people experiencing addiction. Following tenets of evidence-based practice, it is important for workers to assess contextual variables, including religious, spiritual, and cultural beliefs, in addition to research evidence when developing intervention strategies.

Longstanding tensions between religious and secular social services, and fundamental paradigmatic differences regarding the integration of religion in social care activities may complicate the willingness of some practitioners to support 12-step program involvement, especially if they perceive their clients as vulnerable to religious influences. For other practitioners supportive of 12-step program involvement, it is important to recognize the lack of compelling research evidence to support group membership, and to consider alternative treatment approaches when contextual factors indicate their greater congruence with client beliefs and expectations. Like most difficult situations seen in social work practice, individual experiences of addiction are unique and require attention to both research evidence and personal circumstances. Social work scholars concur that primary goals of evidence-based practice must include empowerment and mutuality (Gambrill, 2003; Witkin & Harrison, 2001). In work with clients affiliated with faith communities and faith-related treatment programs, evidence based practice would encourage the enhancement of worker self-awareness of their own positive and negative biases toward faith-related treatment so mutuality could be established. Although addiction may further client vulnerability, it is important that client self-determination and possible choices to enter faith-related treatment programs not be dismissed or underestimated. Social workers may engage clients in discussions of different treatment models, including their treatment philosophies, cultural sensitivity, and empirical effectiveness. Likewise, similar discussions with faith-related service providers may generate models of collaboration that recognized differences, yet share values of support and empowerment. Witkin and Harrison (2001) suggest complementing evidence-based practices with tenets of narrative practice that respect the unique individual story and circumstances brought to the helping encounter. Listening to such stories is crucial to practice effectiveness in the areas of addiction and recovery since empirical evidence provides no clear treatment direction.

To better navigate the complex clinical and ethical issues often associated with 12-step program involvement, workers may engage in the following areas of assessment. (1) Explore with clients the nested cultures of recovery participation. Twelve-step groups often develop their own individual cultures based on participant personalities, social identities, and histories of addiction. Members may share similar cultural backgrounds, live in the same geographic communities, and possibly participate in the same religious institutions. Depending on their own cultural identities, beliefs, and experiences, clients might find group participation validating or exclusionary. (2) Similarly, discuss with clients the influences of social and cultural support on the recovery process, and assess whether the support available in 12-step programs seems favorable or necessary to achieve desired outcomes. (3) Attend to the structure of a client's narrative describing their experience of addiction, and the degree of personal control they perceive in changing behavior. For clients expressing spiritual and/or religious beliefs, examine how these beliefs affect locus of control, self esteem, perceptions of agency and self-efficacy, beliefs about sin and the consequences of sin, relationships with authority. Ways cultural and economic factors affect belief system should also be explored. (4) If clients are unfamiliar with the 12-step program philosophy and interested in learning more about it, practitioners may share AA literature, review the twelve steps, and discuss whether the steps and meeting rituals seem congruent with client beliefs. (5) In addition to assessing the possible risks and benefits of 12-step program participation, workers may want to assess community systems of addiction treatment, and what kinds of options may be available for individuals interested in recovery. The dominance of the 12-step philosophy has been partly attributed to ease of access issues (Wilcox, 1998). Meetings are free, are often scheduled at flexible times, and are to some degree anonymous, though people at meetings often recognize each other. Attending open 12-step meetings and visiting faith-related treatment programs may also enhance worker awareness of service options and related practice effectiveness.

CONCLUSION

Despite a lack of conclusive research evidence supporting their effectiveness, 12-step recovery approaches continue to exert a significant influence on professional treatment programs. For individuals who lack motivation, resources, or opportunities for professional treatment, 12-step meetings may offer opportunities for self-awareness, spiritual development, social support, and behavior change strategies to assist recovery. Principles of evidence-based practice encourage social workers to integrate knowledge of empirical research with awareness of client values and beliefs in clinical decision-making. Client receptivity and responsiveness to 12-step program participation and other spiritually or religiously oriented treatment activities will likely reflect existing spiritual/religious beliefs, cultural backgrounds, addiction experiences, recovery motivation, and willingness to follow the twelve steps, as well as engage in group practices and processes.

Perspectives on addiction and recovery expressed by faith-related providers indicate strong reliance on spiritual and religious faith in treatment programs, and frequent personal experiences of addiction and recovery that motivate assistance to others. Provider narratives of addiction and recovery experiences employ different styles of discourse than empirically based professional literature, and reveal a paradigmatic orientation more allied with faith than science. Although not easily conducive to scientific testing or measurement, narratives of spiritual and personal transformation may facilitate positive connections among individuals sharing similar social backgrounds and experiences. The integration of narrative therapeutic strategies with evidence- based attention to empirical research and client values and beliefs can offer an effective strategy for practitioners navigating complex treatment issues. It is likely that spiritual and scientific views of recovery will never be completely reconciled, though social work attention to person-environment context and evidence-based commitments to empirical evaluation can provide a meaningful synthesis of treatment perspectives, and enhance ethical, effective social work practice in the area of addictions.

REFERENCES

Alcoholics Anonymous World Services (2001). *Alcoholics Anonymous*, (4th ed.) New York City: Alcoholics Anonymous World Services, Inc.

Allahyari, R. (2000). *Visions of charity: Volunteer workers and moral community.* Berkeley: University of California Press.

Bateson, G. (1971). The cybernetics of self: A theory of alcoholism. *Psychiatry, 34*: 1-8.

Bower, B. (1997). Alcoholics synonymous. *Science News, 151*: 62-63.

Brandes, S. (2002). *Staying sober in Mexico City*. Austin, TX: University of Texas Press.

Bufe, C. (1998). *Alcoholics Anonymous: Cult or cure?* Tucson, AZ: See Sharp Press.

Carroll, K. (2001). Constrained, confounded, and confused: Why we really know so little about therapists in treatment outcome research. *Addiction, 96*, 203-206.

Cnaan, R. (2002). *The invisible caring hand: American congregations and the provision of welfare*. New York: New York University Press.

Cook, C. (1988). The Minnesota Model in the management of drug and alcohol dependence: Miracle, method, or myth? Part II. Evidence and Conclusions. *British Journal of Addiction, 83*, 735-748.

Denzin, N. (1987). *The recovering alcoholic*. Newbury Park, CA: Sage Publications.

Fiorentine, R., & Hillhouse, M. (2000). Self-efficacy, expectancies, and abstinence acceptance: Further evidence for the addicted-self model of cessation of alcohol-and drug-dependent behavior. *American Journal of Drug & Alcohol Abuse*, 26(4), 497-521.

Fitzgerald, K. (1996). *Women in AA: Personal stories of recovery*. Lake Forest, IL: Whale's Tale Press.

Forman, R., Bovasso, G., & Woody, G. (2001). Staff beliefs about addiction treatment. *Journal of Substance Abuse Treatment, 21*, 1-9.

Gambrill, E. (2003). Evidence-based practice: Sea change or emperor's new clothes? *Journal of Social Work Education, 39*(1), 3-23.

Gregoire, T. (1995). Alcoholism: The quest for transcendence and meaning. *Clinical Social Work Journal, 23(3)*, 339-359.

Hazelden Foundation (1996). *The twelve steps of Alcoholics Anonymous*. Center City, MN: Hazelden Foundation Press.

hooks, b. (1993). *Sisters of the yam: Black women and self-recovery*. Boston: South End Press.

James, W. (1902). *The varieties of religious experience*. Cambridge, MA: Harvard University Press.

Krestan, J. (2000). *Bridges to Recovery: Addiction, family therapy, and multicultural treatment*. New York: Free Press.

Kurtz, L., & Fisher, M. (2003). Twelve-step recovery and community service. *Health and Social Work, 28*(2), 137-145.

Liberty, H., Johnson, B., Jainchill, N., Ryder, J., Messina, M., Reynolds, S., & Hossain, M. (1998). Dynamic recovery: Comparative study of therapeutic communities in homeless shelters for men. *Journal of Substance Abuse Treatment, 15*(5), 401-423.

Madsen, W. (1974). *The American alcoholic: The nature-nurture controversy in alcoholic research and therapy*. Springfield, IL: Charles C. Thomas Publishers.

Marlatt, A., & Witkiewitz, K. (2002). Harm reduction approaches to alcohol use: Health promotion, prevention, and treatment. *Addictive Behaviors, 27*, 867-886.

Miller, W. (1998). Researching the spiritual dimensions of alcohol and other drug problems. *Addiction, 93*(7), 979-990.

Morell, C. (1996). Radicalizing recovery: Addiction, spirituality, and politics. *Social Work, 41*(3), 306-312.

O'Reilly, E. (1997). *Sobering tales: Narratives of alcoholism and recovery*. Amherst, MA: University of Massachusetts Press.

Project MATCH Research Group (1998). Matching patients with alcohol disorders to treatments: Clinical implications from Project MATCH. *Journal of Mental Health, 7*(6), 589-602.

Raphael, M. (2000). *Bill W., and Mr. Wilson: The legend and life of AA's cofounder.* Amherst, MA: The University of Massachusetts Press.

Saulnier, C. (1996). Images of the twelve-step model, and sex and love addiction in an alcohol intervention group for black women. *Journal of Drug Issues, 26*(1), 95-123.

Sobell, L., Ellingstad, T., & Sobell, M. (2000). Natural recovery from alcohol and drug problems: Methodological review of the research with suggestions for future directions. *Addiction, 95*(5), 749-674.

Stinchfield, R., & Owen, P. (1998). Hazelden's model of treatment and its outcome. *Addictive Behaviors, 23*(5), 669-683.

Strauss, A. (1998). *Basics of qualitative research: Techniques and procedures for developing grounded theory.* Thousand Oaks, CA: Sage Publications.

Tallen, B. (1990). Twelve-step programs: A lesbian feminist critique. *National Women's Studies Association Journal, 2*(3), 390-407.

Tangenberg, K. (2002). *Social work or soul saving: Researching the values of faith-based service programs and their implications for practice.* Paper presented at annual meeting of the Society for Social Work Research. San Diego, CA.

Tangenberg, K. (2001). Surviving two diseases: Addiction, recovery, and spirituality among mothers living with HIV Disease. *Families in Society, 82*(5), 517-524.

Tonigan, J., Connors, G., & Miller, W. (1998). Special populations in Alcoholics Anonymous. *Alcohol Health and Research World, 22*(4), 281-286.

Trimpey, J. (1996). *Rational recovery: The new cure for substance addiction.* New York: Simon and Schuster.

Van Wormer, K. (1995). *Alcoholism treatment: A social work perspective.* Chicago: Nelson-Hall Publishers.

Washington, O., & Moxley, P. (2003). Group interventions with low-income African-American women recovering from chemical dependency. *Health and Social Work, 28*(2), 146-156.

Wilcox, D. (1998). *Alcoholic thinking: Language, culture, and belief in Alcoholics Anonymous.* Westport, CT: Praeger Press.

Williams, C. (1992). *No hiding place: Empowerment and recovery for our troubled communities.* New York: Harper Collins.

Wilson, W. (1939). *Alcoholics Anonymous.* New York: Alcoholics Anonymous World Services, Inc.

Winters, K., Stinchfield, R., Opland, E., Weller, C., & Latimer, W. (2000). The effectiveness of the Minnesota Model approach in the treatment of adolescent drug abusers. *Addiction, 95*(4), 601-613.

Witkin, S., & Harrison, W. (2001). Whose evidence and for what purpose? *Social Work, 46*(4), 293-296.

Implementation of Contingency Management Substance Abuse Treatment in Community Settings

Soo Mi Jang, PhD
Susan L. Schoppelrey, PhD

SUMMARY. Considerable evidence exists regarding the efficacy and cost-effectiveness of contingency management (CM) and related approaches to treating substance use disorders. Despite more than 25 years of research, these interventions are presently underutilized, especially in community settings. This article examines potential barriers related to cost, appropriateness, and effectiveness that may explain the low levels of utilization and proposes strategies for overcoming these barriers. Implications for further research and implementation efforts are also discussed. *[Article copies available for a fee from The Haworth Document Delivery Service: 1-800-HAWORTH. E-mail address: <docdelivery@haworthpress.com> Website: <http://www.HaworthPress.com> © 2005 by The Haworth Press, Inc. All rights reserved.]*

Soo Mi Jang is Visiting Research Associate, and Susan L. Schoppelrey is Assistant Professor, School of Social Work, University of Illinois at Urbana-Champaign.

Address correspondence to: Susan L. Schoppelrey, PhD, Assistant Professor, School of Social Work, University of Illinois at Urbana-Champaign, 1207 West Oregon Street, Urbana, IL 61801 (E-mail: schoppel@uiuc.edu).

[Haworth co-indexing entry note]: "Implementation of Contingency Management Substance Abuse Treatment in Community Settings." Jang, Soo Mi, and Susan L. Schoppelrey. Co-published simultaneously in *Journal of Evidence-Based Social Work* (The Haworth Social Work Practice Press, an imprint of The Haworth Press, Inc.) Vol. 2, No. 1/2, 2005, pp. 41-54; and: *Addiction, Assessment, and Treatment with Adolescents, Adults, and Families* (ed: Carolyn Hilarski) The Haworth Social Work Practice Press, an imprint of The Haworth Press, Inc., 2005, pp. 41-54. Single or multiple copies of this article are available for a fee from The Haworth Document Delivery Service [1-800-HAWORTH, 9:00 a.m. - 5:00 p.m. (EST). E-mail address: docdelivery@haworthpress.com].

http://www.haworthpress.com/web/JEBSW
Digital Object Identifier: 10.1300/J394v02n01_03   *41*

KEYWORDS. Contingency management, substance abuse treatment, community

Contingency management approaches to treating substance use disorders have a solid theoretical base in behavioral principles. Despite decades of research providing convincing evidence of the efficacy of contingency management (CM) and related approaches, these interventions are presently underutilized and are rarely utilized outside of a research setting. Although widely researched in clinical settings, there are relatively few studies examining contingency management in community settings. Given the considerable empirical support for these interventions, it seems prudent to examine the factors preventing a wider adoption of these treatment techniques as well as potential strategies for overcoming these barriers.

Contingency management approaches to substance abuse treatment derive from the operant behavioral psychology perspective of B. F. Skinner and others. The essence of this perspective is the belief that behavior is learned and reinforced by interaction with environmental contingencies (Bigelow & Silverman, 1999, p. 16). Rather than viewing substance abuse as a symptom of underlying psychopathology or a sign of a weak moral character, operant conditioning theory views substance use as the natural result of environmental contingencies that fail to adequately reinforce abstinence or discourage substance abuse (Bigelow & Silverman, 1999). If dysfunctional substance use behavior is acquired through operant conditioning, it is reasoned, those same principles can be utilized to extinguish the substance use.

Contingency management has been called by many names, including incentive therapy (Bigelow, Brooner, & Silverman, 1998), contingency contracting (Boudin et al., 1977), and behavior contracting (Holder, Longabaugh, & Miller, 1991). It has been described as a technique that "organizes treatment delivery, sets specific objective behavioral goals, and attempts to structure the abuser's environment in a manner that is conducive to change" (Stitzer et al., 1989 as cited in Rowan-Szal, Joe, Chatham, & Simpson, 1994, p. 218). Contingency management essentially consists of a system of positive and negative reinforcers designed to make continued substance abuse relatively unattractive and abstinence relatively attractive (Rowan-Szal et al., 1994). Much of the early research on contingency management focused on methadone maintenance programs and used behavioral contingencies such as take-home dosing and increased (or decreased) doses. Contingency management has been successfully applied in drug-free treatment settings by using reinforcers such as vouchers (Higgins, Burdney, & Bickel, 1993), prizes (Petry, 2000), retail items, coupons for gasoline or food, or bus tokens (Rowan-Szal et al., 1994), and even cash (Shaner et al., 1997). This technique has been successfully used in treating addiction to a variety of substances, including dependence on marijuana (Burdney, Higgins, Radonovich, & Novy, 2000), cocaine (Higgins, Burdney, & Bickel, 1993), opiates (Carroll, Sinha, Nich, Babuscio, & Rounsaville, 2002), benzodiazepines (Stitzer, Iguchi & Felch, 1992), and alcohol (Petry, Martin, Cooney, & Kranzler, 2000). In addition, contingency management has been used to treat the homeless (Milby et al., 1996), the seriously mentally ill (Hughes, Hatsukamim, Mitchell, & Dahlgreen, 1986), and pregnant women (Jones, Haug, Silverman, Stitzer, & Svikis, 2001).

EVIDENCE OF EFFICACY

Many studies have demonstrated the efficacy of contingency management and related approaches in treating substance use disorders (Kosten, Poling, & Oliveto, 2003; Preston, Umbricht & Epstein, 2002; Petry & Martin, 2002). Contingency management has consistently shown outcomes superior to traditional substance abuse treatment in terms of retention in treatment and reduction of drug use. For example, Higgins and colleagues (1994) found that 75% of cocaine-dependent clients assigned to the contingency management condition, in which they received counseling as well as vouchers for submission of drug-free urine samples, completed a 24-week trial; in comparison, only 40% of clients who received only counseling did so. Voucher clients were also significantly more likely to achieve at least 2 months of continuous abstinence from cocaine (as verified by urine screens) than those in the counseling-only condition (55% and 15%, respectively). Petry et al. (2000) found that clients receiving contingency management had dramatically higher retention rates over the 8-week period than did clients receiving standard treatment (84% and 22%, respectively). At the end of the treatment period, abstinence was 69% among the contingency management group while 61% of those in the comparison group had relapsed to alcohol use. These and many other studies demonstrate that contingency management affects drug use outcomes and not merely retention in treatment.

In a recent meta-analysis of 30 studies, Griffith et al. (2000) found that contingency management is effective in reducing drug use among methadone maintenance clients. Increases in methadone dose and take-home privileges were associated with larger effect sizes than other reinforcers. Larger effect sizes were associated with shorter time lags between the targeted behavior and the contingency; targeting a single drug or behavior for change rather than multiple behaviors; and more frequent monitoring of behavior (i.e., through urinalysis). One unexpected finding was that studies using non-random assignment of subjects to treatment and control or comparison groups had larger effect sizes than those using random assignment. Whether due to staff expectations, selection bias, or other factors, this finding highlights the importance of considering the research design when interpreting results. It is likely that studies using non-random assignment overestimate the effect size of the intervention.

Perhaps the most frequently cited barrier to the widespread implementation of contingency management is their high cost (Rowan-Szal et al., 1994; Bigelow et al., 1998). Cost concerns relate mainly to the cost of the incentives provided, although biological verification also represents a substantial expense. Contingency management interventions were initially developed in methadone maintenance programs, where incentives were relatively low-cost as they consisted of take-home privileges or increased dosages of methadone, which is itself a strong positive reinforcer (Griffith et al., 2000). Methadone maintenance programs also possess the facilities, staff, and resources necessary to perform routine urinalyses to provide objective verification of abstinence. The marginal cost of adding contingency management interventions and monitoring to methadone maintenance programs is therefore quite low. Incremental costs may be substantially higher for programs that lack the capacity to perform routine biological verification through urinalysis or other methods. Incentives may also represent substantial marginal costs for community-based substance abuse treatment programs.

COST CONSIDERATIONS: INCENTIVES

Although incentive-based treatments such as contingency management have been proven effective, the feasibility of acquiring incentives that are adequate to compete with the reinforcement provided by drug use without being prohibitively expensive remains an issue, particularly in community settings. Aside from the routine facility and staff costs related to counseling and other services, contingency management interventions require adequate funding to provide vouchers or prizes to reinforce abstinence. While it may be possible to obtain time-limited support for research and demonstration programs, the prospects for continued and sustained funding for incentives remains murky. Whether using vouchers or specific prizes, some staff time must also be devoted to purchasing the necessary reinforcers.

While vouchers are effective reinforcers for abstinence, different magnitudes of reinforcement may be required for establishing initial abstinence and for maintaining continued abstinence (Petry & Martin, 2002). Higgins et al. (1994) used an escalating reinforcement schedule whereby vouchers increased in magnitude for each consecutive negative urine screen. Although escalating reinforcement schedules are more effective than fixed schedules, they are complex and can be difficult to implement in a community setting (Jones et al., 2001). Escalating schedules also produce exponential increases in cost and may therefore be of limited utility (Jones et al., 2001).

Two meta-analyses of substance abuse treatment methods have ranked incentive-based treatment relatively high in terms of its efficacy (Miller et al., 1995) and cost-effectiveness (Holder, Longabaugh & Miller, 1991). Contingency management (CM) and the community reinforcement approach (CRA) were ranked at the 81st and 91st percentiles, respectively, in terms of cost-effectiveness (Holder et al., 1991). Only brief interventions and motivational enhancement interventions were found to be equally or more cost-effective than these two incentive-based treatments (CM and CRA; Higgins, 1999, p. 302). Incentive-based treatments may ultimately prove to be cost-effective in reducing revolving-door admissions and societal costs associated with drug dependence; the up-front costs of implementing such a system may preclude its use in many programs (Petry, 2000). The studies examined in these reviews used relatively high-cost reinforcers; it is likely that using lower-intensity reinforcers would increase the cost-effectiveness of incentive-based treatments. While there has been some success in implementing contingency management using relatively low-intensity reinforcers, more research needs to be done to compare the relative efficacy of reinforcers of differing magnitudes.

One suggestion for reducing the cost associated with incentives is the use of on-site retail items (e.g., gift certificates, CDs, baby items) in place of vouchers. This procedure has the advantage of freeing staff from shopping for specific items when clients wish to redeem their vouchers and, in addition, allows greater flexibility in the selection of incentives such that incentives can be solicited via donation from local merchants, thereby further reducing the cost to the program (Amass, 1997). This alternative provides only a modest improvement over the voucher condition, however, as considerable staff time must also be devoted to donation solicitation and management (Petry, 2000) and may still impose an unbearable cost burden for many programs (Kirby, Amass, & McLellan, 1999).

Another option for lowering the incentive-related costs is implementing a lottery system. Rather than rewarding each negative urine screen with a voucher, clients are rewarded with entries in a lottery (Petry & Martin, 2002). Most of the slips in the prize bowl simply contained positive messages, such as "Good job!" Several slips would contain small prizes worth approximately $1 (e.g., fast food coupon), a medium prize worth approximately $20 (e.g., gift certificate, phone card), or a large prize worth $100 (e.g., a TV or stereo). While the reward schedule itself replicated that used in earlier studies, including escalating magnitudes of reinforcers for continued or sustained abstinence, the fact that the rewards were lottery entries rather than vouchers substantially reduced the overall cost of the program without a concomitant reduction in efficacy. The lottery system cost only $137 per client (Petry & Martin, 2002) over a 12-week period, compared to an escalating voucher condition that cost $426 per client over an identical time frame (Silverman et al., 1996).

Rather than manipulating the magnitude of the reinforcer, it has been suggested that the type of reinforcer be modified. Using access to social services as a reinforcer has been suggested and, indeed, has a long history of use on an informal basis. Potential reinforcers might be found in substance abusers' interactions with family, friends, employer, the criminal justice system, and social welfare agencies (Bigelow, Brooner, & Silverman, 1998). Many supportive housing programs impose abstinence as a requirement of participation, for instance. Milby et al. (1996) developed a program that provided employment and housing services to homeless drug abusers contingent upon abstinence. The establishment of a representative payee for disability or other public assistance payments is one potential avenue for establishing a low-cost means of reinforcing abstinence (Jerrel & Ridgely, 1995; Petry, 2000).

COST CONSIDERATIONS: MONITORING

Aside from the cost of incentives, monitoring abstinence through urinalysis or other biological methods imposes additional costs. The consistency and integrity of the monitoring system is key to the success of any contingency management intervention (Schumacher et al., 1999). Staff resources must of course be dedicated to supervising the submission of urine samples or other biological markers of drug use. The considerable costs associated with performing the biological tests themselves and the need for frequent (ideally, at least 3 times per week) testing also pose substantial barriers for many community-based programs (Iguchi, Belding, Morral, Lamb, & Husband, 1997). While biological markers such as breath alcohol levels or saliva nicotine concentrations may be less expensive than urinalysis, these procedures have a briefer detection interval and must be repeated multiple times daily to reliably detect the use of alcohol or nicotine. The use of social contingencies that occur naturally in the client's environment, such as positive interactions with a spouse or children or continued employment in a valued position, is less costly than the use of artificial contingencies such as vouchers or prize drawings. Such a strategy may also have a longer-lasting effect than artificial contingencies. The community reinforcement approach (CRA) is designed to systematically facilitate changes in the client's daily environment to reduce substance abuse and promote a healthier lifestyle (Higgins & Abbott, 2001). Although CM and CRA are based on the same behavioral principles, CRA is generally more broadly geared toward enhancing function in a variety of life domains in addition to substance abuse (Bigelow & Silverman, 1999, p. 24). Thus, CRA represents a potentially cost-effective adjunct to contingency management approaches that utilize artificial incentives such as vouchers or prizes.

Contingency management programs that focus exclusively on abstinence may not modify the behaviors of all participants because many never emit the behavior targeted for reinforcement-the submission of a drug-free urine sample (Morral, Iguchi, & Belding, 1999, p. 205). It may be productive to reinforce behaviors that, while not directly related to abstinence, can indirectly influence important areas of client functioning. It is possible, for instance, to reinforce behaviors such as attendance at group or compliance with goal-related activities (Morral et al., 1999; Iguchi et al., 1997; Petry, Martin, & Finocche, 2001). Such an approach may reduce drug use among those who continue to submit few, if any, drug-free urine samples even after entering methadone maintenance or other forms of drug abuse treatment (Morral et al., 1999). Iguchi et al. (1997) even found that reinforcing goal-oriented behaviors-such as verified attendance at an employment training program-produced outcomes superior to reinforcing negative urine screens. In addition to saving the cost of drug testing, such an approach has other advantages. It relies on positively reinforcing desired behaviors (attendance at a therapy session) rather than reinforcing the absence of an undesirable behavior (drug use). Target behaviors can be made smaller and more achievable, enabling more clients to earn incentives and fostering a feeling of self-efficacy in achieving goals that are denied to clients unable to achieve complete abstinence when urinalysis is used as the criterion behavior (Iguchi et al., 1997).

Using attendance and participation in group treatment rather than abstinence as a criterion behavior provides additional benefits. Petry and colleagues (Petry et al., 2001) demonstrated that improvements in the criterion behaviors of group attendance and compliance with goal-related activities persisted even after the incentives were withdrawn. In addition, there was a spillover effect wherein client attendance at all groups-not just those with incentives-increased (Petry, Martin, & Finocche, 2001). In addition to enhancing attendance, the group environment seemed to improve markedly, as indicated by better group cohesion, a stronger sense of group identity, and a greater ability on the part of all group members to provide verbal reinforcement and support to others (Petry & Simcic, 2002). Reinforcing attendance and participation in treatment groups also makes contingency management interventions more congruent with community-based substance services, which often include group modalities as a central component of treatment (Petry, Martin, & Finocche, 2001) and may improve the cost-effectiveness of contingency management interventions (Kirby et al., 1999).

PERSISTENCE OF TREATMENT EFFECTS

Reductions in substance use achieved through contingency management interventions may be highly dependent upon the availability of artificial contingencies and any treatment effect may degrade rapidly or even reverse once the incentives are withdrawn (Morral et al., 1999). Reversibility is not a phenomena unique to incentive-based treatments, however. Relapse is ubiquitous in the substance abuse field regardless of whether treatment involves CM techniques (Bigelow, Stitzer, Griffiths, & Liebson, 1981, p. 249). Incentive-based therapies, such as contingency management and community reinforcement approach, are essentially indistinguishable from pharmacotherapies and as other psychosocial therapies in that treatment effects tend to be of relatively short duration and to degrade rapidly over time once treatment is withdrawn (Project MATCH Research Group, 1997, as cited in Bigelow et al., 1998).

Early attrition is a substantial problem in all substance abuse treatment programs, regardless of setting or theoretical orientation (Higgins & Abbott, 2001). Even if the effects of contingency management are not long-lived, they may be useful in increasing retention in treatment if timed correctly (Bigelow et al., 1998). CM interventions can also be useful in enhancing client motivation to change, which can, in turn, enhance the efficacy of any subsequent treatment provided (Bien et al., 1993; Brown & Miller, 1993; Lincourt, Kuettel, & Bombardier, 2002). Achieving drug abstinence may be a necessary first step prior to improving outcomes in other domains. Consequently, the use of CM in the initial stages of treatment may enhance the efficacy of later stages as well as enhancing outcomes in domains other than substance use. Once drug abstinence is achieved, patients may begin to work on other areas of concern, such as alleviating depression, improving legal problems, finding employment, and reducing family conflict (Petry & Martin, 2002).

The community reinforcement approach (CRA), used in conjunction with contingency management or sequentially, is an ideal mechanism for ensuring the long-term maintenance of treatment effects. CRA is one of the most effective interventions for treating alcohol dependence (Miller et al., 1995). Although originally developed more than thirty years ago to treat alcoholism (Hunt & Azrin, 1973, as cited in Meyer & Miller, 2001), the community reinforcement approach has been combined with explicit CM procedures (Higgins et al., 1993, 1994; Bickel, Amass, Higgins, Badger, & Esch, 1998). While CM has traditionally focused on substance use outcomes, CRA typically includes a number of functional domains such as work family, and social and recreational areas. CRA attempts to increase the frequency and amount of reinforcement clients receive from prosocial activities such as work and family in order to make alcohol and drug use relatively less appealing (Higgins & Abbott, 2001).

The goal of CRA is to systematically alter the drug user's environment, so that reinforcement density from non-drug sources is relatively high during sobriety and low during drug use (Higgins et al., 1999, p. 36). Because CM is an integral component of CRA, it is important to devise process measure to assess the integrity of its administration (Pantalon & Schottenfeld, 1999, p. 311). CRA can potentially be used to sustain the effects of CM by focusing on broader client concerns (e.g., about family relationships) rather than narrowly focusing on urine toxicology or treatment attendance (Kosten et al., 2003, p. 670).

It would appear that CM, which is quite useful in achieving initial abstinence and preventing early drop-outs, is an ideal complement to CRA, which utilizes natural rather than artificial incentives and focuses on a broad range of problem areas relevant to the client's psychosocial functioning in areas beyond substance use. Indeed, several studies have demonstrated the efficacy of combining CRA with vouchers (Higgins & Abbot, 2001). Another study illustrated that the combination of CM and cognitive-behavioral treatment (CBT) produced outcomes superior to either intervention alone (Epstein, Hawkins, Covi, & Umbricht, 2003).

CONCLUSION

In a 1981 review, Bigelow and colleagues noted several limitations related to the use of contingency management approaches in treating drug abuse and dependence (Bigelow, Stitzer, Griffiths, and Liebson, 1981). Among the limitations they noted were the cost of biological verification and incentives, acceptability of contingency management approaches to staff and clients, and the high rates of relapse to drug use upon withdrawal of positive contingencies. Although notable progress has been made, these barriers remain largely intact today. The present article has reviewed several of the most pressing reasons for the low utilization of CM and proposed methods for making these interventions more feasible.

Future research must move out of the laboratory and into the community to examine the costs, barriers, and effectiveness of CM approaches as they are implemented in "real world" community settings. It may also be advantageous to examine ways in which the organizational culture of specific community programs may facilitate or impede the implementation of CM and other novel approaches to substance abuse treatment. An examination of staff attitudes on an individual level and as a function of occupational subcultures (e.g., social work, paraprofessional substance abuse counselors) may shed light on resistance from program staff to implementing incentive-based treatment in general. Ultimately, it is important to develop educational and other strategies to address these systematic barriers to the implementation of evidence-based practice within community agencies that treat substance abuse and related problems.

REFERENCES

Amass, L. (1997). Financing voucher programs for pregnant substance abusers through community donations. In L.S. Harris (Ed.), *Problems of drug dependence: Proceedings of the 58th Annual Scientific Meeting* (p. 60; NIH Pub. No. 174). Washington, DC: GPO.

Bickel, W., Amass, L., Higgins, S.T., Badger, G.J., & Esch, R. (1997). Behavioral treatment improves outcomes during opioid detoxification with buprenorphine. *Journal of Consulting & Clinical Psychology, 65,* 803-810.

Bien, T., Miller, W., and Borough, J. (1993). Motivational interviewing with alcohol outpatients. *Behavioral Psychotherapy, 21,* 347-356.

Bigelow, G., Brooner, R., and Silverman, K. (1998). Competing motivations: Drug reinforcement vs. non-drug reinforcement. *Journal of Psychopharmacology, 12*(1), 8-14.

Bigelow, G., and Silverman, K. (1999). Theoretical and empirical foundations of contingency management for drug abuse. In S.T. Higgins, & K. Silverman (Eds.), *Motivating behavior change among illicit-drug abusers: Research on contingency management interventions* (pp. 15-31). Washington, DC: American Psychological Association.

Bigelow, G., Stitzer, M., Griffiths, R., and Liebson, I. (1981). Contingency management approaches to drug self-administration and drug abuse: Efficacy and limitations. *Addictive Behaviors, 6,* 241-252.

Boudin, H., Valentine, V., Inghram, R., Brantly, J., Ruiz, M., Smith, G., Caltin, R., and Regan, E. (1977). Contingency contracting with drug abusers in the natural environment. *International Journal of the Addictions, 12*(1), 1-16.

Brown, J., and Miller, W. (1993). Impact of motivational interviewing on participation and outcome in residential alcoholism treatment. *Psychology of Addictive Behaviors, 7,* 211-218.

Burdney, A.J., Higgins, S.T., Radonovich, K.J., and Novy, P.L. (2000). Adding voucher-based incentives to coping skills and motivational enhancement improves outcomes during treatment for marijuana dependence. *Journal of Consulting & Clinical Psychology, 68,* 1051-1061.

Carroll, K.M., Sinha, R., Nich, C., Babuscio, T., and Rounsaville, B. (2002). Contingency management to enhance naltrexone treatment of opioid dependence: A randomized clinical trial of reinforcement magnitude. *Experimental and Clinical Psychopharmacology, 10*(1), 54-63.

Epstein, D.H., Hawkins, W.E., Covi, L., and Umbricht, A. (2003) Cognitive-Behavioral Therapy plus contingency management for cocaine use: Findings during treatment and across 12-month follow-up. *Psychology of Addictive Behavior, 17*(1), 73-82.

Griffith, J.D., Rowan-Szal, G.A., Roark, R.R., and Simpson, D. (2000). Contingency management in outpatient methadone treatment: A meta-analysis. *Drug and Alcohol Dependence, 58,* 55-66.

Higgins, S.T. (1999). Potential contributions of the community reinforcement approach and contingency management to broadening the base of substance abuse treatment. In J.A. Turner, D.M. Donovan, and G.A. Marlatt (Eds.), *Changing addic-*

tive behavior: Bridging clinical and public health strategies (pp. 283-306). New York: The Guilford Press.

Higgins, S.T., and Abbott, P.J. (2001). CRA and treatment of cocaine and opioid dependence. In R.J. Meyer, & W.R. Miller (Eds.), *A community reinforcement approach to addiction treatment* (pp. 123-146). New York: Cambridge University Press.

Higgins, S.T., Burdney, A.J., and Bickel, W.K. (1993). Achieving cocaine abstinence with a behavioral approach. *American Journal of Psychiatry, 150,* 763-769.

Higgins, S.T., Burdney, A.J., Bickel, W.K., Foerg, F.E., Donham, R., and Badger, G.J. (1994). Incentives improve outcome in outpatient behavioral treatment of cocaine dependence. *Archives of General Psychiatry, 51,* 568-576.

Higgins, S.T., Roll, J.H., Wong, C., Tidey, J.W., and Dantona, R. (1999). Clinic and laboratory studies on the use of incentives to decrease cocaine and other substance use. In S.T. Higgins, and K. Silverman (Eds.), *Motivating behavior change among Illicit-drug abusers: Research on contingency management interventions* (pp. 35-56). Washington, DC: American Psychological Association.

Holder, H., Longabaugh, R., and Miller, W.R. (1991). The cost-effectiveness of treatment for alcoholism: A first approximation. *Journal of Studies on Alcohol, 52,* 517-540.

Hughes, J.R., Hatsukamim, D.K., Mitchell, J.E., and Dahlgren, L.A. (1986). Prevalence of smoking among psychiatric outpatients. *American Journal of Psychiatry, 143,* 993-997.

Iguchi, M.Y., Belding, M.A., Morral, A.R., Lamb, R.F., and Husband, S.D. (1997). Reinforcing operants other than abstinence in drug abuse treatment: Effective alternatives for reducing drug use. *Journal of Consulting & Clinical Psychology, 65*(3), 421-428.

Jerrel, J.M., and Ridgely, M.S. (1995). Comparative effectiveness of three approaches to serving people with severe mental illness and substance use disorders. *Journal of Nervous & Mental Disease, 183,* 566-576.

Jones, H.E., Haug, N., Silverman, K., Stitzer, M., and Svikis, D. (2001). The effectiveness of incentives in enhancing treatment attendance and drug abstinence in methadone-maintained pregnant women. *Drug and Alcohol Dependence, 61,* 297-306.

Kirby, K.C., Amass, L., and McLellan, A.T. (1999). Disseminating contingency management research to drug abuse treatment practitioners. In S.T. Higgins, and K. Silverman (Eds.), *Motivating behavior change among illicit-drug abusers: Research on contingency management interventions* (pp. 329-344). Washington, DC: American Psychological Association.

Kosten, T., Poling, J., and Oliveto, A. (2003). Effects of reducing contingency management values on heroin and cocaine use for buprenorphine- and desipramine-treated patients. *Addiction, 98,* 665-671.

Lincourt, P., Kuettel, T., and Bombardier, C.H. (2002). Motivational interviewing in a group setting with mandated clients: A pilot study. *Addictive Behaviors, 27,* 381-391.

Meyer, R.J., and Miller, W.R. (Eds.). (2001). *A community reinforcement approach to addiction treatment.* New York: Cambridge University Press.

Milby, J.B., Schumacher, J.E., Raczynski, J.M. Caldwell. E., Engle, M., Michael, M., and Carr, J. (1996). Sufficient conditions for effective treatment of substance abusing homeless. *Drug and Alcohol Dependence, 43,* 39-47.

Miller, W.R., Brown, J.M., Simpson, T.L., Handmaker, N.S., Bien, T.H., Luckie, L.F., Montgomery, H.A., Hester, R.K., and Tonigan, J.S. (1995). What works? A methodological analysis of the alcohol treatment outcome literature. In R.K. Hester, & W.R. Miller (Eds.), *Handbook of alcoholism treatment approaches: Effective alternatives* (2nd ed.) (pp. 221-241). Boston: Allyn & Bacon.

Morral, A., Iguchi, M., and Belding, M. (1999). Reducing drug use by encouraging alternative behaviors. In S.T. Higgins, and K. Silverman (Eds.), *Motivating behavior change among illicit-drug abusers: Research on contingency management interventions* (pp. 203-220). Washington, DC: American Psychological Association.

Pantalon, M.V., and Schottenfeld, R.S. (1999). Monitoring therapist and patient behavior during behavioral interventions for illicit-drug use: Process research perspectives. In S.T. Higgins, and K. Silverman (Eds.), *Motivating behavior change among illicit-drug abusers: Research on contingency management interventions* (pp. 309-326). Washington, DC: American Psychological Association.

Petry, N.M. (2000). A comprehensive guide to the application of contingency management procedures in clinical settings. *Drug and Alcohol Dependence, 58*, 9-25.

Petry, N.M., and Martin, B. (2002). Low-cost contingency management for treating cocaine-and opioid-abusing methadone patients. *Journal of Consulting & Clinical Psychology, 70*(2), 398-405.

Petry, N.M., Martin, B., Cooney, J.L., and Kranzler, H.R. (2000). Give them prizes, and they will come: Contingency management for treatment of alcohol dependence. *Journal of Consulting & Clinical Psychology, 68*(2), 250-257.

Petry, N.M., Martin, B., and Finocche, C. (2001). Contingency management in group treatment: A demonstration project in an HIV drop-in center. *Journal of Substance Abuse Treatment, 21*, 89-96.

Petry, N., Petrakis, I., Trevisanm L., Wiredu, G., Boutros, N., Martin, B., and Kosten, T. (2001). Contingency management interventions: From research to practice. *American Journal of Psychiatry, 158*(5), 694-702.

Petry, N., and Simcic, F. (2002). Recent advances in the dissemination of contingency management techniques: Clinical and research perspectives. *Journal of Substance Abuse Treatment, 23*(2), 81-86.

Preston, K., Umbricht, A., and Epstein, D.H. (2002). Abstinence reinforcement maintenance contingency and one-year follow-up. *Drug and Alcohol Dependence, 67*, 125-137.

Rowan-Szal, G., Joe, G., Chatham, L., and Simpson, D. (1994). A simple reinforcement system for methadone clients in a community-based treatment program. *Journal of Substance Abuse Treatment*, 11(3), 217-223.

Schumacher, J.E., Milby, J.B., McNamara. C.L., Wallace, D., Michael, M., Popkin, S., and Usdan, S. (1999). Effective treatment of homeless substance abusers: The role of contingency management. In S.T. Higgins, and K. Silverman (Eds.), *Motivating behavior change among illicit-drug abusers: Research on contingency management interventions* (pp. 77-94). Washington, DC: American Psychological Association.

Shaner, A., Roberts, L.J., Eckman, T.A., Tucker, D.E., Tsuang, J.W., Wilkins, J.N., and Mintz, J. (1997). Monetary reinforcement of abstinence from cocaine among mentally ill patients with cocaine dependence. *Psychiatric Services, 48*, 807-810.

Silverman, K., Higgins, S.T., Brooner, R.K., Montoya, I.D., Cone, E.J., Schuster, C.R., and Preston, K.L. (1996). Sustained cocaine abstinence in methadone maintenance patients through voucher-based reinforcement therapy. *Archives of General Psychiatry, 53,* 409-415.

Stitzer, M.L., Iguchi, M.Y., and Felch, L.J. (1992). Contingent take-home incentives: Effects on drug use of methadone maintenance patients. *Journal of Consulting & Clinical Psychology, 60,* 927-934.

Motivational Interviewing
and Behavior Change:
How Can We Know How It Works?

Deborah Nahom, PhD

SUMMARY. This article describes the process of 60 Motivational Interviewing (MI) or Adapted Motivational Interviewing (AMI) interventions reported in the literature between 1986 and 2002. Examination of the articles revealed a gap in our understanding of whether or not MI/AMI is effective and the *process by which* it is effective. An intervention-process research framework is suggested for future research in order to reduce this gap in our knowledge of psychotherapeutic and addiction treatment techniques. *[Article copies available for a fee from The Haworth Document Delivery Service: 1-800-HAWORTH. E-mail address: <docdelivery @haworthpress.com> Website: <http://www.HaworthPress.com> © 2005 by The Haworth Press, Inc. All rights reserved.]*

Deborah Nahom was affiliated with the School of Social Work, University of Washington, and is now affiliated with the South Lanarkshire Council, Scotland, UK.

Address correspondence to: Deborah Nahom, PhD, G/1 73 Cartside Street, Glasgow G42 9TL, Scotland, UK (E-mail: dnahom@u.washington.edu).

Special thanks are given to Elizabeth Wells, Diane Morrison, and Lewayne Gilchrist for encouragement and expertise.

This work was funded in part by the Grant 5RO1-DA08625 from the National Institute of Drug Abuse.

This article is based on the author's dissertation, submitted in partial fulfillment of the requirements for a doctoral degree in social work at the University of Washington.

[Haworth co-indexing entry note]: "Motivational Interviewing and Behavior Change: How Can We Know How It Works?" Nahom, Deborah. Co-published simultaneously in *Journal of Evidence-Based Social Work* (The Haworth Social Work Practice Press, an imprint of The Haworth Press, Inc.) Vol. 2, No. 1/2, 2005, pp. 55-78; and: *Addiction, Assessment, and Treatment with Adolescents, Adults, and Families* (ed: Carolyn Hilarski) The Haworth Social Work Practice Press, an imprint of The Haworth Press, Inc., 2005, pp. 55-78. Single or multiple copies of this article are available for a fee from The Haworth Document Delivery Service [1-800-HAWORTH, 9:00 a.m. - 5:00 p.m. (EST). E-mail address: docdelivery@haworthpress.com].

KEYWORDS. Motivational interviewing, treatment effectiveness research, process research, addiction treatment, literature review

Though many different types of interventions have been found to lead to a certain type of behavioral change, most intervention research fails to explain precisely how the intervention worked to produce this change. As such, questions remain as to what parts of the intervention are necessary to produce behavioral change and what parts may not be essential. Each of a number of different therapeutic techniques, grounded in different theoretical backgrounds, implies a path a client takes to reach a certain behavioral outcome. Simplistically speaking, client-centered techniques imply that in order for a client to change, the clinician must be accepting and empathic, and that the client must feel accepted and understood in order to change behaviors. Cognitive behavioral techniques imply that clinicians must help clients increase their coping skills and self-efficacy, and that once clients do increase these things, their behavior will change. Regardless of these implied paths, much intervention research fails to document the mechanisms by which any one of these techniques produces behavioral outcomes (Longabaugh, 2001). For example, even though cognitive behavioral techniques focus on increasing coping skills and/or self-efficacy, there is little empirical support suggesting that these types of interventions were effective due to the fact that they increased coping skills or self-efficacy (Longabaugh, 2001).

A SPECIFIC INTERVENTION

One field of well-documented intervention research that provides a specific example of this lack of understanding of the mechanisms by which an intervention is effective is that of motivational interviewing. Motivational interviewing (MI) is one of a plethora of treatment techniques developed in the addictions field for helping people work through ambivalence about behavior change (Rollnick, Heather, & Bell, 1992). Most recently described as "a method of communication rather than a set of techniques" (Miller & Rollnick, 2002, p. 25), motivational interviewing has been widely studied over the past 20 years. It is a style of intervention that uses ideas from a wide range of psychotherapeutic perspectives. MI is a client-centered technique, and is considered an evolution of the humanistic therapy developed by Carl Rogers, as well as "fundamentally a way of being with and for people-a facilitative approach that evokes natural change" (Miller & Rollnick, 2002, p. 25). At the same time, the clinician maintains a strong sense of purpose and direction, and actively chooses the right moment to intervene in incisive ways (Miller & Rollnick, 1991). Confrontation becomes the goal of the intervention, not the technique to instigate behavior change. For example, the clinician confronts the client by exposing the reality of the situation (e.g., "Using drugs isn't working for you because you never have any money leftover for food and rent") instead of being directly confrontational (e.g., "You need to stop using drugs so you will be able to use your money to pay for food and rent"). The purpose of the confrontation in motivational interviewing is for one to see and accept reality, so that one can change accordingly (Miller & Rollnick, 1991).

THE GAPS

Processes. Although there is evidence suggesting MI is effective at bringing about behavior change, especially in relation to substance abuse behaviors (Bien, Miller, & Boroughs, 1993; Bien, Miller, & Tonigan, 1993; Brown & Miller, 1993; Handmaker, 1993; Miller, Benefield, & Tonigan, 1993; Miller, Sovereign, & Krege, 1988), the underlying reasons and mechanisms that make it successful in these cases remain a mystery (Burke, Arkowitz, & Dunn, 2002; Dunn, Deroo, & Rivera, 2001; Miller, 1996; Miller & Rollnick, 2002). In fact, Miller (1996) has suggested we are only beginning to understand the links between the processes of motivational interviewing and outcomes. Several ideas in this regard have been put forth by various researchers and scholars. For example, Frank Logan (1993) suggests that, in order to change patterns of addictive behavior, people must go through the process of valuing the change in behavior, choosing the change in behavior, and then deciding to change their behavior. Others have suggested that the process of motivational interviewing challenges a person's core identity, giving rise to dissonance between one's self-concept and one's behavior, which in turn motivates one to instigate a behavior change (Downey, Donovan, & Rosengren, 2000).

One place to look for the answer to this puzzle about the process by which motivational interviewing leads to certain outcomes is the theoretical basis from which this technique stems. Although principles from perspectives such as motivational, social, and cognitive psychology, the Transtheoretical Model of Change (TMC) suggested by Prochaska and his colleagues (Prochaska & DiClemente, 1983; Prochaska, DiClemente, & Norcross, 1992), and the client-centered philosophy of Carl Rogers (1951, 1954) form the foundation of motivational interviewing, there is no distinct theory regarding how and why motivational interviewing should work. Thus, it is not surprising that, at this point in time, our understanding of how MI produces certain behavioral outcomes is limited.

Outcomes. There is also a gap in our understanding of the efficacy of MI. Research evidence suggests that MI is no more effective than, or maybe even less effective than cognitive behavioral skill training or 12-step facilitation techniques (Project MATCH Research Group, 1998). In their qualitative review of the MI literature, Burke et al. (2002) suggest that the difficulty in drawing firm conclusions about the efficacy of MI is due to the fact that virtually all of the published empirical studies deal with the efficacy of Adapted Motivational Interviewing interventions (AMIs), as opposed to MI in relatively pure form. They also suggest that the AMI treatments under investigation are often vague and imprecise making treatment fidelity difficult to ascertain. Their review concludes there is a dearth of evidence regarding how and why interventions related to motivational interviewing might work and there is little direct evidence thus far to suggest that AMIs actually work by enhancing motivation or readiness for change. A later meta-analytic review of 30 controlled clinical trials found that AMIs were equivalent to other active treatments, superior to no-treatment or placebo controls in terms of efficacy for problems involving drugs, alcohol and diet and exercise, and clinically impactful (Burke, Arkowitz, & Menchola, 2003). Yet it was still concluded that we are far from understanding the precise links between the processes and outcomes of this intervention.

Understanding the mechanisms that make motivational interviewing (or AMIs, or any other psychotherapeutic intervention style) effective would be useful in improving practice by identifying core elements needed in the intervention to ensure successful behavior change. An in-depth understanding of these mechanisms may also help identify which populations are most suited for MI interventions and why. Furthermore, an understanding of the necessary and sufficient elements of MI interventions may enrich our understanding of how interventions work in general, or could at least provide alternative hypotheses about the nature of successful interventions. This information would be useful not only to researchers and those who develop interventions, but also for clinicians who work directly with clients, who many times are asked to implement interventions that may or may not be well-suited to their personal style. This article aims (a) to examine the literature reporting evaluations of motivational interviewing and adapted motivational interviewing interventions, (b) to point out where the gap is in our understanding of links between processes and outcomes in MI and AMIs, and (c) to provide a framework from which future research on the efficacy and effectiveness of motivational interviewing can begin to fill in the gaps of our current understanding of this intervention.

CURRENT KNOWLEDGE ABOUT MI

What we do know about the potentially "necessary and sufficient ingredients" of MI related interventions is based on the writings of Miller and Rollnick (1991, 2002), the originators of MI. From these writings, researchers and interventionists conducting studies of the efficacy of MI/AMI develop interventions that use either the six core elements of effective brief interventions (FRAMES; see Bien, Miller, & Tonigan, 1993; Miller & Rollnick, 1991), the four basic principles of MI (Miller & Rollnick, 2002), or both. The six core elements of brief interventions are: (a) feedback, (b) responsibility, (c) advice, (d) menu of options, (e) empathy, and (f) self-efficacy. The four basic principles of MI are: (a) express empathy, (b) develop discrepancy, (c) roll with resistance, and (d) support self-efficacy. As Noonan and Moyers (1997) point out, brief interventions have often been confused with MI because they share some of the same effective ingredients. This probably accounts for the recent distinction between "pure" MI and "AMIs." However, when attempting to determine the process by which interventions are effective, it is important to include hypothesized effective ingredients. From this body of literature, then, it can be presumed (however inaccurately) that these elements and principles must be present for the intervention to be effective and for behavior change to take place.

LINKING PROCESSES TO OUTCOMES

Unfortunately, to date, the literature reporting about the effectiveness of MI has focused almost exclusively on client outcomes as opposed to intervention process. This makes it difficult to reach conclusions about *how* these principles and elements invoked as encompassing the MI or AMI studied operate when the intervention delivered produces successful behavior change. Ideally, in the efficacy and effectiveness trials, the principles of MI and elements of brief interventions would be measured along with behavioral outcomes, and the process of change would become more evident. However, in reality, this is impossible, particularly because there are no agreed upon, theoretically driven, empirically validated "core" elements of MI.

METHOD

A Descriptive Review

For the purposes of providing an in depth look at the potential process of MI/AMI, the presence of FRAME elements and core MI principles were examined in a comprehensive review of the literature. It must be stressed that this was a qualitative review as opposed to a statistical, meta-analytic review, attempting to describe what authors and researches who have studied MI/AMI as an intervention style have written and concluded about how and if the intervention works. The review was also intended to illuminate the gaps in this literature and elucidate a way forward. Given the lack of a specific theoretical model of the process of MI/AMI as well as the lack of empirical data of processes involved in the interventions, a meta-analysis was deemed inappropriate for the purposes of this review.

This review included 60 articles written between 1986 to 2002 that evaluated the effectiveness of motivational interviewing in empirical studies, smaller pilot studies, or case studies. Lists of articles were obtained from the Motivational Interviewing website (http://motivational interview.org/library/biblio.html) and from a search on PsycINFO. Articles were included if they described a particular study of a motivational interviewing intervention, an adapted motivational interviewing intervention or a motivational enhancement intervention (MET-a manualized form of MI). Meta-analyses and reviews including more that one MI/AMI intervention were excluded. Because intervention processes were of interest, this review did not exclude smaller, non-clinically controlled trials as is typically the case in meta-analytic reviews. Of these 60 articles, 45 were empirical studies evaluating the efficacy of MI/AMI in relation to myriad behavioral outcomes such as alcohol, tobacco, and other drug use; risky sexual behavior; and health care treatment compliance. Eleven articles were identified as pilot studies and these articles described the use of MI/AMI with a number of different substance using populations (e.g., those with dual diagnoses, street sex workers, teen smokers, mandated clients, and military personnel), and to facilitate a number of different outcomes (e.g., increasing asthma medication adherence, marital satisfaction, and contraception use). The remaining four articles provided case examples of the use of MI/AMI in different populations: (a) older veterans with alcohol and other illicit drug use (Royer et al., 2000), (b) men who have sex with men and may engage in risky sexual behavior (Rutledge et al., 2001), (c) people experiencing acute psychotic disorders (Kemp, David, & Hayward, 1996), and (d) adolescents with conduct problems (Greenwald, 2002). Because MI/AMI interventions have been developed using FRAMES and/or the core principles of MI (as is commonly stated in the introductions to the studies), the interventions included in this review were examined for both the six common elements of brief interventions as well as the four principles of MI to determine potential processes of MI interventions. Table 1 lists the articles reviewed by study category (e.g., empirical, pilot or case study), each element and principle, and whether or not the specific element or principle was discussed in the article. If the element or principle was discussed at any point in the article in terms of being part of the MI intervention, this information was noted and considered "present." Any measurement of the element or principle (or lack thereof) was also noted. Information is also given about the outcome of the study in relation to MI/AMI's effectiveness as a behavior change intervention. For example, studies listed in boldface are those in which an MI/AMI intervention is compared to other behavior change intervention techniques (e.g., cognitive behavioral treatment or risk reduction) and both types of intervention produced significant changes in behavior.

RESULTS

Brief Intervention Elements

Feedback. When looking at specific components of the interventions, almost two-thirds of the studies (regardless of type) provided some form of feedback. Although a majority of the time, feedback was given based on an earlier assessment and compared to some normative data, sometimes feedback was given in the form of reflections about progress (Kemp et al., 1996; Saunders, Wilkinson, & Phillips, 1995). In one case, feedback was considered somewhat of a summary of an initial consultation and was pro-

TABLE 1. Articles Reviewed, Elements, Principles, and Outcomes

		Brief Intervention Elements						MI Principles			
Reference	Year	F	R	A	M	E	S	1	2	3	4
Empirical Studies/Clinical Trials											
*Van Bilsen &Van Ernst	1986		x			x		x	x		x
Kuchipudi, Hobein, Flickinger, & Iber	1990	x		x	x	x					
*Anderson & Scott	1992	x		x							
Baker, Heather, Wodak, Dixon, & Holt	1993	x	x	x	x	x		x		x	x
*Miller, Benefield, & Tonigan	1993	x				x		x			
Baker, Kochan, Dixon, Heather, & Wodak	1994	x	x								x
*Agnostinelli, Brown, & Miller	1995	x									x
*Saunders, Wilkinson, & Philips	1995	x	x			x		x	x	x	x
Woollard, Beilin, Lord, Puddey, MacAdam, & Rouse	1995	x			x						
*Carey, Maisto, Kalichman, Forsyth, Wright, & Johnson	1997	x	x	x	x	x		x	x		x
Senft, Polen, Freeborn, & Hollis	1997	x		x	x				x		
*Smith, Kratt, Heckemeyer, & Mason	1997	x		x	x	x		x	x	x	x
Booth, Kwiatkowski, Iguchi, Pinto, & John	1998			x	x	x		x			x
Colby et al.	1998	x	x	x	x	x		x	x	x	x
Butler, Rollnick, Cohen, Bachman, Russell, & Stott	1999		x	x	x	x		x	x	x	
*Hanmaker, MIller, & Manicke	1999	x		x	x	x		x	x		x
*Longshore, Grills, & Anon	1999		x	x	x	x		x	x	x	x

Study	Year								
*Ludman, Curry, Meyer, & Taplin	1999	×		×	×	×	×		
*Monti et al.	1999	×	×	×	×	×	×		×
*Swanson, Pantalon, & Cohen	1999	×	×	×	×	×	×	×	×
*Treasure, Katzman, Schmidt, Troop, Todd, & deSilva	1999								
*Bosari & Carey	2000	×			×		×	×	×
Carey et al.[a]	2000			×	×	×	×		×
*Harper & Hardy	2000								
*Kelly, Halford, & Young	2000	×							
*Martino, Carroll, O'Malley, & Rounsaville	2000	×	×		×	×	×		×
*Schneider, Casey, & Kohn	2000	×	×	×	×	×	×	×	×
*Stephens, Roffman, & Curtin	2000	×	×	×	×	×	×	xx	×
Tappin et al.	2000		×	×	×	×	×	xx	
*Thevos, Quick, & Yanduli[b]	2000								
*Baer, Kivlahan, Blume, McKnight, & Marlatt	2001	×		×	×	×		×	
*Baker, Boggs, & Lewin[c]	2001								
*Barrowclough et al.	2001		×	×	×	×	×	×	×

TABLE 1 (continued)

Reference	Year	Brief Intervention Elements						MI Principles			
		F	R	A	M	E	S	1	2	3	4
Empirical Studies/Clinical Trials											
*Carroll, Libby, Sheehan, & Hyland	2001					×		×		×	×
*Emmons, Hammond, Fava, Velicer, Evans, & Monroe	2001	×	×		×	×	×	×	×	×	×
*Murphy et al.[d]	2001	×				×		×		×	
*Resnicow et al.	2001		×	×		×		×		×	×
*Safren et al.[e]	2001			×		×		×			
*Sellman, Sullivan, Dore, Adamson, & MacEwan[f]	2001	×		×		×		×			×
Smith et al.	2001			×	×	×	×	×			×
*Hulse & Tait	2002	×				×		×			×
*Humfress, Igel, Lamont, Tanner, Morgan & Schmidt	2002	×	×		×	×	×	×		×	×
*Schilling, El-Bassel, Finch, Roman, & Hanson[g]	2002	×	×	×		×		×	×	×	×
*Stein, Charuvastra, Maksdad, & Anderson	2002	×		×		×	×	×	×	×	×
*Stotts, DiClemente, & Dolan-Mullen	2002	×	×	×	×	×		×		×	×

Study	Year								
*+Cordova, Warren, & Gee	2001							×	
*+Picciano, Roffman, Kalichman, Rutledge, & Berghuis[h]	2001	×		×	×			×	×
+Schmaling, Blume, & Afari	2001	×						×	
*Stotts, Schmits, Rhoades, & Grabowski	2001	×		×	×			×	×
Van Horn & Bux	2001			×	×			×	×
*Woodruff, Edwards, Conway, & Elliot	2001			×	×			×	×
*Carey, Carey, Maisto, & Purnine	2002	×	×	×	×			×	×
*Cigrang, Severson, & Peterson	2002			×	×			×	×
Cowley, Farley, & Beamis	2002	×	×	×	×			×	×
*Lincourt, Kuettel, & Bombardier	2002	×	×					×	×
*Yahne, Miller, Irvin-Vitela, & Tonigan	2002	×		×	×			×	×

TABLE 1 (continued)

Reference	Year	Brief Intervention Elements						MI Principles			
		F	R	A	M	E	S	1	2	3	4
Case Studies											
*Greenwald	2002										
*Kemp, David, & Hayward	1996	x		x	x	x	x	x	x	x	x
*Royer, Dickson-Fuhrmann, McDermott, Taylor, Rosansky, & Jarvik	2000		x	x	x	x	x	x	x	x	x
*Rutledge, Roffman, Mahoney, Picciano, Berghuis, & Kalichman	2001	x	x		x	x	x	x	x	x	x

Note. Brief Intervention Elements: F (Feedback); R (Responsibility); A (Advice); M (Menu of Options); E (Empathy); S (Self-Efficacy). MI Principles: 1 (Express empathy); 2 (Support self-efficacy); 3 (Roll with resistance); 4 (Develop discrepancy). "xx" in Roll with resistance column indicates this was reported as "avoiding argumentation." * = positive behavior change in the study; + = change in something other than behavior (i.e., attitude, motivation, knowledge, satisfaction). **Authors in bold** indicate behavior change that was not specific only to the MI intervention.

[a]Significant results were found among those in the intervention group with imperfect intentions. [b]In one of two studies reported. [c]Significant group differences were found in percent abstinent at 6 months. [d]Changes seen in intervention group when pulling out heavy drinkers.

[e]Changes in adherence seen at week 2 but not at week 12. [f]Significant behavior change specific to MI compared to other conditions seen among heavy drinkers only. [g]Change in only one outcome measure. [h]Intervention efficacy demonstrated for Non-Whites.

66

vided in an individual letter (Humfress et al., 2002), and in another, the feedback was given in terms of the probability of pregnancy occurring in the next few months (Cowley, Farley, & Beamis, 2002). Two studies did not specify what was contained within the feedback (Hulse & Tait, 2002; Stein, Charuvastra, Maksdad, & Anderson, 2002). The provision of feedback of any sort was neither necessary nor sufficient to instigate behavior change, since feedback was present in both studies evidencing positive behavior change attributed to the MI/AMI intervention and those evidencing positive behavior change that was not specific to the MI/AMI intervention condition. Also, feedback was present in studies in which no behavior change took place.

Responsibility. Responsibility was mentioned in 40% of these studies, and many times it was implied with letting participants know that it was up to them if they wanted to change behavior or not, follow through with appointments or not, or by asking participants to come up with their own solutions. "Responsibility for change" was explicitly mentioned in three studies (Carey et al., 1997; Carey et al., 2000; Stephens, Roffman, & Curtin, 2000). In one case, this happened when participants in the delayed treatment control group would ask whether to stop or continue use of marijuana during the delay period (Stephens et al.). These participants were told that it was their decision. In another case, participants were encouraged to choose risk reduction practices that were consistent with their values, relationships, supports and life circumstances (Carey et al., 2000). Responsibility was also neither necessary nor sufficient to the behavior change process as it was mentioned in those studies with behavior change attributed to the MI-related intervention, those with behavior change not specific to the MI-related intervention, and those in which no behavior change was found. There were also studies in which behavior change occurred and responsibility was not mentioned.

Advice. Advice was given in almost half (47%) of the studies examined, usually in the form of referrals, discussion of goals, or with the introduction of specific behavioral skills (such as coping strategies). However, advice was not restricted to MI-related interventions alone; it was also given in a risk reduction intervention (Booth, Kwiatkowski, Iguchi, Pinto, & John, 1998), a brief advice condition (Butler et al., 1999; Colby et al., 1998), a confrontational intervention (Schneider, Casey, & Kohn, 2000), and a relapse prevention condition (Stephens et al., 2000). In some cases, advice was given in the form of a pamphlet (Sellman, Sullivan, Dore, Adamson, & MacEwan, 2001; Smith et al., 2001). Advice was also found in studies reflecting all three behavioral change conditions: behavioral change attributed to MI/AMI, behavioral change not specific to MI/AMI, and no behavior change. Also, advice was not present in cases when behavioral change was seen.

Menu of Options. A menu of options was evident in most of the same studies in which advice was given (42% of all studies), as that too came in the form of referrals, practicing behavioral skills, and discussing change plans and goals. Providing a menu of options was not restricted to MI/AMI interventions, but was evident in comparison interventions as well (Booth et al., 1998; Handmaker, Miller, & Manicke, 1999; Schneider et al., 2000; Stephens et al., 2000). As with the three previous brief intervention elements, providing a menu of options was neither necessary nor sufficient to produce positive behavioral outcomes and was found in studies in which behavior change took place and those in which no behavior change took place.

Common Brief Intervention Elements and MI Principles

Express Empathy. Empathy was discussed in three-quarters of the studies reviewed (45 of 60), and many times was referred to as reflective listening, paraphrasing, and/or summarizing. In one case (Booth et al., 1998), empathy was not restricted to the MI-related intervention condition, but was also found in the risk reduction intervention. Of all the times empathy was either implied or explicitly mentioned, it was measured (in various ways) in only eight cases (Carey, Carey, Maisto, & Purnine, 2002; Humfress et al., 2002; Monti et al., 1999; Murphy et al., 2001; Picciano, Roffman, Kalichman, Rutledge, & Berghuis, 2001; Saunders et al., 1995; Smith et al., 2001; Stein et al., 2002). In one case (Saunders et al.), participants were asked to rate clinician empathy at a 3-month follow-up point, and the researchers found no significant differences in ratings of empathy for clinicians in the control group and clinicians in the MI-related intervention group. In another study (Monti et al. 1999), participants in the MI/AMI intervention group rated clinicians empathy very highly (3.7 on a 4-point scale), while participants in the Standard Care (control) group were not asked to rate clinician empathy at all. Another study found that clients in the experimental group (MI/AMI) felt more listened to than clients in the control group (Standard Treatment; Humfress et al. 2002). Other studies used Likert scale ratings by the client on clinician attributes such as "helpful, accepting and understanding" (Smith et al. 2001), "competence" (Murphy et al. 2001), and "caring" (Carey et al. 2001). Only one study had clinicians rate the degree to which the key elements of motivational enhancement occurred (including reflective listening techniques and expressing empathy) on a Likert scale (Picciano et al., 2001); however, these ratings were never reported in relation to client outcomes. In fact, none of the studies measuring clinician attributes such as empathy reported the relationship between perceived clinician empathy and client outcome. Also, since empathy was found in studies in which no behavior change took place, it cannot be determined how it relates to the behavior change process.

Support Self-Efficacy. Self-efficacy was mentioned in almost three-quarters of the studies examined (72%), and was measured within the intervention in only three cases (Longshore, Grills, & Anon, 1999; Monti et al., 1999; Picciano et al., 2001). Other times it was implied in that clinicians "affirmed participants' commitment to change," or "built confidence." Self-efficacy was also not restricted to MI/AMI interventions alone (Stephens et al., 2000). Here again, it is difficult to assess how self-efficacy is related to behavioral change outcomes, since it was mentioned in both studies finding positive behavioral changes as well as those finding no behavior change. As was the case with empathy, even when self-efficacy was measured within the intervention, its relationship to client outcome was never reported.

Motivational Interviewing Principles

Roll with Resistance. Clinicians were said to have rolled with resistance in 25 of the studies examined (42%) and to have avoided argumentation in 24 of the studies examined. However, in many cases, it was not noted how exactly this was done, nor was it ever measured. Most times it was implied by the fact that clinicians were listening reflectively. In two cases, avoiding argumentation was referred to without a reference to rolling with resistance (Stephens et al., 2000; Tappin et al., 2000), and, as was the case with rolling with resistance, was implied by clinicians using reflective listening strategies. One study (Smith, Kratt, Heckemeyer, & Mason, 1997) explicitly mentioned avoiding argumentation by refraining from confronting clients, and a minority of others mentioned avoiding argumentation by reflective listening (Schneider et al., 2000; Rutledge et al., 2001). However, rolling with resistance and avoiding argumentation, like all the constructs mentioned so far, do not seem to be related to behavioral change, as these techniques were reportedly used in studies finding positive behavior changes and those with no such findings.

Develop Discrepancies. Finally, the development of discrepancies was evident in over two-thirds of these studies (68%), and was most often identified as discussing the pros and cons of the specific behavior, or as filling out a decisional balance worksheet. In one case (Stephens et al., 2000), it was present in both the MI/AMI intervention and the comparison intervention (Relapse Prevention). This construct was measured only when intervention adherence was being measured. In these cases (Picciano et al., 2001; Stein et al., 2002) the clinician would fill out a checklist or rate the extent to which ambivalence was discussed. It was never measured explicitly from the client's perspective, nor related to intervention outcomes. This, too, was found in studies reporting no behavior change, so its relationship to the process of behavior change is unclear.

DISCUSSION

Summary of Results

Overall, these articles suggest that MI/AMI interventions result in positive behavioral change for participants (49 of the 60; 82%), though these types of interventions may not be any more effective than other types of treatment (such as relapse prevention, non-directive listening or brief advice; Booth et al., 1998; Colby et al., 1998; Harper & Hardy, 2000; Hulse & Tait, 2002; Schneider et al., 2000; Sellman et al., 2001; Stephens et al., 2000; Treasure et al., 1999), or even no treatment at all (Ludman, Curry, Meyer, & Taplin, 1999). Also, the use of MI/AMI alone versus in combination with other treatments and in varying amounts did not always result in significant differences between treatment conditions (Baker, Boggs, & Lewin, 2001; Stein et al., 2002). More significantly, as can be seen from the discussion above, it is no more clear how this behavior change, when it occurs, comes about. While the six common elements of brief interventions as well as the four principles of motivational interviewing were mentioned in many of these evaluation studies, there is no evidence of the way in which they operated within each specific intervention group. For the most part, they were neither measured, nor operationally defined, and in some cases, were only implied to be part of the MI/AMI intervention (e.g., one report states, ". . . the intervention followed the MI style described by Miller & Rollnick (1991)") (Kelly, Halford, & Young, 2000, p. 1540). Even though positive behavioral outcomes were obtained in many of these studies and with a variety of treatments, there is still no evidence as to how these came about. Thus, the core elements of MI, as well as the core elements of many other treatment modalities, remain a mystery, and the lack of measurement of these principles and elements makes it impossible to explain how the intervention process did or did not result in significant changes in behavior.

Where Do We Go from Here?

There has been a call, not only in the MI intervention literature, but also in the psychotherapy literature writ large, for a more thorough investigation of the complex relationships between process, technique and outcome in psychotherapeutic interventions (Burke et al., 2002; Carroll, Nich, & Rounsaville, 1997; Dunn et al., 2001; Longabaugh, 2001; Miller, 1996; Miller & Rollnick, 2002). There is the question of common ingredients versus unique factors specific to individual types of treatments that needs to be answered (e.g., do therapies work more because of the ingredients common to each therapy or is there something unique to each therapy that makes it effective?). This question is leftover from the "dodo bird verdict" (a phrase borrowed from *Alice in Wonderland* stating, "Everyone has won and so all must have prizes." [Hubble, Duncan, & Miller, 1999, p. 6]). In other words, we know psychotherapy is effective, and we also know that one type of psychotherapy is no more effective than all the rest (Llewelyn & Hardy, 2001). With well over three hundred different types of psychotherapy, ranging alphabetically from Active Analytical Psychotherapy to Zaraleya Psychoenergetic Technique (Gordon, 2000), and with the number of psychotherapy approaches and theories having grown by approximately 600% in 40 years (Hubble et al., 1999), it can be difficult for helping professionals to know what kind of intervention to use. This is especially true in the case of clinicians working with clients who have persistent and complex issues, such as substance dependence.

This paper, though not using empirical means, begins to describe one specific intervention, what is thought to encompass its process, and whether or not these processes are related to outcomes. Though there are clearly limitations to this approach, such as the lack of empirical rigor or the questionable reliability of the author's findings (e.g., would another author reach the same decisions?), this paper did not set out to answer the question of whether or not MI is efficacious and, if so, by what process. Rather, it set out to illuminate gaps in our current understanding and to propose an additional way of investigating interventions so our understanding can be enhanced. What is clear from this exercise is that, if nothing else, the literature describing and testing the efficacy of MI/AMI does not allow for conclusions to be drawn regarding relationships between intervention processes and outcomes. Further, the procedures reported within this body of literature in regard to the intervention include a wide range of strategies (for example, to develop discrepancies, strategies such as the Decisional Balance Exercise, values clarification, feedback on behavior are used). Not much is known about how these methods bring about change in motivation. Analyses that lead to an increased understanding about the relative efficacy of MI strategies and the processes that underlie them would enhance clinical practice. It is in this way that we will begin to understand what it is about different therapies that do or do not make them effective. To determine the means by which MI is successful and to better understand the process of change, the intervention process needs to be taken into account, explicitly measured, and reported. For example, Nahom (2003) designed a study describing a theoretical model of the process of change, and then empirically examined this model using tape ratings of intervention sessions. Tape raters were asked to determine to what extent each of the proposed variables in the hypothesized process of change model was present in the intervention. These ratings were then used to predict the extent of behavior change (in this case, a reduction of cocaine use). Also, in a recently published study, Amrhein, Miller, Yahne, Palmer, and Fulcher (2003) examined client commitment language during MI and its prediction of drug use outcomes. They found client commitment language did predict future drug use behavior over and above the predictive ability of past drug use behavior (Amrhein et al., 2003). Theirs is a seminal study in that it provides the first clear empirical evidence consistent with hypothesized mechanisms of the efficacy of MI. It also moves us closer as a field to understanding what might be happening within the intervention to foster a process of behavior change.

These two examples provide two different ways to begin to examine the processes operating within an intervention that may or may not contribute to the overall goal of behavior change. Clearly, in order to clarify our understanding of not only *if* interventions work, but also *how* interventions work, models of behavior change (e.g., Prochaska and DiClemente's (1983) Transtheoretical Model of Change; Orlinsky and Howard's (1986) generic model of the psychotherapy process; Henry and Strupp's (1994) interpersonal process model) need to be explicitly incorporated into intervention research, adequately measured and empirically validated. Understanding processes of interventions and being explicit about them will help us as a social service field to develop effective interventions, to train people adequately in delivering effective interventions, and to answer more detailed questions about how and why interventions are successful, what part is due to the actual intervention, the specific clinician, and the individual client involved.

REFERENCES

References marked with an asterisk indicate studies included in the review.

*Agostinelli, G., Brown, J. M., & Miller, W. R. (1995). Effects of normative feedback on consumption among heavy drinking college students. *Journal of Drug Education, 25,* 31-40.

Amrhein, P. C., Miller, W. R., Yahne, C. E., Palmer, M., & Fulcher, L. (2003). Client commitment language during motivational interviewing predicts drug use outcomes. *Journal of Consulting & Clinical Psychology, 71,* 862-878.

*Anderson, P., & Scott, E. (1992). The effect of general practitioners' advice to heavy drinking men. *British Journal of Addictions, 87,* 891-900.

*Baer, J. S., Kivlahan, D. R., Blume, A. W., McKnight, P., & Marlatt, G. A. (2001). Brief interventions for heavy-drinking college students: 4-year follow-up and natural history. *American Journal of Public Health, 91,* 1310-1316.

*Baker, A., Boggs, T. G., & Lewin, T. J. (2001). Randomized controlled trial of brief cognitive-behavioural interventions among regular users of amphetamine. *Addiction, 96,* 1279-1287.

*Baker, A., Heather, N., Wodak, A., Dixon, J., & Holt, P. (1993). Evaluation of a cognitive-behavioural intervention for HIV prevention among injecting drug users. *AIDS, 7,* 247-256.

*Baker, A., Kochan, N., Dixon, J., Heather, N., & Wodak, A. (1994). Controlled evaluation of a brief intervention for HIV prevention among injecting drug users not in treatment. *AIDS Care, 6,* 559-570.

*Barrowclough, C., Haddock, G., Tarrier, N., Lewis, S. W., Moring, J., O'Brien, R., et al. (2001). Randomized controlled trial of motivational interviewing, cognitive behavior therapy, and family intervention for patients with comorbid schizophrenia and substance use disorders. *American Journal of Psychiatry, 158,* 1706-1713.

*Barrowclough, C., Haddock, G., Tarrier, N., Moring, J., & Lewis, S. (2000). Cognitive behavioral intervention for individuals with severe mental illness who have a substance misuse problem. *Psychiatric Rehabilitation Skills, 4,* 216-233.

Bien, T. H., Miller, W. R., & Boroughs, J. M. (1993). Motivational interviewing with alcohol outpatients. *Behavioral Psychotherapy, 21,* 347-356.

Bien, T. H., Miller, W. R., & Tonigan, J. S. (1993). Brief interventions for alcohol problems: A review. *Addiction, 88,* 315-336.

*Booth, R. E., Kwiatkowski, C., Iguchi, M. Y., Pinto, F., & John, D. (1998). Facilitating treatment entry among out-of-treatment injection drug users. *Public Health Reports, 111*(Suppl. 1), 116-128.

*Bosari, B., & Carey, K. B. (2000). Effects of a brief motivational intervention with college student drinkers. *Journal of Consulting & Clinical Psychology, 68,* 728-733.

Brown, J. M., & Miller, W. R. (1993). Impact of motivational interviewing on participation and outcome in residential alcoholism treatment. *Psychology of Addictive Behaviors, 7,* 211-218.

Burke, B. L., Arkowitz, H., & Dunn, C. (2002). The efficacy of motivational interviewing and its adaptations. In W. R. Miller, & S. Rollnick (Eds.), *Motivational interviewing: Preparing people for change* (2nd ed., pp. 217-251). New York: The Guilford Press.

Burke, B. L., Arkowitz, H., & Menchola, M. (2003). The efficacy of motivational interviewing: A meta-analysis of controlled clinical trials. *Journal of Consulting & Clinical Psychology, 71*, 843-861.

*Butler, C. C., Rollnick, S., Cohen, D., Bachmann, M., Russell, I., & Stott, N. (1999). Motivational consulting versus brief advice for smokers in general practice: A randomized trial. *British Journal of General Practice, 49*, 611-616.

*Carey, K. B., Carey, M. P., Maisto, S. A., & Purnine, D. M. (2002). The feasibility of enhancing psychiatric outpatients' readiness to change their substance use. *Psychiatric Services, 53*, 602-608.

*Carey, M. P., Braaten, L. S., Maisto, S. A., Gleason, J. R., Forsyth, A. D., Durant, L. E., et al. (2000). Using information, motivational enhancement, and skills training to reduce the risk of HIV infection for low-income urban women: A second randomized clinical trial. *Health Psychology, 19*, 3-11.

*Carey, M. P., Maisto, S. A., Kalichman, S. C., Forsyth, A. D., Wright, E. M., & Johnson, B. T. (1997). Enhancing motivation to reduce the risk of HIV infection for economically disadvantaged urban women. *Journal of Consulting & Clinical Psychology, 65*, 531-541.

*Carroll, K. M., Libby, B., Sheehan, J., & Hyland, N. (2001). Motivational interviewing to enhance treatment initiation in substance abusers: An effectiveness study. *The American Journal on Addictions, 10*, 335-339.

Carroll, K. M., Nich, C., & Rounsaville, B. J. (1997). Contribution of the therapeutic alliance to outcome in active versus control psychotherapies. *Journal of Consulting & Clinical Psychology, 65*, 510-514.

*Cigrang, J. A., Severson, H. H., & Peterson, A. L. (2002). Pilot evaluation of a population-based health intervention for reducing use of smokeless tobacco. *Nicotine and Tobacco Research, 4*, 127-131.

*Colby, S. M., Monti, P. M., Barnett, N. P., Rohsenow, D. J., Weissman, K., Sprito, A., et al. (1998). Brief motivational interviewing in a hospital setting for adolescent smoking: A preliminary study. *Journal of Consulting & Clinical Psychology, 66*, 574-578.

*Cordova, J. V., Warren, L. Z., & Gee, C. B. (2001). Motivational interviewing as an intervention for at-risk couples. *Journal of Marital & Family Therapy, 27*, 315-326.

*Cowley, C. B., Farley, T., & Beamis, K. (2002). "Well, maybe I'll try the pill for just a few months . . ." Brief motivational and narrative-based interventions to encourage contraceptive use among adolescents at high risk for early childbearing. *Families, Systems, and Health, 20*, 183-204.

Downey, L., Donovan, D. M., & Rosengren, D. B. (2000). To thine own self be true: Self-concept and motivation for abstinence among substance abusers. *Addictive Behaviors, 25*, 743-757.

Dunn, C., Deroo, L., & Rivera, F. P. (2001). The use of brief interventions adapted from motivational interviewing across behavioral domains: A systematic review. *Addiction, 96*, 1725-1742.

*Emmons, K. M., Hammond, K., Fava, J. L., Velicer, W. F., Evans, J. L., & Monroe, A. D. (2001). A randomized trial to reduce passive smoke exposure to low-income households with young children. *Pediatrics, 108*, 18-24.

Gordon, N. S. (2000). Researching psychotherapy, the importance of the client's view: A methodological challenge. *The Qualitative Report, 4*(3/4). Retrieved May 15, 2001, from http://www.nova.edu/ssss/QR/QR4-3/gordon.html.

*Greenwald, R. (2002). Motivation-Adaptive Skills-Trauma Resolution (MASTR) therapy for adolescents with conduct problems: An open trial. *Journal of Aggression, Maltreatment, & Trauma, 6*, 237-261.

Handmaker, N. S. (1993). Motivating pregnant drinkers to abstain: Prevention in prenatal care clinics (Doctoral dissertation, University of New Mexico, 1993). *Dissertation Abstracts International, 45*, 3619.

*Handmaker, N. S., Miller, W. R., & Manicke, M. (1999). Findings of a pilot study of motivational interviewing with pregnant drinkers. *Journal of Studies on Alcohol, 60*, 285-287.

*Harper, R., & Hardy, S. (2000). An evaluation of motivational interviewing as a method of intervention with clients in a probation setting. *British Journal of Social Work, 30*, 393-400.

Henry, W. P., & Strupp, H. H. (1994). The therapeutic alliance as interpersonal process. In A. O. Horvath, & L. S. Greenberg (Eds.), *The working alliance: Theory, research, and practice* (pp. 51-84). New York: John Wiley & Sons, Inc.

Hubble, M. A., Duncan, B. L., & Miller, S. D. (1999). Introduction. In M. A. Hubble, B. L. Duncan, & S. D. Miller (Eds.), *The heart and soul of change: What works in therapy* (pp. 1-19). Washington DC: American Psychological Association.

*Hulse, G. K., & Tait, R. J. (2002). Six-month outcomes associated with a brief alcohol intervention for adult in-patients with psychiatric disorders. *Drug and Alcohol Review, 21*, 105-112.

*Humfress, H., Igel, V., Lamont, A., Tanner, M., Morgan, J., & Schmidt, U. (2002). The effect of a brief motivational intervention on community psychiatric patients' attitudes to their care, motivation to change, compliance, and outcome: A case control study. *Journal of Mental Health, 11*, 155-166.

*Kelly, A. B., Halford, W. K., & Young, R. M. (2000). Maritally distressed women with alcohol problems: The impact of a short-term alcohol focused intervention on drinking behaviour and marital satisfaction. *Addiction, 95*, 1537-1549.

*Kemp, R., David, A., & Hayward, P. (1996). Compliance therapy: An intervention targeting insight and treatment adherence in psychotic patients. *Behavioural and Cognitive Psychotherapy, 24*, 331-350.

*Kuchipudi, V., Hobein, K., Flickinger, A., & Iber, F. L. (1990). Failure of a 2-hour motivational intervention to alter recurrent drinking behavior in alcoholics with gastrointestinal disease. *Journal of Studies on Alcohol, 31*, 356-360.

*Lincourt, P., Kuettel, T. J., & Bombardier, C. H. (2002). Motivational interviewing in a group setting with mandated clients: A pilot study. *Addictive Behaviors, 27*, 381-391.

Llewelyn, S., & Hardy, G. (2001). Process research in understanding and applying psychological therapies. *British Journal of Clinical Psychology, 40*, 1-12.

Logan, F. M. (1993). Animal learning and motivation and addictive drugs. *Psychological Reports, 73*, 291-306.

Longabaugh, R. (2001). Why is motivational interviewing effective? *Addiction, 96*, 1773-1774.

*Longshore, D., Grills, C., & Annon, K. (1999). Effects of a culturally congruent intervention on cognitive factors related to drug-use recovery. *Substance Use and Misuse, 34*, 1223-1241.

*Ludman, E. J., Curry, S. J., Meyer, D., & Taplin, S. H. (1999). Implementation of outreach telephone counseling to promote mammography. *Health Education and Behavior, 26*, 689-702.

*Martino, S., Carroll, K. M., O'Malley, S. S., & Rounsaville, B. J. (2000). Motivational interviewing with psychiatrically ill substance abusing patients. *The American Journal on Addictions, 9*, 88-91.

Miller, W. R. (1983). Motivational interviewing with problem drinkers. *Behavioural Psychotherapy, 11*, 147-172.

Miller, W. R. (1996). Motivational interviewing: Research, practice, and puzzles. *Addictive Behaviors, 21*, 835-842.

*Miller, W. R., Benefield, R. G., & Tonigan, J. S. (1993). Enhancing motivation to change in problem drinking: A controlled comparison of two therapist styles. *Journal of Consulting & Clinical Psychology, 61*, 455-461.

Miller, W. R., & Rollnick, S. (1991). *Motivational interviewing: Preparing people to change addictive behaviors.* New York: The Guilford Press.

Miller, W. R., & Rollnick, S. (2002). *Motivational interviewing: Preparing people for change* (2nd ed.). New York: The Guilford Press.

Miller, W. R., Sovereign, R. G., & Krege, B. (1988). Motivational interviewing with problem drinkers: II. The Drinker's Check-up as a preventive intervention. *Behavioural Psychotherapy, 16*, 251-268.

*Monti, P. M., Colby, S. M., Barnett, N. P., Sprito, A., Rohsenow, D. J., Myers, M., et al. (1999). Brief intervention for harm reduction with alcohol-positive older adolescents in a hospital emergency department. *Journal of Consulting & Clinical Psychology, 67*, 989-994.

*Murphy, J. G., Duchnick, J. J., Vuchinich, R. E., Davison, J. W., Karg, R. S., Olson, A. M., et al. (2001). Relative efficacy of a brief motivational intervention for college student drinkers. *Psychology of Addictive Behaviors, 15*, 373-379.

Nahom, D. (2003). The process of change in helping relationships. (Doctoral dissertation, University of Washington, 2003). *Dissertation Abstracts International, 64*, 1849.

Orlinsky, D. E., & Howard, K. I. (1986). Process and outcome in psychotherapy. In S. L. Garfield, & A. E. Bergin (Eds.), *Handbook of psychotherapy and behavior change* (pp. 311-381). New York: John Wiley & Sons.

*Picciano, J. F., Roffman, R. A., Kalichman, S. C., Rutledge, S. E., & Berghuis, J. P. (2001). A telephone based brief intervention using motivational enhancement to facilitate HIV risk reduction among MSM: A pilot study. *AIDS and Behavior, 5*, 251-262.

Prochaska, J. O., & DiClemente, C. C. (1983). Stages and processes of self-change of smoking: Toward an integrative model of change. *Journal of Consulting & Clinical Psychology, 51*, 390-395.

Prochaska, J. O., DiClemente, C. C., & Norcross, J. C. (1992). In search of how people change: Applications to addictive behaviors. *American Psychologist, 47*, 1102-1114.

Project MATCH Research Group. (1998). Therapist effects in three treatments for alcohol problems. *Psychotherapy Research, 8*, 455-474.

*Resnicow, K., Jackson, A., Wang, T., De, A.K., McCarty, F., Dudley, W. N., et al. (2001). A motivational interviewing intervention to increase fruit and vegetable intake through black churches: Results of the Eat for Life trial. *American Journal of Public Health, 91,* 1686-1693.

Rogers, C. R. (1951). *Client-centered therapy.* Boston: Houghton Mifflin Company.

Rogers, C. R. (1954). Introduction. In C. R. Rogers, & R. F. Dymond (Eds.), *Psychotherapy and personality change* (pp. 3-11). Chicago: The University of Chicago Press.

Rollnick, S., Heather, N., & Bell, A. (1992). Negotiating behaviour change in medical settings: The development of brief motivational interviewing. *Journal of Mental Health, 1,* 25-37.

*Royer, C. M., Dickson-Fuhrmann, E., McDermott, C. H., Taylor, S., Rosansky, J. S., & Jarvik, L. F. (2000). Portraits of change: Case studies from an elder-specific addiction program. *Journal of Geriatric Psychiatry & Neurology, 13,* 130-133.

*Rutledge, S. E., Roffman, R. A., Mahoney, C., Picciano, J. F., Berghuis, J. P., & Kalichman, S. (2001). Motivational enhancement counseling strategies in delivering a telephone-based brief HIV prevention intervention. *Clinical Social Work Journal, 29,* 291-306.

*Safren, S. A., Otto, M. W., & Worth, J. L. (1999). Life-Steps: Applying cognitive behavioral therapy to HIV medication adherence. *Cognitive and Behavioral Practice, 6,* 332-341.

*Safren, S. A., Otto, M. W., Worth, J. L., Salomon, E., Johnson, W., Mayer, K., et al. (2001). Two strategies to increase adherence to HIV antiretroviral medication: Life-Steps and medication monitoring. *Behaviour Research and Therapy, 39,* 1151-1162.

*Saunders, B., Wilkinson, C., & Phillips, M. (1995). The impact of a brief motivational intervention with opiate users attending a methadone programme. *Addiction, 90,* 415-424.

*Schilling, R. F., El-Bassel, N., Finch, J. B., Roman, R. J., & Hanson, M. (2002). Motivational interviewing to encourage self-help participation following alcohol detoxification. *Research on Social Work Practice, 12,* 711-730.

*Schmaling, K. B., Blume, A. W., & Afari, N. (2001). A randomized controlled pilot study of motivational interviewing to change attitudes about adherence to medications for asthma. *Journal of Clinical Psychology in Medical Settings, 8,* 167-172.

*Schneider, R. J., Casey, J., & Kohn, R. (2000). Motivational versus confrontational interviewing: A comparison of substance abuse assessment practices at employee assistance programs. *The Journal of Behavioral Health Services & Research, 27,* 60-74.

*Sellman, J. D., Sullivan, P. F., Dore, G. M., Adamson, S. J., & MacEwan, I. (2001). A randomized controlled trial of motivational enhancement therapy (MET) for mild to moderate alcohol dependence. *Journal of Studies on Alcohol, 62,* 389-396.

*Senft, R. A., Polen, M. R., Freeborn, D. K., & Hollis, J. F. (1997). Brief intervention in a primary care setting for hazardous drinkers. *American Journal of Preventive Medicine, 13,* 464-470.

*Smith, S. S., Jorenby, D. E., Fiore, M. C., Anderson, J. E., Mielke, M. M., Beach, K. E., et al. (2001). Strike while the iron is hot: Can stepped-care treatments resurrect relapsing smokers? *Journal of Consulting & Clinical Psychology, 69,* 429-439.

*Smith, D. E., Kratt, P. P., Heckemeyer, C. M., & Mason, D. A. (1997). Motivational interviewing to improve adherence to a behavioral weight-control program for older obese women with NIDDM: A pilot study. *Diabetes Care, 20*, 52-54.

*Stein, M. D., Charuvastra, A., Maksdad, J., & Anderson, B. J. (2002). A randomized trial of a brief alcohol intervention for needle exchangers (BRAINE). *Addiction, 97*, 691-700.

*Stephens, R. S., Roffman, R. A., & Curtin, L. (2000). Comparison of extended versus brief treatments for marijuana use. *Journal of Consulting & Clinical Psychology, 68*, 898-908.

*Stotts, A. L., DiClemente, C. C., & Dolan-Mullen, P. (2002). One-to-One: A motivational intervention for resistant pregnant smokers. *Addictive Behaviors, 27*, 275-292.

*Stotts, A. L., Schmitz, J. M., Rhoades, H. M., & Grabowski, J. (2001). Motivational interviewing with cocaine-dependent patients: A pilot study. *Journal of Consulting & Clinical Psychology, 69*, 858-862.

*Swanson, A. J., Pantalon, M., & Cohen, K. R. (1999). Motivational interviewing and treatment adherence among psychiatric and dually diagnosed patients. *The Journal of Nervous & Mental Disease, 187*, 630-635.

*Tappin, D. M., Lumsden, M. A., McIntyre, D., McKay, C., Gilmour, W. H., Webber, R., et al. (2000). A pilot study to establish a randomized trial methodology to test the efficacy of a behavioural intervention. *Health Education Research: Theory and Practice, 15*, 491-502.

*Thevos, A. K., Quick, R. E., & Yanduli, V. (2000). Motivational interviewing enhances the adoption of water disinfection practices in Zambia. *Health Promotion International, 15*, 207-214.

*Treasure, J. L., Katzman, M., Schmidt, U., Troop, N., Todd, G., & deSilva, P. (1999). Engagement and outcome in the treatment of bulimia nervosa: First phase of a sequential design comparing motivation enhancement therapy and cognitive behavioural therapy. *Behavior Research and Therapy, 37*, 405-418.

*Van Bilsen, H. P. J. G., & van Emst, A. J. (1986). Heroin addiction and motivational milieu therapy. *The International Journal of the Addictions, 21*, 707-713.

*Van Horn, D. H. A., & Bux, D. A. J. (2001). A pilot test of motivational interviewing groups for dually diagnosed inpatients. *Journal of Substance Abuse Treatment, 20*, 191-195.

*Woodruff, S. I., Edwards, C. C., Conway, T. L., & Elliot, S. P. (2001). Pilot test of an internet virtual world chat room for rural teen smokers. *Journal of Adolescent Health, 29*, 239-243.

*Woollard, J., Beilin, L., Lord, T., Puddey, I., MacAdam, D., & Rouse, I. (1995). A controlled trial of nurse counselling on lifestyle change for hypertensives treated in general practice: Preliminary results. *Clinical and Experimental Pharmacology and Physiology, 22*, 466-468.

*Yahne, C. E., Miller, W. R., Irvin-Vitela, L., & Tonigan, J. S. (2002). Magdalena Pilot Project: Motivational outreach to substance abusing women street sex workers. *Journal of Substance Abuse Treatment, 23*, 49-53.

Iatrogenic Effects of Group Treatment on Adolescents with Conduct and Substance Use Problems: A Review of the Literature and a Presentation of a Model

Mark J. Macgowan, PhD, LCSW
Eric F. Wagner, PhD, LCSW

SUMMARY. Group therapy is the most popular approach in the treatment of adolescent substance use problems. Recently, concerns have mounted about possible iatrogenic effects of group therapy based on studies on adolescents with conduct disorder. This paper reviews three possible contributors to response to group treatment among adolescents, and proposes a model of the relations among these variables, specifically

---

Mark J. Macgowan and Eric F. Wagner are affiliated with the Community-Based Intervention Research Group, Florida International University.

Address correspondence to: Mark J. Macgowan, PhD, LCSW, Community-Based Intervention Research Group, Florida International University, University Park, MARC 310, Miami, FL 33199 (E-mail: Macgowan@fiu.edu).

Partial support for this article came from the U.S. National Institute on Alcohol Abuse and Alcoholism grant RO1 AA13369.

[Haworth co-indexing entry note]: "Iatrogenic Effects of Group Treatment on Adolescents with Conduct and Substance Use Problems: A Review of the Literature and a Presentation of a Model." Macgowan, Mark J. and Eric F. Wagner. Co-published simultaneously in *Journal of Evidence-Based Social Work* (The Haworth Social Work Practice Press, an imprint of The Haworth Press, Inc.) Vol. 2, No. 1/2, 2005, pp. 79-90; and: *Addiction, Assessment, and Treatment with Adolescents, Adults, and Families* (ed: Carolyn Hilarski) The Haworth Social Work Practice Press, an imprint of The Haworth Press, Inc., 2005, pp. 79-90. Single or multiple copies of this article are available for a fee from The Haworth Document Delivery Service [1-800-HAWORTH, 9:00 a.m. - 5:00 p.m. (EST). E-mail address: docdelivery@haworthpress.com].

http://www.haworthpress.com/web/JEBSW
Digital Object Identifier: 10.1300/J394v02n01_05

in regard to how they independently and interactively contribute to outcomes among youth with conduct and substance use problems. *[Article copies available for a fee from The Haworth Document Delivery Service: 1-800-HAWORTH. E-mail address: <docdelivery@haworthpress.com> Website: <http://www.HaworthPress.com> © 2005 by The Haworth Press, Inc. All rights reserved.]*

KEYWORDS. Conduct disorder, adolescent substance abuse, group treatment, adolescents

INTRODUCTION

Group therapy is the most commonly used approach in the treatment of alcohol and other drug (AOD) use problems (Khantzian, 2001; Stinchfield, Owen, & Winters, 1994). It is especially popular in the treatment of adolescents with AOD use problems because (a) of the importance of the peer-group during this developmental period (Nowinski, 1990), (b) adolescents seem to like it (O'Leary et al., 2002), and (c) it is cost-effective (French et al., 2002). Although there is considerable evidence that group therapy can be effective in reducing a range of adolescent problems including AOD use (e.g., Hoag & Burlingame, 1997; Kaminer & Burleson, 1999; Panas, Caspi, Fournier, & McCarty, 2003; Waldron, Slesnick, Brody, Turner, & Peterson, 2001), research also has documented unanticipated iatrogenic effects of group therapy when conducted with youth with conduct problems (e.g., Catterall, 1987; Dishion, McCord, & Poulin, 1999; Feldman & Caplinger, 1977). Adolescents with AOD use problems commonly demonstrate co-occurring conduct problems; a recent study found that 89% of youth in treatment for substance use problems also have a diagnosis of conduct disorder (Clark & Bukstein, 1998). Thus, there is reason to be concerned about possible iatrogenic effects of group treatment on adolescent with AOD use problems. Considering the apparently conflicting evidence about group therapy's efficacy with youth having conduct problems, it is crucial for AOD researchers to examine group factors and processes to understand what can make treatment groups harmful.

Studies of iatrogenic effects have found that aggregating youth with conduct disorder (CD) created environments in which youth exhibited negative behavior that was positively reinforced by other group members (i.e., "deviancy training," Dishion et al., 1999). However, other studies have suggested that antisocial behavior and deviancy training also were affected by group leader behaviors (Dishion, Poulin, & Burraston, 2001; Feldman, Caplinger, & Wodarski, 1983). These findings collectively suggest that (a) group composition, (b) member-reinforced disruptive behavior in groups, and (c) leadership behavior may have independent effects on outcomes for substance abusing adolescents who participate in group treatment. The purpose of this article is to review research on each of these three possible contributors to treatment response among teenagers who receive group treatment for AOD problems, many of whom also have associated conduct disorder. In addition, we introduce a model of the relations among these variables, specifically in regard to how they may independently and interactively contribute to AOD outcomes among substance abusing adolescents. This model is intended to guide future research on possible iatrogenic effects of group treatment on adolescents with substance use problems.

GROUP COMPOSITION

Group composition plays a major role in outcomes in group-based treatment research (Bertcher & Maple, 1974; Burlingame, Fuhriman, & Mosier, 2003; Feldman et al., 1983). An important compositional variable linked to retention and outcomes in groups is the presence of youth with conduct disorder (CD). Adolescent AOD treatment studies suggest that a diagnosis of CD is significantly related to negative outcomes such as treatment dropout (Galaif, Hser, Grella, & Joshi, 2001; Kaminer, Burleson, & Goldberger, 2002; Kaminer, Tarter, Bukstein, & Kabene, 1992). However, most studies have treated CD as a pre-group, individual-level variable; no study to date has examined the compositional mix of conduct disorder on outcomes. If CD is a factor in explaining outcomes, it is likely that aggregating youths with CD in groups may compound the likelihood of poor outcomes.

A review of 28 group-based treatments involving juvenile offenders reported that in most cases, group counseling did not result in significant behavior changes (Romig, 1978). The author of the review concluded that it was the aggregation of CD youths in such groups that led to the lack of treatment effects. Another study examined the effects of a group counseling workshop involving high school students at risk of dropping out (Catterall, 1987). Students who participated in the program were more likely to drop out of school by the following semester than those in the comparison group. Catterall concluded that the negative findings were due to within-group bonding among antisocial teens.

Recent studies by Dishion and colleagues have provided further evidence supporting the negative influence of CD adolescents on one another. These researchers found that youth who participated in the Teen Focus Groups had increased smoking and delinquency at 1- and 3-year follow-ups (Dishion & Andrews, 1995; Poulin, Dishion, & Burraston, 2001). The studies by Dishion and colleagues identified subtle processes in the groups, which resulted in the disruptive processes leading to poor outcomes. Specifically, youths used these groups to showcase their problematic behavior, and reinforcing responses from peers ("deviancy training") increased antisocial behavior (Dishion et al., 1999; Eddy, Dishion, & Stoolmiller, 1998). Dishion and associates found that aggregating youths with conduct problems provides the basis for group processes that result in poor outcomes.

Feldman and colleagues also examined the elements and processes of group treatment when conducted with youth with conduct problems (Feldman & Caplinger, 1977; Feldman et al., 1983). However, theirs is the only study in which researchers experimentally manipulated the number of youths with conduct problems in groups to assess outcomes. Homogeneous groups consisting of boys with conduct problems demonstrated no improvements in antisocial behavior. These researchers demonstrated that groups with higher concentrations of youth with conduct problems would likely have poorer outcomes, particularly in the absence of experienced leadership or proper treatment implementation.

A recent meta-analysis of skills training groups examined whether there were differences in treatment effects for interventions that differed in group composition (Ang & Hughes, 2002). The study reported a respectable overall effect size ($d = .55$) for skills training groups composed exclusively of adolescents with conduct problems. However, this effect size was significantly lower than that reported for skills training interventions delivered in the context of either individual treatment or non-aggregated compositions ($d = .70$). Homogeneous groups of antisocial youths tended to have reduced effects on outcomes when compared with mixed groups.

Collectively, this body of research suggests that groups with a higher percentage of youth with conduct problems will display greater antisocial behavior in groups, which will lead to poorer outcomes. Although the research reviewed does not directly address the degree of conduct disorder within groups, it is plausible that groups with higher percentages of youth with conduct disorder and/or youth with more severe conduct disorder will more likely exhibit antisocial behavior in the group, leading to poorer outcomes, than groups with fewer youth with conduct problems and less severe conduct problems. In sum, it appears that a diagnosis of conduct disorder may be an important factor in explaining outcomes in adolescent AOD treatment research, but no research has been done that examines the compositional mix of conduct disorder in AOD treatment groups. Furthermore, group composition is hypothesized to be a necessary but insufficient variable in influencing outcomes. The studies by Dishion, Feldman and associates, reviewed above, clearly indicate that composition alone did not adequately explain outcomes. These studies found that within-group factors (e.g., deviancy training, leadership behaviors) explained the effects. Composition thus sets the stage for the expression of antisocial behavior and deviancy training in groups, which leads to poor outcomes.

ANTISOCIAL BEHAVIOR AND DEVIANCE TRAINING IN GROUP

The previously described studies by Feldman and Dishion and colleagues (i.e., Dishion & Andrews, 1995; Dishion et al., 1999; Eddy et al., 1998; Feldman & Caplinger, 1977; Feldman et al., 1983; Poulin et al., 2001) reported that conduct disordered youths in groups displayed antisocial behavior and deviancy training. *Antisocial behavior* in group is "any action that serves to disrupt, hurt, annoy, or otherwise prevent members from participating in the group's tasks or activities" (Feldman & Caplinger, 1977, p. 15). *Deviancy training* within groups is "the process of contingent positive reactions to rule-breaking discussions" (Dishion et al., 1999, p. 756).

Although research on this topic is limited, studies performed to date clearly and consistently indicate that groups in which such disruptive behaviors occur have poorer outcomes (Dishion & Andrews, 1995; Dishion et al., 2001; Feldman & Caplinger, 1977; Feldman et al., 1983; Rose, 1998). Stated simply, groups whose members display more disruptive, hurtful, or annoying behaviors demonstrate less response to treatment than groups whose members display lower levels of these behaviors.

In their recent investigations, Dishion and colleagues found that the sequences of rule breaking talk reinforced by laughter predicted increases in self-reported smoking and teacher-reported delinquency years later. These researchers have labeled this phenomenon "deviance training," and they have suggested that the aggregation of delinquent youth in treatment groups may both exacerbate normative social pressures for conformity during adolescence and reduce access to the protective effects of less deviant peers. Dishion, McCord, and Poulin (1999) have argued that adolescent peer networks formed because of deviance, such as treatment groups for adolescents with conduct and AOD problems, provide a context where these problem behaviors may be reinforced. While the presence of disruptive behavior in groups and the process of deviance training are expected to have significant impacts on outcomes, these effects appear to be moderated by group leader behaviors, as described in the next section.

GROUP LEADER BEHAVIORS

Small group researchers have noted that leadership is one of the most important factors in explaining the functioning of small groups and predicting group therapy outcomes (e.g., Burlingame, Mackenzie, & Strauss, 2004; Cartwright & Zander, 1968; Dies, 1994). Yet, therapist variables and their relations to key outcomes have been left "virtually unstudied in the substance abuse treatment field" (Stinchfield et al., 1994, p. 469). An important unanswered question is how leader behaviors affect disruptive behavior within groups to impact outcomes. The effects of leadership behaviors on outcomes can be examined from two perspectives: immediate outcomes after the leader's intervention, and long-term outcomes (Greene, 2000). Examination from both perspectives is essential for understanding of the impact of group leader behaviors on response to group treatment.

The classic studies by Lewin, White, and Lippitt demonstrated the effects of three forms of leadership (authoritarian, democratic, and laissez-faire) on children's behavior in group (Lewin & Lippitt, 1938; Lewin, Lippitt, & White, 1939; White & Lippitt, 1968). The studies revealed that there was more aggression (about 30 times more) and more scape- goating in authoritarian-led groups than in democratically led groups. In addition, authoritarian leadership was likely to develop disruptive sub- groupings. These early studies revealed that leader behaviors had a direct impact on disruptive behavior in the groups.

An important finding from Feldman and colleagues was that group leadership was influenced by group compositional variables (Feldman & Caplinger, 1977; Feldman et al., 1983). Although experienced leaders (e.g., those with graduate level coursework in group methods) were more effective than inexperienced leaders in fostering positive behavior change, there were differential effects based on group composition. Leader experience was "significantly influenced by contextual variables and, especially, by the compositional nature of the treatment group" (Feldman & Caplinger, 1977, p. 5). However, group composition was only weakly related to outcomes when groups were led by experienced leaders, but was very influential when groups were led by less experienced leaders.

Further details from the Feldman studies revealed that leader *behaviors* accounted for more of the variance in explaining behavior within the groups than leader *experience* (Feldman et al., 1983). Leader experience accounted for 2% of the variance, but leader behaviors accounted for an average of 80% of the explained variance in youths' antisocial behavior in-group. Thus, leader behaviors appear to have much greater impact on member behaviors in-group than leader experience. Furthermore, *negative* leader behaviors (i.e., criticism, threats, or negative attention) were significantly associated with antisocial behavior in groups. For example, a leader's negative attention to member behavior was the best predictor of antisocial behavior, accounting for an average of 11% of the variance in observed antisocial behavior over treatment (Feldman et al., 1983, p. 235).

Additionally, the effects of leader behaviors were substantially increased when analyses were done at the group level. When the variables were aggregated to examine the effects at the group level, negative leader interventions such as negative attention explained an average of 42% of the variance in antisocial behavior during the first two treatment phases (16 weeks). Criticism accounted for 22% of the variance during the first phase of treatment. Positive attention was inversely associated with antisocial behavior across all phases of treatment, explaining an average of 11% of the variance in group antisocial behavior. The researchers concluded that "the data reveal clearly that the *direct* effects of leader interventions are manifested primarily at the *group* level, and not at the individual level of analysis" (Feldman et al., 1983, p. 250, emphasis in the original).

Dishion and colleagues did not examine the specific effects of leader behaviors on outcomes. However, they concluded that leaders have an important influence in reducing deviancy training noting that "skilled group leadership that could orchestrate a dynamic group environment that does *not* provide group attention for deviance would reduce or eliminate the iatrogenic effect" (Dishion et al., 2001, p. 89, emphasis in the original). This quote underscores the importance of the interaction between leader behavior and disruptive behavior in groups in determining response to adolescent AOD group treatment.

In sum, leader behaviors have a clear influence on member disruptive behavior in group, which in turn, affect outcomes. In particular, leadership seems to have a stronger impact on group-level behavior than on individuals within the group. However, no study to date has examined the effects of leader behaviors in reducing disruptive behavior in group, and the ultimate effects that leader behaviors have on AOD outcomes.

Proposed Model

Given the foregoing, we would like to propose the model depicted in Figure 1 to guide future research on the possible iatrogenic effects of group treatment on adolescents with substance use problems. The variables include in the model are hypothesized to have little influence on their own (i.e., they have little direct effect) and their influence on outcomes is hypothesized to change over the life of the group. Group composition, disruptive behavior in group, and leader behaviors are hypothesized to work together to affect outcomes. Disruptive behavior in

FIGURE 1. Proposed model of relations among group composition, disruptive behavior, and leader behaviors in predicting response to AOD group treatment.

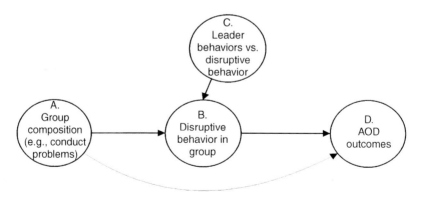

Note. Left to right positioning reflects temporal order. Dashed arrow indicates a correlation that weakens when the other variable is considered.

group (B) is viewed as a mediator of AOD outcomes in group (D), explaining how group composition (A) affects AOD outcomes (D). Full mediation is proposed; disruptive behavior (B) is expected to dominate the effects of group composition (A). The direct effects of group composition (dashed arrow) weakens when disruptive behavior in group is considered (Finney, 1995; Kraemer, Stice, Kazdin, Offord, & Kupfer, 2001). However, it is proposed that the effects of this part of the model are influenced by leader behaviors. Once disruptive behavior is displayed in group, leader behaviors related to the presence of disruptive behavior in the group (C) are expected to influence the effect of disruptive behavior in groups. Thus, leader behaviors affect the strength of the relationship between disruptive behavior and AOD outcomes (Finney, 1995, p. 137; Kraemer et al., 2001, p. 852). The elements are hypothesized to work together to explain AOD outcomes.

CONCLUSIONS

Research concerning possible iatrogenic effects of group treatment on adolescents with AOD use problems is important for a number of reasons. First, identifying the factors that contribute to iatrogenic effects will help develop effective group treatment approaches. With the high co-occurrence of AOD abuse/dependence and conduct disorder, many group interventions potentially could have unintended iatrogenic effects. Without research into the "side effects" of treatment, "interventions that produce iatrogenic effects propagate" (Eddy et al., 1998, p. 58). Second, no study had appeared in the literature that examined possible iatrogenic effects with adolescents in group treatment for AOD problems. The literature thus far has been devoted to iatrogenic effects with adolescent in group treatment for conduct problems. Third, there has been no research on the independent, combined, and longitudinal influences of group composition, disruptive behavior, and leader behaviors on outcomes among adolescents who participate in group therapy, regardless of the presenting problems. Given (a) the prevalence of group treatment for adolescents with AOD problems and (b) the field's interest in improving the interventions that we provide, it is our hope that the literature review and proposed model presented herein will inspire and guide future research on the topic of possible iatrogenic effects of group treatment on adolescents with AOD use problems.

REFERENCES

Ang, R. P., & Hughes, J. N. (2002). Differential benefits of skills training with antisocial youth based on group composition: A meta-analytic investigation. *School Psychology Review, 31*(2), 164-185.

Bertcher, H. J., & Maple, F. F. (1974). Elements and issues in group composition. In P. H. Glasser, R. C. Sarri, & R. D. Vinter (Eds.), *Individual change through small groups* (pp. 186-208). New York: The Free Press.

Burlingame, G. M., Fuhriman, A., & Mosier, J. (2003). The differential effectiveness of group psychotherapy: A meta-analytic perspective. *Group Dynamics: Theory, Research, and Practice, 7*(1), 3-12.

Burlingame, G. M., Mackenzie, K. R., & Strauss, B. (2004). Small group treatment: Evidence for effectiveness and mechanisms of change. In M. J. Lambert (Ed.), *Bergin and Garfield's handbook of psychotherapy and behavior change* (5th ed., pp. 647-696). Hoboken, NJ: Wiley.

Cartwright, D., & Zander, A. F. (Eds.). (1968). *Group dynamics: Research and theory* (3d ed.). New York, NY: Harper & Row.

Catterall, J. S. (1987). An intensive group counseling dropout prevention intervention: Some cautions on isolating at-risk adolescents within high schools. *American Education Research Journal, 24,* 521-540.

Dies, R. R. (1994). Therapist variables in group psychotherapy research. In A. Fuhriman, & G. M. Burlingame (Eds.), *Handbook of group psychotherapy: An empirical and clinical synthesis* (pp. 114-154). New York: Wiley.

Dishion, T. J., & Andrews, D. (1995). Preventing escalation in problem behaviors with high risk young adolescents: Immediate and 1-year outcomes. *Journal of Consulting & Clinical Psychology, 63*(4), 538-548.

Dishion, T. J., McCord, J., & Poulin, F. (1999). When interventions harm-Peer groups and problem behavior. *American Psychologist, 54*(9), 755-764.

Dishion, T. J., Poulin, F., & Burraston, B. (2001). Peer group dynamics associated with iatrogenic effects in group interventions with high-risk young adolescents. In D. W. Nangle, & C. A. Erdley (Eds.), *The role of friendship in psychological adjustment* (pp. 79-92). San Francisco: Jossey-Bass.

Eddy, J. M., Dishion, T. J., & Stoolmiller, M. (1998). The analysis of intervention change in children and families: Methodological and conceptual issues embedded in intervention studies. *Journal of Abnormal Child Psychology, 26*(1), 53-69.

Feldman, R. A., & Caplinger, T. E. (1977). Social work experience and client behavioral change: Multivariate analysis of process and outcome. *Journal of Social Service Research, 1*(1), 5-33.

Feldman, R. A., Caplinger, T. E., & Wodarski, J. S. (1983). *The St. Louis conundrum: The effective treatment of antisocial youths.* Englewood Cliffs, NJ: Prentice-Hall.

Finney, J. W. (1995). Enhancing substance abuse treatment evaluations: Examining mediators and moderators of treatment effects. *Journal of Substance Abuse, 7*(1), 135-150.

French, M. T., Roebuck, M. C., Dennis, M. L., Diamond, G., Godley, S. H., Tims, F., et al. (2002). The economic cost of outpatient marijuana treatment for adolescents: findings from a multi-site field experiment. *Addiction, 97*(s1), 84-97.

Galaif, E. R., Hser, Y.-I., Grella, C. E., & Joshi, V. (2001). Prospective risk factors and treatment outcomes among adolescents in DATOS-A. *Journal of Adolescent Research, 16*(6), 661-678.

Greene, L. R. (2000). Process analysis of group interaction in therapeutic groups. In A. P. Beck, & C. M. Lewis (Eds.), *The process of group psychotherapy: Systems for analyzing change* (pp. 23-47). Washington, DC: American Psychological Association.

Hoag, M. J., & Burlingame, G. M. (1997). Evaluating the effectiveness of child and adolescent group treatment: A meta-analytic review. *Journal of Clinical Child Psychology, 26*(3), 234-246.

Kaminer, Y., & Burleson, J. A. (1999). Psychotherapies for adolescent substance abusers: 15-month follow-up of a pilot study. *American Journal on Addictions, 8*(2), 114-119.

Kaminer, Y., Burleson, J. A., & Goldberger, R. (2002). Cognitive-behavioral coping skills and psychoeducation therapies for adolescent substance abuse. *Journal of Nervous & Mental Disease, 190*(11), 737-745.

Kaminer, Y., Tarter, R. E., Bukstein, O. G., & Kabene, M. (1992). Comparison between treatment completers and noncompleters among dually diagnosed substance-abusing adolescents. *Journal of the American Academy of Child & Adolescent Psychiatry, 31*(6), 1046-1049.

Khantzian, E. J. (2001). Reflections on group treatments as corrective experiences for addictive vulnerability. *International Journal of Group Psychotherapy, 51*(1), 11-20.

Kraemer, H. C., Stice, E., Kazdin, A., Offord, D., & Kupfer, D. (2001). How do risk factors work together? Mediators, moderators, and independent, overlapping, and proxy risk factors. *American Journal of Psychiatry, 158*(6), 848-856.

Lewin, K., & Lippitt, R. (1938). An experimental approach to the study of autocracy and democracy: A preliminary note. *Sociometry, 1*, 292-300.

Lewin, K., Lippitt, R., & White, R. K. (1939). Patterns of aggressive behavior in experimentally created "social climates." *Journal of Social Psychology, 10*, 271-299.

Nowinski, J. (1990). *Substance abuse in adolescents & young adults: A guide to treatment*. New York: W. W. Norton.

O'Leary, T. A., Brown, S. A., Colby, S. M., Cronce, J. M., D'Amico, E. J., Fader, J. S., et al. (2002). Treating adolescents together or individually? Issues in adolescent substance abuse interventions. *Alcoholism, Clinical, and Experimental Research, 26*(6), 890-899.

Panas, L., Caspi, Y., Fournier, E., & McCarty, D. (2003). Performance measures for outpatient substance abuse services: Group versus individual counseling. *Journal of Substance Abuse Treatment, 25*(4), 271-278.

Poulin, F., Dishion, T. J., & Burraston, B. (2001). 3-Year iatrogenic effects associated with aggregating high-risk adolescents in cognitive-behavioral preventive interventions. *Applied Developmental Science, 5*(4), 214-224.

Rose, S. D. (1998). *Group therapy with troubled youth: A cognitive behavioral interactive approach*. Thousand Oaks: Sage Publications.

Stinchfield, R., Owen, P. L., & Winters, K. C. (1994). Group therapy for substance abuse: A review of the empirical literature. In A. Fuhriman, & G. M. Burlingame (Eds.), *Handbook of group psychotherapy: An empirical and clinical synthesis* (pp. 458-488). New York: John Wiley and Sons.

Waldron, H. B., Slesnick, N., Brody, J. L., Turner, C. W., & Peterson, T. R. (2001). Treatment outcomes for adolescent substance abuse at 4-and 7-month assessments. *Journal of Consulting & Clinical Psychology, 69*(5), 802-813.

White, R., & Lippitt, R. (1968). Leader behaviors and member reaction in three "social climates." In D. Cartwright, & A. F. Zander (Eds.), *Group dynamics: Research and theory* (3d ed., pp. 318-335). New York, NY: Harper & Row.

Empirical and Theoretical Support for the Inclusion of Non-Abstinence-Based Perspectives in Prevention Services for Substance Using Adolescents

Samuel A. MacMaster, PhD
Lori K. Holleran, PhD
Katherine Chaffin, MSSW

SUMMARY. The purpose of this article is to present the Harm Reduction Model and its potential as a framework from which to provide prevention services for adolescents. While it may be uncomfortable for service providers to acknowledge, the vast majority of adolescents in the United States will have used mood-altering substances sometime during their teen years. While non-abstinence-based prevention services have existed for some time, they are not without controversy. This article pro-

---

Samuel A. MacMaster (E-mail: smacmast@utk.edu) is Assistant Professor, and Katherine Chaffin (E-mail: kmcclern@utk.edu) is Graduate Research Assistant, the University of Tennessee, College of Social Work-Nashville, 193 East Polk Avenue, Nashville, TN 37210 . Lori K. Holleran is Assistant Professor, The University of Texas at Austin School of Social Work, 1925 San Jacinto Boulevard, Austin, TX 78712 (E-mail: lorikay@mail.utexas.edu).

[Haworth co-indexing entry note]: "Empirical and Theoretical Support for the Inclusion of Non-Abstinence-Based Perspectives in Prevention Services for Substance Using Adolescents." MacMaster, Samuel A., Lori K. Holleran, and Katherine Chaffin. Co-published simultaneously in *Journal of Evidence-Based Social Work* (The Haworth Social Work Practice Press, an imprint of The Haworth Press, Inc.) Vol. 2, No. 1/2, 2005, pp. 91-111; and: *Addiction, Assessment, and Treatment with Adolescents, Adults, and Families* (ed: Carolyn Hilarski) The Haworth Social Work Practice Press, an imprint of The Haworth Press, Inc., 2005, pp. 91-111. Single or multiple copies of this article are available for a fee from The Haworth Document Delivery Service [1-800-HAWORTH, 9:00 a.m. - 5:00 p.m. (EST). E-mail address: docdelivery@haworthpress.com].

http://www.haworthpress.com/web/JEBSW
Digital Object Identifier: 10.1300/J394v02n01_06

poses Harm Reduction as a complimentary or alternative perspective for work with adolescents for whom abstinence may not be immediately possible and/or may not be a realistic outcome for services. This article outlines the abstinence-oriented and Harm Reduction perspectives, as well as the Stages of Change model; utilizing empirical support, it then discusses how these perspectives can work together in social work practice in the adolescent substance abuse prevention arena. *[Article copies available for a fee from The Haworth Document Delivery Service: 1-800-HAWORTH. E-mail address: <docdelivery@haworthpress.com> Website: <http://www.HaworthPress. com> © 2005 by The Haworth Press, Inc. All rights reserved.]*

KEYWORDS. Adolescence, substance abuse prevention, harm reduction

Complete abstinence from all non-medical drugs has been the understood goal of most substance abuse prevention programs in the United States of America. Although non-abstinence based interventions have always existed as a service possibility, the Harm Reduction Model provides a new and important perspective on adolescent substance abuse prevention. This development is being increasingly utilized within the substance abuse treatment community (MacMaster, 2004; Clapp & Burke, 1999) and should receive the attention of individuals working with adolescents in prevention realms. When viewed from the perspective of the Stages of Change model (Prochaska & DiClemente, 1982; Prochaska, DiClemente, & Norcross, 1992) and the Adolescent Psychosocial Developmental models (Erickson, 1968), the utility of strict adherence to an abstinence-only perspective is brought into question. This article briefly outlines the abstinence-oriented and Harm Reduction perspectives, as well as the Stages of Change model; utilizing empirical support, it then discusses how these perspectives can work together in social work practice in the adolescent substance abuse prevention arena.

ADOLESCENT SUBSTANCE USE

It has become a de facto norm for adolescents to experiment with substances (Kaplow, Curran, & Dodge, 2002). The vast majority of adolescents in the United States will have used mood-altering substances sometime during their teen years. The Monitoring the Future survey of approximately 50,000 8th, 10th, and 12th graders in about 420 public and private secondary schools supports this point concluding that the majority (78.4%) of high school seniors responded that they had tried alcohol and a smaller majority (53%) had tried an illicit drug (Johnston, O'Malley & Bachman, 2003a). Notably, almost one-third (29%) had tried some drug other than marijuana. These percentages are somewhat consistent over time, since the survey began in 1975 (Johnston, O'Malley & Bachman, 2003b). The Youth Risk Behavior Survey, an annual survey of high school students provides similar results. This national study also found that a nearly identical percentage of youth (78%) has experimented with alcohol during their lifetime, and additionally nearly half (47%) had a drink within the prior month (CDC, 2003).

Despite the discomfort that social workers may experience, it is critical that the acknowledgement is made that, although illegal, experimentation with alcohol and drugs during adolescence has been found to be statistically normative (Kaplow, Curran, & Dodge, 2002). Substance use in and of itself constitutes a potential risk for a myriad of other problems for adolescents. It is also important to note that most adolescents navigate through this use without major consequences to their ongoing development. Longitudinal studies of substance use suggest that the vast majority of adolescents will eliminate destructive patterns of use, and simply "mature out" of these patterns as they take on adult roles and responsibilities (Bachman, Wadsworth, O'Malley, Johnston, & Schulenberg, 1997; Labouvie, 1996).

Similarly, it is also important to acknowledge that use of a substance does not in and of itself constitute a substance abuse problem. In addition to the "maturing out" process noted above, most youth who experiment with illicit drug and alcohol use do not develop drug abuse or dependence problems either in adolescence or in adulthood (Newcomb, 1997). In fact, the overwhelming majority of adolescents who use substances do not develop a substance use disorders (Newcomb, 1997). Additionally, experimental use may actually be indicative of psychological health. Shelder and Block (1990) found that adolescents who experimented with drug use, (were neither frequent users nor abstainers), experienced higher levels of good psychological health and were better psychologically adjusted than their peers.

SUBSTANCE USE WITHIN THE CONTEXT
OF ADOLESCENT DEVELOPMENT

Development of Self Concept

Adolescent development is a matter of biology, culture, and psychology. Archambault (1992) makes the critical point that adolescents are forced into this period of great change by culture and biology, regardless of how well their environment has prepared them for this change, and that their sense of worth is unsure at best (Lawson & Lawson, 1992, p. 11). Adolescence is marked by a progression towards separation and individuation via a shift from primary closeness with parents to increasing intimacy with peers (Savin-Williams & Berndt, 1990). This shift in importance and intensity of peer relations affects the level of influence peers have on each other regarding substance use. Researchers have identified peer influence as one of the strongest risk factors for substance abuse among majority and minority youth (Beauvais, 1992; 1998).

Adolescents create themselves by trying on new selves, and by associating with groups of peers that reflect who they are and want to be. Eccles and colleagues have done extensive work on the extent to which young people engage in activities that fit into the image of the kind of person they want to be (Eccles & Barber, 1999). This image, or self-schema, may also influence the meaning of engaging in risky behaviors. In this research, a group of high school students active in student activities and organized school athletics tended to have high alcohol use, although they were doing well in school and had a high likelihood of going to college. A second group of young people engaged in similar amounts of alcohol consumption but were also engaged in other risky behaviors and were doing poorly in school. A third group was highly anxious beginning around 6th grade; they became increasingly anxious as they proceeded through high school and increased their drinking, presumably to calm their anxiety. The meaning of alcohol use and the relevant consequences are different for each of these groups. Eccles (1999) pointed out that telling the first group of young people that alcohol use would have dire consequences for them might be ineffective because their experiences contradict this message. For them, it is suggested that encouraging designated drivers and other tactics to avoid negative consequences of drinking might be more effective than preaching abstinence.

In relation to identity formation in adolescents, youth use substances for three primary reasons: (1) a sense that they will understand themselves and their environment better, (2) to increase experiences and activity, and (3) because it has the effect of producing a "high" or greater sense of social ease (Segal, Cromer, Stevens, & Wasserman, 1982).

OVERVIEW OF THEORETICAL MODELS

Trans-Theoretical Stages of Change Model

We begin our theoretical discussion by first considering the Trans-Theoretical Stages of Change Model (Prochaska & DiClemente, 1982; Prochaska, DiClemente & Norcross, 1992). This perspective provides an important background, as (1) 'change' (specifically substance abuse behavior change) is the ultimate outcome that we seek to achieve, and (2) the Stage of Change Model has become an increasingly utilized perspective in substance abuse treatment (Miller, 1999). The Stages of Change Model suggests a five-stage process that individuals must cycle through, including: precontemplation, contemplation, preparation, action, and maintenance (Prochaska, DiClemente, & Norcross, 1992). Change within this model is viewed as a long-term cyclical process and not as a linear process. Prochaska, DiClemente, and Norcross (1992) suggest that the vast majority (85%-90%) of addicted people are not in the action stage. Thus, abstinence-based substance abuse prevention services would not necessarily be appropriate to the individual's current stage.

While the Stages of Change Model has been widely accepted, its utility is largely heuristic in providing a dynamic view of substance abuse treatment and recovery. While emphasizing the need to target an individual's current stage of change is useful, what is lacking in the Stages of Change Model is a clear specification of mechanisms, which drive the change process. The model does posit different processes of change (strategies or techniques) used as individuals progress through different stages, with more cognitive/experiential processes used in the earlier stages and more behavioral strategies used in the later stages. These processes suggest general guidelines for intervention strategies, though specific mechanisms are not yet delineated.

Abstinence Oriented Models

Although the federal government did not regulate drug use until passage of the Harrison Act in 1914, abstinence and prohibition of most substance use (with the obvious exception of some substance, i.e., alcohol, nicotine and caffeine), has undergirded drug policy for most of this century (Zimring & Hawkins, 1992). Although alcohol remains legal for those over the age of twenty-one, there are similar "zero-tolerance" mandates for under-age drinking (ONDCP, 1999). Thus the Drug Free Schools and Communities Act Amendment of 1989 requires elementary, secondary and all colleges to implement and enforce abstinence-based policies related to substance use by students (USDOE, 1999). At the federal level, the Anti-Drug Abuse Act of 1988 currently mandates abstinence-based drug policy. Current drug policy is based specifically on section 6201 of this act, which established the goal of a drug-free America and provided Congressional requirements to reduce drug abuse and its consequences (ONDCP, 1999). This policy states that all non-medical drug use is illegal, there are fines and imprisonment for substance abuse, and help is only extended to those who have a desire to abstain from all use (Brown, 1995).

Traditional Prevention Models

Historically, drug prevention has most commonly consisted of the information education approach, which assumes that once adults make adolescents aware of the health hazards of substances and reinforce abstinence, they will develop anti-drug attitudes and subsequently make choices not to use. Research which questions the effectiveness of "information only" prevention programs (Botvin, Baker, & Dusenbury, 1995; Bukoski, 1985; Tobler, 1986, 1989) finds that not only does this form of intervention fail to produce reduction in drug use, but some programs led to a subsequent increase in use of substances afterwards (Falck & Craig, 1988). For example, Drug Abuse Resistance Education (DARE) is the most widespread drug prevention program in the United States with well over three million participants ("Project DARE," 1990). In some cases, DARE has not only failed to reduce drug use, but some researchers have found that there was a subsequent increase in students' substance use afterwards (Clayton, 1991; Harmon, 1993). Despite this lack of empirical support, millions of government dollars and hundred of hours of school time have been spent on this one program every year.

With the contributions of social theorists including Bandura (1977), Jessor and Jessor (1975, 1977), and McGuire (1974), models began to consider the interplay of individual, social and environmental factors (Falck & Craig, 1988). These models incorporated the complex, multi-level interaction of children with their environment and social and family systems. The ecological model stresses the concept of multiple levels of influence on child development and the complex interaction of child and environment (Lorion, 1987; Tolan, Guerra, & Kendall, 1995). They focus on social skills and general functioning rather than on substances alone.

Programmatic Exemplars. SAMHSA has identified programs with core components, which designate empirically grounded, theoretically-based, with positive outcomes. They all have the following elements (SAMHSA, 2002):

1. Program content addressing life skills or knowledge and skills related to substances (noting that substance-related content alone is inadequate).
2. Opportunities to practice/use new knowledge.
3. Community building beyond individual-level change.
4. Structured curricula with clear and easy directions.
5. Consistent messages sent through multiple channels.
6. Emphasis on relationship building as a precursor to the delivery of program content.
7. Utilization of naturally occurring social networks and parental or social system involvement wherever possible.
8. Emphasis on integrating programs into clients real lives.
9. Strengths focus and asset rather than deficit modeling.
10. Continuity through high fidelity to the program, dosage adequacy, and consistency.

Key programs identified as having all these components include LifeSkills Training (Botvin, 1990, 1995, 1997), Project ALERT (Ellikson, 1998; Ellikson, Bell, & McGuigan, 1993), and Project Northland (Pentz, 1990), to name a few. Instead of information provision, recent research supports the efficacy of a combination of life skills (skills related to successful functioning regarding achievements and interpersonal relationships) and resistance training interventions (i.e., skills related to effectively refraining from risky behaviors). All of these, and most other programs adopted by schools, are abstinence-based prevention models aiming at the goal of preventing use of substances. The historical "Just Say No" campaigns were initially determined by preventionists to be unsuccessful due to the need for more specific prevention and resistance strategies (i.e., HOW to say NO). It is time to further scrutinize this prevention goal of abstinence.

Harm Reduction Model

A conceptual framework that provides for individuals willing to be engaged in services, but not immediately seeking abstinence is Harm Reduction. Based on a public health model of social problems, Harm Reduction seeks to eliminate the negative consequences of given phenomena for the members of a society without necessarily eliminating the phenomena (Des Jarlais, 1995). Primarily seen as a policy level framework, it is not synonymous with legalization, although the two are often confused (UNIDCP, 1997). Practitioners utilizing this perspective attempt to develop interventions that reduce drug-related harm without necessarily promoting abstinence as the only solution. Common to discussions of Harm Reduction (Des Jarlais, 1995; Drucker, 1995; Harm Reduction Coalition, 1996; Scavuzzo, 1996; van Laar, Dezwart, & Mensink, 1996; Springer, 1991, 1996) are the following five assumptions.

1. Substance use has and will be part of our world; accepting this reality leads to a focus on reducing drug-related harm rather than reducing drug use itself.
2. Abstinence from substances is clearly effective at reducing substance related harm, however it is only one of many possible objectives of services to substance users.
3. Substance use inherently causes harm, however many of the most harmful consequences of substance use, (HIV/AIDS, Hepatitis-C, overdoses, automobile accidents, etc.), can be effectively eliminated without complete abstinence.
4. Services to substance users must be provided in a relevant, "user-friendly" manner if they are to be effective in helping people to minimize their substance-related harm.
5. Substance use must be understood from a broad perspective and not solely as an individual act; accepting this idea moves interventions away from the use of coercion of individuals and criminal justice solutions and towards a public health/social work perspective.

Harm Reduction has served as the basis of substance abuse polices and practices in several Western European countries. Specifically, Harm Reduction was originally suggested in the 1920s in the United Kingdom, as part of the Rolleston Committee's recommendations regarding drug policy and later emerged as a pragmatic response to a rise in Hepatitis-C rates related to injection drug use in the early 1980s (Scavuzzo, 1996). Harm Reduction currently has served as the underpinning to drug policy and practice in the Netherlands for almost thirty years (van Laar, Dezwart, & Mensink, 1996). The Dutch have utilized Harm Reduction since the recommendations of the 1971 Hulsman Report became the base for Dutch Harm Reduction strategies in the Revised Opium Act of 1976 (Cohen, 1994). Several other Western European countries (Switzerland and Germany) have also used Harm Reduction as a base for some or all of their substance use policy (UNIDCP, 1997).

A recent development has been the rapid adoption of Harm Reduction among HIV/AIDS related service providers in the United States in response to the clear association between HIV/AIDS risk and injection drug use (Clapp & Burke, 1999). Within this context, HIV/AIDS prevention has taken priority over preventing substance use. The preventable harm caused by HIV/AIDS clearly outweighs the need to maintain adherence to the abstinence-based perspective. Quite simply, "dead addicts don't recover" (Vail & Stokes, 1999).

A Larger Continuum of Prevention Models

The Stages of Change model suggests that complete abstinence may not be a reasonable initial expectation for many adolescents. While abstinence oriented services certainly fit for those individuals who have either never used substances, or have used and are ameliorable to eliminating use, they do not provide meaningful interventions for all adolescents who have used substances. It is therefore more important to provide services that target the individual's current stage of change and to work to increase motivation to make continued changes. Thus, Harm Reduction provides a potential framework for service provision to potential service users at earlier stages.

Comparisons between abstinence-oriented and Harm Reduction based services are often made on a mutually exclusive basis (McCafferty, 2000). This is an artificial contention, as these two perspectives can be incorporated together to provide a more comprehensive continuum of services. Progression through the Stages of Change model can continue for individuals that access non-abstinence based services. Rather than stopping or slowing this progression, involvement in Harm Reduction services would quite likely accelerate an individual's potential for continued change. Harm Reduction based services can also fill the void for service recipients who are not yet at the action stage and are by definition not eligible and/or appropriate for abstinence based services. These individuals continue to have service needs despite their lack of expressed desire to remain substance free. Programs based on an abstinence-only perspective simply do not provide services to these individuals, as this would be seen as enabling their using behaviors.

Empirical Support for the Use
of Harm Reduction Based Prevention Services

While there have been several articles written about the need to broaden the framework on which prevention services are based, none have included empirical support for these interventions (Beck, 1998; Bonomo, & Bowes, 2001; Duncan, Nicholson, Clifford, Hawkins, & Petosa, 1994). The following section of this article provides evidence of the efficacy of Harm Reduction based services for a range of substance use related prevention needs.

Alcohol Skills Training for College Aged Drinking

Harm Reduction specific strategies have been shown to decrease problems associated with alcohol use for college-aged drinkers. For example, the Alcohol Skills Training Program (ASTP), a 6-week program for young adult drinkers, uses a cognitive behavioral approach to the prevention of alcohol problems by stressing the moderate use of, or abstinence from, addictive substances (Fromme, Marlatt, Baer, & Kivlahan, 1994). The program provides skill-based training around setting drinking limits, monitoring one's own drinking, rehearsing drink refusal, and practicing other useful behaviors through role play (Dimeff, Baer, Kivlahan, & Marlatt, 1998). The Brief Alcohol Screening and Intervention for College Students (BASICS), based on the original ASTP model, (Dimeff, Baer, Kivlahan, & Marlatt, 1998) involves a non-confrontational Harm Reduction approach to help students reduce their alcohol consumption and decrease the behavioral and health risks associated with heavy drinking. As with all Harm Reduction programs, the goal of the program is not to necessarily eliminate all alcohol use but facilitate change that will reduce the negative consequences associated with drinking, particularly binge drinking.

There is some evidence supporting the effectiveness of alcohol skills training programs. Evaluations of ASTP have found it to be superior to educational interventions in a one-year follow-up measure of alcohol consumption rates (Kivlahan, Marlatt, Fromme, Coppel, & Brand, 1990). Participants in the BASICS program at the University of Washington reduced the amount of alcohol consumed each time they drank to a larger extent than a control group of other high-risk drinkers. Program participants also reported that their alcohol-related problems (fighting, vandalism, driving under the influence, having blackouts, missing classes and/or having unprotected sex) were also reduced to a larger extent when compared to a control group (Marlatt, Baer, Kivlahan, Dimeff, Larimer, Quigley, Somers, & Williams, 1998). In keeping with the Stages of Change perspective and a larger continuum of services, participants in these programs were also referred to traditional abstinence based programs if deemed necessary. This, again, exemplifies the ability of participants to progress within the Stages of Change model despite the use of non-abstinence based strategies.

Brief Motivational Interviews for Alcohol Involved Youth in Emergency Rooms

Monti, Spirito, Myers, Colby, Barnett, Rohsenow, Woolard, and Lewnader (1999) conducted a study of 18- and 19-year-old individuals with either a positive blood alcohol concentration or a report of alcohol prior to trauma who were admitted to a hospital emergency room. The 94 participants were selected randomly to be either in the experimental group (consisting of standard care plus motivational interviewing focused on empathy and developing a goals to reduce alcohol related harm) or standard care (consisting of typical urgent care as well as handouts on avoiding drinking and driving and a list of local treatment agencies). All participants were interviewed at 3 and 6 months post intervention. Results indicated that adolescents who were exposed to a Harm Reduction concept were significantly less likely to drink and drive and were significantly less likely to have alcohol related injuries or problems than those adolescents who were in the standard care group.

Substance User Education

While the harm reduction-based programs targeting adolescents that inform substance users about choices in their use and improve decision-making skills have been provided in the United States, e.g., Drug Consumer Safety Education program in Oregon (Beck, 1998) and the What is Really Going on Program in California (de Leon, 2000), recent research from Australia supports the use of this modality (Bonomo, & Bowes, 2001). The School Health Harm Reduction Project (SHAHRP) is a school-based package of complementary interventions that assists 13-17-year-old Australians identify and develop plans for reducing the harm in high risk drinking situations (McBride, Farringdon, & Midford, 2000). Outcome data based on a three-year longitudinal quasi-experimental designed outcome study utilizing a sample of 2,329 participants in fourteen schools in experimental and comparisons groups suggests that the program was successful. Specifically, participants experienced significantly higher rates of increased knowledge about alcohol use, improved attitudes regarding alcohol use, and a reduction in harm associated with alcohol use when compared to students who did participate. Of particular interest was the finding that there were significant differences in alcohol consumption, as well as harm, for those students who participated in the intervention (McBride, Farringdon, & Midford, 2000; McBride, Midford, & Farringdon, 2000; McBride, Midford, Farringdon, & Phillips, 2000; Midford, McBride, & Munro, 1998).

Syringe Exchange and Services to Injection Drug Users

Of all interventions for active users, syringe exchange has gained the most notoriety. This Harm Reduction strategy has been employed with increasing regularity within this country despite a ban on federal funding (Paone, Des Jarlais, Singh, Grove, & Shi, 1998; Paone, Des Jarlais, Clark, Shi, Krim, & Purchase, 1997). Syringe exchange attempts to remove the agent through which HIV/AIDS is spread (the shared syringe), this high-risk behavior can be eliminated without necessarily eliminating the drug use itself. Due to the fact that eighty to ninety percent of all injection drug users are out of treatment at any given point in time (Sisk, Hatziandreu, & Hughes, 1990), interventions to the vast majority of injection drug users are necessary regardless of their motivation towards abstinence. There are currently over one hundred and seventy-one SEPs operating in the United States (MacMaster & Womack, 2002), however only eighteen of these programs provide services to youth under the age of eighteen (Harm Reduction Coalition, 2004).

There is growing evidence that this strategy is effective at facilitating positive changes for injection drug users who are not seeking absti-

nence. The targeted outcome, HIV infection rates, ha
decrease (Des Jarlais, Marmor, Paone, Titus, Shi, Perli:
man, 1996; Heimer, Kaplan, & Cadman, 1992; Kap
1994; Hurley, Jolley, & Kaldor, 1997). In addition, these
also been shown to facilitate other positive changes in in
behaviors. The prevalence of sharing of injection equip
shown to decrease (Bluenthal, Kral, Erringer, & Edlin, 1998; Robles,
Colon, Matos, Finlinson, Munzo, Marrero, Garcia, & Reyes, 1998;
Guydish, Bucardo, Young, Grinstead, & Clark, 1993; Hagan, Des
Jarlais, Purcase, Friedman, Reid, & Bell, 1993; Watter, Estilo, Clark, &
Lorvick, 1994; Heimer, Khosnod, Bigg, Guydish, & Junge, 1988;
Guydish, Clark, Garcia, & Bucardo, 1995) and prevalence of the disin-
fection of injection equipment has been shown to increase (Hagan, Des
Jarlais, Purcase, Friedman, Reid, & Bell, 1993). Needle exchanges have
also been found to serve as conduits for abstinence based drug treatment
for program participants (Heimer, 1998; Brooner, Kidorf, King,
Eilenson, Svikis, & Vlahov, 1998; Vlahov, Junge, Brookmeyer, Cohn,
Riley, Armenian, & Beilenson, 1997). This exemplifies the ability of
progress within the Stages of Change model despite the use of non-abstinence based strategies.

Adulterant Screening

As part of a program that promotes health and safety within the rave
and nightclub communities Dance Safe provides chemical analyses of
drugs provided by an affiliated laboratory. These services are directed
primarily towards non-addicted, recreational drug users as part of a
larger continuum of peer-based educational programs to reduce drug
abuse and empower young people to make healthy, informed lifestyle
choices (Santamour, Martin, Scott, Ford, Messer, & Schmidt, 2002).
While specific outcome data is not available to determine the effectiveness of this intervention in terms of who uses the information and how it
is utilized, the program has been successful at providing both web-
based analyses for substances sent in to the organization and home-
based testing kits mailed anonymously to individuals.

IMPLICATIONS FOR PRACTICE

Acknowledgement of the high number of adolescents who report experimenting and even using substances regularly can lead to more real-

...c and effective prevention messages. Holleran, Taylor-Seehafer, Pomeroy, & Neff, in press) note that youth are not open to prevention efforts that they perceive are not "reality-based." The failure to acknowledge the aforementioned reality of youth experimentation and high rates of substance use undoubtedly would prohibit youth engagement with programming. On the other hand, if substance use is realistically depicted in program and curriculum development, it is much more likely to resonate with the recipients and to have the desired impact. In fact, many prominent prevention scientists maintain that the key to effective prevention is the targeted audiences sense of ownership of the program (Price & Lorion, 1987; Kelly, 1987). This is not likely if they do not agree with the content and aims of the program.

The other important aspect of social work in the prevention realm is the concepts of "client centeredness" and "meeting the client where he/she is." While it is distasteful to accept that not only are many youth experimenting with substances, or using them sporadically or regularly, one must recognize that most youth who are at risk are not looking to abstain and may tune out vehement abstinence messages. Many adolescents have rejected or minimized prevention interventions, which touted drugs as "dangerous," "deadly," and "bad" in lieu of their own perceptions to the contrary.

One of the important considerations is that while abstinence may be the best intervention for those youth who are chemically predisposed for addiction or dependence, there is actually a continuum of youth between those that need abstinence and those who are considering use and those who are already using in small amounts to those who are in need of intervention. In the substance abuse and mental health field, there is awareness of the continuum of health care including universal, selective, indicated, case identification, standard treatment, long-term treatment, and aftercare (SAMSHA, 2002), Presently, universal prevention interventions focus only on the individuals who are not using in this continuum. There must be more attention paid to the gray areas between prevention and treatment. Harm Reduction Models serve as a bridge between these two erroneously dichotomized arenas.

CONCLUSIONS

This article describes Harm Reduction as a new perspective that provides an alternative to strict adherence to an abstinence-based perspective for social workers working with adolescents on issues of substance use. The traditional abstinence-based perspective clearly provides an appropriate treatment approach for many individuals who are experiencing problems associated with their substance use. This paper provides a complimentary or alternative perspective for work with those individuals for whom abstinence may not be immediately appropriate or useful. When used in conjunction with the Stages of Change model, Harm Reduction and abstinence-based interventions can be seen as informing separate portions of the same continuum. An important skill in the art of the social work practice is determining the best fit when matching client needs with interventions. In some instances, Harm Reduction based services potentially provide a better fit with clients' needs than the traditional abstinence-based interventions. In other instances, abstinence-based programming may be the more appropriate choice.

The use of the Harm Reduction services has been found to be a useful perspective from which effective interventions have been developed. These interventions did not remove the possibility of future abstinence-based interventions and engaged clients with services by meeting them where they are. This perspective can be used with other similar populations who could benefit from low threshold programs, i.e., individuals whose motivation for change has not yet at the action stage in the Stages of Change model. This would include groups of individuals, like the college-aged drinkers, who have experienced only minimal harmful consequences due to their substance use and may not recognize their use as a problem and may be inappropriate for abstinence-based interventions. Similarly, groups of individuals, like the active injection drug users, who may be aware of the consequences of their use, but lack the motivation to make major changes, will benefit from programs whose goal is to foster any positive change. The key to any successful social work program is the matching of client needs with the appropriate intervention. Practioners need to be aware of their clients' motivation and utilize the best fitting model to provide appropriate services. The Harm Reduction perspective is one such model. Just as there are groups who will benefit from Harm Reduction-based programming, highly motivated adolescents who are seeking to maintain abstinence or could quickly move into the action stage of the Stages of Change model would not be appropriate candidates for these interventions.

Importantly, there does not appear to be an ethical dilemma created by the use of this perspective. In fact, it could be suggested that Harm Reduction actually provides a better fit than an abstinence-only perspective to social workers' mandates to maintain a commitment to clients' needs and to facilitate self-determination. As social workers become more familiar with perspective, it is hoped that other innovative interventions will be developed, both in work with individuals experiencing problems related to their substance use and in work with many other social problems.

REFERENCES

Archambault, D.L. (1992). Adolescence: A physiological, cultural, and psychological no man's land. In G. W. Lawson, & A.W. Lawson (Eds.), *Adolescent Substance Abuse: Etiology, Treatment, & Prevention.* Gaithersburg, MD: Aspen Publishers.

Bachman, J.G., Wadsworth, K.N., O'Malley, P.M., Johnston, L.D., & Schulenberg, J.E. (1997). *Smoking, drinking, and drug use in young adulthood: The impacts of new freedoms and new responsibilities.* Mahwah, NJ: Lawrence Erlbaum Associates.

Bandura, A. (1977). *Social learning theory.* Englewood Cliffs, NJ: Prentice Hall.

Beauvais, F. (1992). An integrated model for prevention and treatment of drug abuse among American Indian youth. *Journal of Addictive Diseases, 11,* 63-80.

Beauvais, F. (1998). Cultural identification and substance use in North America: An annotated bibliography. *Substance Use and Misuse, 33,* 1315-1336.

Beck, J. (1998). 100 Years of "Just Say No" Versus "Just Say Know" Reevaluating Drug Education Goals for the Coming Century. *Evaluation Review, 22* (1), 15-45.

Bluenthal, R., Kral, A., Erringer E., & Edlin, B. (1998). Use of illegal syringe exchange and injection-related risk behaviors among street-recruited injection drug users in Oakland, CA, 1992-1995. *Journal of AIDS, 18,* 505.

Bonomo, Y., &. Bowes, G. (2001). Annotation: Putting Harm Reduction into an adolescent context. *Child Health 37,* 5-8.

Botvin, G.J., Baker, E., & Dusenbury, L. (1995). Long-term followup results of a randomized drug abuse prevention trial in a white middle class population. *Journal of the American Medical Association, 273* (14), 1106-1112.

Botvin, G. J., Baker, E., Dusenbury, L., Tortu, S., & Botvin, E. M. (1990). Preventing adolescent drug abuse through a multimodal cognitive-behavioral approach: Results of a 3-year study. *Journal of Consulting & Clinical Psychology, 58*(4), 437-446.

Botvin, G.J. (1997). Preventing adolescent cigarette smoking. *Journal of Developmental & Experimental Pediatrics, 18*(1), 47-48.

Brooner, R., Kidorf, M., King, V., Beilson, P., Svikis, D., & Vlahov, D. (1998). Drug abuse treatment success among needle exchange participants. *Public Health Reports, 113,* 129-139.

Brown, L. (1995). *Reducing the impact of drugs on American society.* Washington, DC: Office of National Drug Control Policy.

Bukoski, W.J. (1985). School-based substance abuse prevention: A review of program research. In S. Ezekoye, K. H. Kumpfer, & W. J. Bukoski (Eds.), *Childhood and chemical abuse: Prevention and intervention.* New York: The Haworth Press, Inc.

Centers for Disease Control (CDC). (2003). *National Youth Risk Behavior Survey: Trends in the Prevalence of Alcohol Use.* Washington DC: DHHS.

Clapp, J., & Burke, A. (1999). Discriminant analysis of factors differentiating among substance abuse treatment units in their provision of HIV/AIDS Harm Reduction services. *Social Work Research*, 23, 69-76.

Clayton, S. (1991). Gender differences in psychosocial determinants of adolescent smoking. *Journal of School Health*, 61, 115-120.

Cohen, P. (1994, March). *The case of two Dutch drug policy commissions: An exercise in Harm Reduction 1968-1976.* Paper presented at the 5th International Conference on the Reduction of Drug Related Harm, Addiction Research Foundation, Toronto.

De Leon, A. (2000). *What is really going on? Exploring a Harm Reduction approach to drug education: A curriculum for school based groups.* Alameda, CA: Xanthos.

Des Jarlais, D. (1995). Harm reduction: A framework for incorporating science into drug policy. *American Journal of Public Health*, 85, 10-12.

Des Jarlais, D., Marmor, M., Paone, D., Titus, S., Shi, Q., Perlis, T., Jose, B., & Friedman, S. (1996). HIV incidence among injecting drug users in New York City syringe exchange programmes. *Lancet*, 348, 987-991.

Dimeff, L., Baer, J., Kivlahan, D., & Marlatt G. (1998). *Brief alcohol screening and intervention for college students: A Harm Reduction approach.* New York: The Guilford Press.

Drucker, E. (1995). Harm reduction: A public health strategy. *Current Issues in Public Health*, 1, 64-70.

Duncan, D. F., Nicholson, T., Clifford, P., Hawkins, W., & Petosa. R. (1994). Harm Reduction: An emerging new paradigm for drug education. *Journal of Drug Education* 24 (4), 281-290.

Eccles, J. S., & Barber, B. L. (1999). Student council, volunteering, basketball, or marching band: What kind of extracurricular involvement matters? *Journal of Adolescent Research 14*, 10-43.

Ellickson, P. L. (1998). Preventing adolescent substance abuse: Lessons from the Project ALERT program. In J. Crane (Ed.), *Social programs that work*. New York: Russell Sage Foundation.

Ellickson, P. L., Bell, R. M., & McGuigan, K. (1993). Preventing adolescent drug use: Long-term results of a junior high program. *American Journal of Public Health*, 83(6), 856-861.

Erikson, E. H. (1968). *Identity youth and crisis.* New York: W. W. Norton.

Falck, R., & Craig, R. (1988). Classroom-oriented, primary prevention programming for drug abuse. *Journal of Psychoactive Drugs*, 20(4), 403-408.

Fromme, K., Marlatt, G., Baer, J., & Kivlahan, D. (1994). The Alcohol Skills Training Program: A group intervention for young adult drinkers. *Journal of Substance Abuse Treatment*, 11, 143-154.

Guydish, J., Bucardo, J., Young, M., Grinstead, O., & Clark, W. (1993). Evaluating needle exchange: Are there negative effects? *AIDS*, 7, 871-876.

Guydish, J., Clark, G., Garcia, D., & Bucardo, J. (1995). Evaluation of needle exchange using street-based survey methods. *Journal of Drug Issues*, 25, 33-41.

Hagan, H., Des Jarlais, D., Purchase, D., Friedman, S., Reid, T., & Bell, T. (1993). An interview study of participants in the Tacoma, Washington, syringe exchange. *Addiction*, 88, 1691-1697.

Harm Reduction Coalition. (1996). *Mission and principles of harm reduction*. Oakland, CA: Author.

Harm Reduction Coalition. (2004). *Harm Reduction youth services survey*. Oakland, CA: Author.

Harmon, M. A. (1993). Reducing the risk of drug involvement among early adolescents: An evaluation of drug abuse resistance education (DARE). *Evaluation Review, 17,* 221-239.

Hay Group. (1998). *Substance abuse benefit cost trends 1988-1998.* Report commissioned by The American Society on Addiction Medicine: Arlington VA.

Heimer, R. (1998). Can syringe exchange serve as a conduit to substance abuse treatment? *Journal of Substance Abuse Treatment, 15,* 183-191.

Heimer, R., Kaplan E., & Cadman, E. (1992). Prevalence of HIV-infected syringes during a syringe exchange program. *New England Journal of Medicine, 327,* 1883-1884.

Heimer, R., Khosnod, K., Bigg, D., Guydish, J., & Junge, B. (1988). Syringe use and reuse effects of syringe exchange programs in four cities. *Journal of AIDS & Human Retrovirology, 18,* S37.

Holleran, L. K., Taylor-Seehafer, M. A., Pomeroy, E. C., & Neff, J. A. (in press). Substance abuse prevention for high risk youth: Exploring culture and alcohol and drug use. *Alcoholism Quarterly, special edition on Latinos and substance abuse,* Melvin Delgado (Ed.).

Hurley, S., Jolley, D., & Kaldor, J. (1997). Effectiveness of needle exchange programmes for prevention of HIV infection. Lancet, 349, 1797-1800.

Jessor, R. & Jessor, S. L. (1975). Adolescent development and the onset of drinking. *Journal of Studies on Alcohol, 36,* 27-51.

Jessor, R., & Jessor. S. L. (1977). *Problem behavior and psychosocial development. A longitudinal study of youth.* New York: Academic Press.

Johnston, L. D., O'Malley, P. M., & Bachman, J. G. (2003a). *Monitoring the Future national survey results on adolescent drug use: Overview of key findings, 2002* (NIH Publication No. 03-5374). Bethesda, MD: National Institute on Drug Abuse

Johnston, L. D., O'Malley, P. M., & Bachman, J. G. (2003b). *Monitoring the Future national survey results on drug use, 1975-2002. Volume I: Secondary school students* (NIH Publication No. 03-5375). Bethesda, MD: National Institute on Drug Abuse.

Kaplan E., & Heimer, R. (1994). HIV incidence among needle exchange participants. *Journal of AIDS & Human Retrovirology, 10,* 175-176.

Kaplow, J.B., Curran, P.J., & Dodge, K.A. (2002). Child, parent, and peer predictors of early-onset substance use: A multisite longitudinal study. *Journal of Abnormal Child Psychology, 30*(3), 199-216.

Kelly, J. G. (1987). Seven Criteria When Conducting Community-Based Prevention Research: A Research Agenda and Commentary. In J. A. Steinberg, & M.M. Silverman (Eds.), *Preventing Mental Disorders: A Research Perspective* (DHHS Publication No. ADM 87-1492). Washington DC: U.S. Government Printing Office.

Kivlahan, D., Marlatt, G., Fromme, K., Coppel D., & Brand, E. (1990). Secondary prevention with college drinkers: Evaluation of an alcohol skills training program. *Journal of Consulting & Clinical Psychology, 58,* 805-810.

Labouvie, E. (1996). Maturing Out of Substance Use: Selection and Self-Correction. *Journal of Drug Issues, 26,* 457-476.

Lawson, G. W., & Lawson, A. W. (1992). *Adolescent substance abuse: Etiology treatment, and prevention*. Gaithersburg, MD: Aspen Publishers.

Lorion, R. (1987). Methodological challenges in prevention research. In D. Shaffer, I. Philips, & N. B. Enzer (Eds.), *Prevention of Mental Health Disorders, Alcohol and Other Drug Use in Children and Adolescents*. OSAP Prevention Monograph-2. (DHHS Pub. No. ADM 90-1646). Washington, DC: U.S. Government Printing Office.

MacMaster, S.A. (2004). Harm Reduction: A new perspective on substance abuse services. *Social Work, 49*: 356-363.

MacMaster, S. A., & Womack, B. G. (2002). Preventing HIV transmission among injection drug users: A brief history of syringe exchange programs *Journal of HIV/AIDS & Social Services, 1*, 95-112.

Marlatt, G. A., Baer, J. S., Kivlahan, D. R., Dimeff, L. A., Larimer, M. E., Quigley, L. A., Somers, J. M., & Williams, E. (1998). Screening and brief intervention for high-risk college student drinkers: Results from a two-year follow-up assessment. *Journal of Consulting & Clinical Psychology, 66*, 604-615.

McBride, N., Farringdon, F., & Midford, R. (2000). What harms do young Australians experience in alcohol-use situation? *Australian and New Zealand Journal of Public Health, 24* (1), 54-59.

McBride, N. T., Midford, R., & Farringdon, F. (2000). Alcohol Harm Reduction in schools: planning an efficacy study in Australia. *Drug and Alcohol Review, 19*, 83-93.

McBride, N. T., Midford, R., Farringdon, F., & Mike Phillips. (2000). Early results from a school alcohol harm minimization study: The School Health and Alcohol Harm Reduction Project. *Addiction, 95*(7), 1021-1042.

McCafferty, B. (2000). *Decriminalizing drugs is wrong: Why wreck more lives with drug abuse?* Reprint of an Editorial appearing in the Cincinnati Enquirer, August 6, 1998. Washington, DC: Office of National Drug Control Policy.

McGuire, W. J. (1974). Communication-persuasion models for drug education: Experimental findings. In M. S. Goodstadt (Ed.), *Research on methods and programs of drug education*. Toronto: Addictions Research Foundation.

Midford, R., McBride, N., & Munro, G. (1998). Harm Reduction in school drug education: Developing an Australian approach. *Drug and Alcohol Review, 17*, 319-328.

Miller, W. (1999). *Enhancing motivation for change in substance abuse treatment. Treatment Improvement Protocol, 35*. Washington, DC: DHHS.

Monti, P. M., Spirito, A., Myers, M., Colby, S. M., Barnett, N. P., Rohsenow, D. J., Woolard, R. & Lewnader, W. (1999). Brief intervention for Harm Reduction with alcohol-positive older adolescents in a hospital emergency department. *Journal of Consulting & Clinical Psychology, 67*(6), 989-994.

Newcomb, M. D. (1997). Psychosocial predictors and consequences of drug use: A developmental perspective within a prospective study. *Journal of Addictive Diseases, 16*(1), 51-89.

Office of National Drug Control Strategy. (1999). *The national drug control strategy, 1999: budget summary*. Washington, DC: Office of National Drug Control Policy.

Paone, D., Des Jarlais, D., Clark, J., Shi, Q., Krim, M., & Purchase, D. (1997). Update: Syringe exchange programs-United States, 1997. *Morbidity and mortality weekly report, 46*, 565-568.

Paone, D., Des Jarlais, D., Singh, M., Grove, D., & Shi, Q. (1998). Update: Syringe exchange programs-United States, 1997. *Morbidity and mortality weekly report, 47,* 684-5, 691.

Pentz, M. A., Trebow, E. A., & Hansen, W. B. (1990). Effects of program implementation on adolescent drug use behavior: The Midwestern Prevention Program (MPP). *Evaluation Review, 14* (3), 264-89.

Price, R. H., & Lorion, R. P. (1987). Prevention programming as organizational reinvention: From research to implementation. In D. Shaffer, I. Philips, & N. B. Enzer (Eds.), *Prevention of Mental Health Disorders, Alcohol, and Other Drug Use in Children and Adolescents.* OSAP Prevention Monograph-2. (DHHS Pub. No. ADM 90-1646). Washington, DC: U.S. Government Printing Office.

Prochaska, J. O., & DiClemente, C.C. (1982). Trans-theoretical therapy: Towards a more integrative model of change. *Psychotherapy theory research and practice, 19,* 276-288.

Prochaska, J. O., DiClemente, C. C., & Norcross, J. C. (1992). In search of how people change. *American Psychologist, 47,* 1102-1114.

Robles, R., Colon, H., Matos, T., Finlinson, H., Munzo, A., Marrero, C., Garcia, M., & Reyes, J. (1998). Syringe and needle exchange as HIV/AIDS prevention for injection drug users in Puerto Rico. *Health Policy, 45,* 209-220.

Santamour, T., Martin, M., Scott, T., Ford, K., Messer, N., & Schmidt, J. (2002, December). *Dance Safe Up off the Floor.* Paper presented at the 4th National Harm Reduction Conference, Seattle, WA.

Savin-Williams, R. C., & Berndt, T. J. (1990). Friendship and peer relations. In S. S. Feldman, & G. R. Elliott (Eds.), *At the threshold: The developing adolescent.* Cambridge, MA: Harvard University Press.

Scavuzzo, M. (1996). *Harm reduction: a work in progress.* Minneapolis, MN: Safe Works AIDS Project.

Segal, B., Cromer, F., Hobfoll, S. (1982). Reasons for alcohol use by detained and adjudicated juveniles. *Journal of Alcohol & Drug Education, 28,* 53-58.

Shedler, J., & Block, J. (1990). Adolescent drug use and psychological health: A longitudinal inquiry. *American Psychologist, 45,* 612-630.

Sisk, J., Hatziandreu, E., & Hughes, R. (1990). *The effectiveness of drug abuse treatment: Implications for controlling AIDS/HIV infections.* Washington, DC: Office of Technology Assessment, Congress of the United States, Background Paper, 6.

Springer, E. (1991). Effective AIDS prevention with active drug users: The Harm Reduction model. *Journal of Chemical Dependency Treatment, 4,* 141-157.

Steinberg, J. A., & Silverman, M. M. (1987. Preventing mental disorders: A research perspective (DHHS Pub. No. ADM 87-1492). Washington, DC: U.S. Government Printing Office.

Substance Abuse and Mental Health Services Administration (SAMHSA). (2003). Science-Based Prevention Programs and Principles: Effective Substance abuse and mental health programs for every community (USDHHS publication number SMA 03-3764). Washington, DC: U.S. Government Printing Office.

Tobler, N. S. (1986). Meta-analysis of 143 adolescent drug prevention programs: Quantitative outcome results of program participants compared to a control comparison group. *Journal of Drug Issues, 4,* 537-567.

Tobler, N. S. (1989, October). *Drug prevention programs can work: Research findings*. Paper presented at the meeting of on "What Works: An International Perspective on Drug Abuse Treatment and Prevention Research," New York.

Tolan, P. H., Guerra, N. G., & Kendall, P. C. (1995). A developmental-ecological perspective on antisocial behavior in children and adolescents: Toward a unified risk and intervention framework. *Journal of Consulting & Clinical Psychology, 63,* 579-584.

United Nations International Drug Cntrol Programme. (1997). *World drug report.* New York: Oxford University Press.

United States Department of Education. (1999). *Safe and drug-free schools and communities act of 1994: Project overview.* Washington, DC: Author.

Vail, K.V., & Stokes, S. (1999, October). *Needle exchange and non-abstinence based drug treatment.* Paper Presented at the Northeast-Midwest Regional Conference on Heroin and Other Opiate Treatment, Best Practices and Futuristic Models for the New Millennium, Cleveland, Ohio.

van Laar, M., de Zwart, W., & Menisk, C. (1996). *Netherlands alcohol and drug report (4): Addiction care and assistance.* Utrecht: Trimbos Institute.

Vlahov, D., Junge, B., Brookmeyer, R., Cohn, S., Riley, E., Armenian, H., Beilenson, P. (1997). Reductions in high-risk drug use behaviors among participants in the Baltimore needle exchange program. *Journal of Acquired Immune Deficiency Syndrome, 16,* 400-406.

Watter, J. Estilo, M., Clark, G., & Lorvick, J. (1994). Syringe and needle exchange as HIV/AIDS prevention for injection drug users. *Journal of the American Medical Association, 271,* 115-120.

Wenger, L., & Rosenbaum, M. (1994). Drug treatment on demand-not. *Journal of Psychoactive Drugs, 26,* 1-11.

Zimring, F., & Hawkins, G. (1992). *The search for rational drug control.* New York: Cambridge University Press.

Detecting Serious Mental Illness Among Substance Abusers: Use of the K6 Screening Scale

James A. Swartz, PhD
Arthur J. Lurigio, PhD

SUMMARY. Serious mental illnesses (SMIs) commonly co-occur with substance-use disorders and, if undetected and untreated, adversely affect their clinical course. This paper describes the use and scoring of the K6 scale, a brief and valid screening tool for SMI, in a large general population sample derived from the 2001 National Household Survey on Drug Abuse (NHSDA). Analyses examine the demographic characteris-

James A. Swartz is affiliated with the Jane Addams College of Social Work, University of Illinois at Chicago.

Arthur J. Lurigio is affiliated with the Department of Criminal Justice, Loyola University of Chicago.

Address correspondence to: James A. Swartz, PhD, Jane Addams College of Social Work, University of Illinois at Chicago, 1040 West Harrison Street (M/C 309), Chicago, IL 60607 (E-mail: jaswartz@uic.edu).

The authors gratefully acknowledge support for this research from the Robert Wood Johnson Foundation's Substance Abuse Policy Research Program under grant 049629 and from the National Institute on Drug Abuse under grant R01 DA013943-02.

[Haworth co-indexing entry note]: "Detecting Serious Mental Illness Among Substance Abusers: Use of the K6 Screening Scale." Swartz, James A., and Arthur J. Lurigio. Co-published simultaneously in *Journal of Evidence-Based Social Work* (The Haworth Social Work Practice Press, an imprint of The Haworth Press, Inc.) Vol. 2, No. 1/2, 2005, pp. 113-135; and: *Addiction, Assessment, and Treatment with Adolescents, Adults, and Families* (ed: Carolyn Hilarski) The Haworth Social Work Practice Press, an imprint of The Haworth Press, Inc., 2005, pp. 113-135. Single or multiple copies of this article are available for a fee from The Haworth Document Delivery Service [1-800-HAWORTH, 9:00 a.m. - 5:00 p.m. (EST). E-mail address: docdelivery haworthpress.com].

tics and patterns of substance use disorders among persons with and without a co-occurring SMI. *[Article copies available for a fee from The Haworth Document Delivery Service: 1-800-HAWORTH. E-mail address: <docdelivery@haworthpress.com> Website: <http://www.HaworthPress.com> © 2005 by The Haworth Press, Inc. All rights reserved.]*

KEYWORDS. Mental illness, substance abuse, assessment, MICA

Data from the Epidemiological Catchment Area Study (ECA) and the National Comorbidity Survey (NCS) show that individuals with substance use disorders have very high rates of co-occurring psychiatric disorders and vice versa (Kessler et al., 1994; Kessler & Walters, 2002; Regier et al., 1990). Although the comorbidity rates for serious mental illnesses (SMI) are high among non-institutionalized, drug-dependent individuals, they are even higher among individuals in drug or psychiatric treatment programs. For example, one study found that 226 of 420 patients in psychiatric and drug treatment programs (54%) met DSM-IV (American Psychiatric Association, 2002) diagnostic criteria for a past-year, co-occurring disorder (Havassy, Alvidrez, & Owen, 2004). These and findings from other studies suggest that persons afflicted with only one kind of disorder (either a psychiatric or substance use disorder) are the exception in treatment settings (Substance Abuse and Mental Health Services Administration [SAMHSA], 2002).

Clients with co-occurring disorders are challenging to the drug and mental health treatment systems because of their prevalence in both systems and the complex symtomatology they present to treatment providers. Effective treatment for this heterogeneous population requires addressing numerous issues. In comparison to single-disorder clients, those with co-occurring disorders have higher rates of recidivism, criminal involvement, suicide, and homelessness, more frequent psychiatric hospitalizations, and lower rates of treatment and medication adherence. They are also more costly to the health care system (Dickey, Normand, Weiss, Drake, & Azeni, 2002; Lacro, Dunn, Dolder, Leckband, & Jeste, 2002; Mueser, Drake, & Wallach, 1998; Ries & Comtois, 1997; SAMSHA, 2002; Soyka, 2000). Several studies have found that individuals with co-occurring disorders can be especially prone to violent behavior when off medication (e.g., Arseneault, Moffitt, Caspi, Taylor, & Silva, 2000; Swartz et al., 1998). Additionally, such individuals tend to exercise poor judgment and participate in risky behaviors such as, unprotected sexual intercourse and needle sharing. As a result, they are at increased risk relative to the general population for HIV-infection and other sexually transmitted infections such as, gonorrhea and syphilis, and for medical conditions related to injection drug use such as, endocarditis and Hepatitis C (Cournos & McKinnon, 1997; Kalichman, Kelly, Johnson, & Bulto, 1994).

The prevalence, severity, and complexity of co-occurring disorders underscore the need for comprehensive and fully integrated treatment services for such conditions. However, because comprehensive treatment means that services must span what have historically been two parallel but disparate systems of care, considerable challenges exist to reshaping the existing mental health and substance abuse treatment systems as well as the administrative and funding structures that support them (Drake et al., 2001).

Closely related to the need for integrated systems of care is the need to conduct comprehensive screenings and assessments for detecting the presence of co-occurring disorders. Valid diagnostic data are especially critical for social workers, who often are the gatekeepers for treatment referral and entry. Stiffman and her colleagues (Stiffman et al., 2001) have found that the gatekeeper's knowledge and endorsement of services explains a large portion of the variation in accessing care. In many instances, the gatekeepers for treatment services work outside drug or psychiatric treatment settings, including schools, private offices, primary health care clinics, or in managed care organizations. In such settings, time constraints are common, and it is impossible or undesirable to administer lengthy and complex instruments (e.g., the Diagnostic Interview Schedule [DIS]: Robins, Helzer, Croughan, & Ratcliff, 1981; the Structured Clinical Interview for DSM-IV [SCID]: First, Spitzer, Gibbon, & Williams, 1997) to render psychiatric diagnoses. Nonetheless, it is also undesirable to rely solely on clinical judgment. Abundant research has shown that diagnosis made on the basis of clinical judgment alone is subject to bias and less likely to adhere to the use of established diagnostic criteria (e.g., Wood, Garb, Lilienfeld, & Nezworski, 2002). An optimal assessment strategy would involve short and easy-to-administer-screening tools that are diagnostically valid and provide data to inform and complement a clinical interview.

Although several relatively brief and easy-to-administer screening tools have been developed for substance-use disorders (e.g., the CAGE, MAST, and DAST), few comparably brief instruments have been developed to screen for psychiatric disorders. Brief screening tools for psychiatric disorders are complicated to construct simply because the number of DSM-IV Axis I non-substance-use disorders far exceeds the number of substance-use disorders. Thus, whereas it is feasible to briefly screen for all substances or simply for any substance abuse or dependence disorder, it is not feasible to screen for every Axis I psychiatric disorder. Moreover, even if it were possible to screen for every DSM-IV Axis I disorder, not everyone with a co-occurring psychiatric disorder needs treatment for the disorder. Clinical severity and treatment lie on a gradient; even some persons with severe psychiatric disorders are able to function adequately without clinical intervention (Regier et al., 1998). Hence, the diagnostic challenge is to determine which psychiatric disorders require screening and to define when a disorder is severe enough to warrant clinical intervention or further assessment. In the next section, we compare the relative merits of different brief instruments for SMI that are severe enough to warrant clinical intervention.

Candidate Screening Instruments

Two different approaches have been taken to make screening for psychiatric disorders more manageable and accurate. One approach determines if an individual meets the diagnostic criteria for a limited number of diagnoses by focusing on those more likely to be clinically severe and to require treatment or other interventions. The restricted subset of all DSM-IV diagnoses usually includes those defined as SMI (see Johnson, 1997): disorders of the schizophrenic spectrum (i.e., schizophrenia, schizoaffective disorder, and schizophreniform disorder), bipolar disorder, and major depressive disorder. Tools that adopt a diagnostic approach to screening include the Composite International Diagnostic Interview-Short Form (CIDI-SF; Kessler, Andrews, Mroczek, Üstün, & Wittchen., 1998); the Mini-Neuropsychiatric Interview (MINI; Sheehan et al., 1998); and the Referral Decision Scale (RDS; Teplin and Swartz, 1989).

The MINI, the CIDI-SF and, to a lesser extent, the RDS are modular. Each module consists of a self-contained sequence of questions for diagnosing a specific disorder or class of disorders. This modularity resembles the structure of longer assessment instruments for psychiatric diagnosis such as, the DIS (Robins et al., 1981) and the newer Composite International Diagnostic Interview (CIDI; Robins et al., 1988), from which the MINI and cognate tools were derived. For example, one module of the MINI screens for psychotic disorders while another screens for bipolar disorders. Administration time can be shortened by omitting modules that screen for disorders that are of no current interest to researchers or clinicians. Despite this administrative flexibility, there are problems with all of these instruments specifically and with this class of instruments generally that limit their usefulness.

The diagnostic approach to screening equates diagnosis with illness severity and need for clinical intervention. Only those persons who are deemed to have one or more of the screened-for diagnoses are referred for further assessment and treatment. The potential drawback is that the approach misses individuals who have a severe manifestation of a disorder that is not included in the screening (e.g., post-traumatic stress disorder, generalized anxiety disorder) and who might require clinical intervention (i.e., false negatives). The converse is also true; as we already noted, not everyone meeting the criteria for a DSM-IV psychiatric diagnosis requires treatment for that disorder (Regier et al., 1998). Moreover, despite the administrative flexibility of selecting diagnoses for specific screening purposes, the necessity of obtaining valid DSM-IV diagnoses adds a level of complexity to the instruments that involves skip patterns and probes that can make these instruments complex to administer, especially for lay interviewers.

The problems related to screening for psychiatric disorders using a diagnostic approach has recently led to a second approach that de-emphasizes diagnosis and focuses on symptom severity and level of impairment (Kessler et al., 2002). Although it is based on a notion of what constitutes a psychiatric illness that is not new (see Murphy, 2002), this approach has gained more currency of late because large-scale epidemiological surveys have found surprisingly high prevalence rates of psychiatric disorders, with 20 to 30 percent of the general population meeting DSM criteria for at least one past-year Axis I disorder (Regier et al., 1990; Kessler et al., 1994). It is unlikely that such a large proportion of the general population requires mental health treatment services. Thus, the findings of these surveys have limited utility for guiding federal and state treatment resource allocation. This conclusion focused attention on screening for the symptom severity and level of functional impairment given the presence of a DSM-IV Axis I diagnosis as a better way of discriminating the need for psychiatric treatment (see Regier et al., 1998; Slade & Andrews, 2002). Examples of screening tools that adopt a symptom severity approach includes the section of the Addiction Severity Index that screens for psychological problems (ASI; McLellan et al., 1992); the Brief Psychiatric Rating Scale (BPRS; Overall & Gorham, 1962); the Symptom Checklist 90 (SCL-90; Derogatis, Lipman, & Covi, 1973); and the recently developed K6/K10 scales (Kessler et al., 2002).

Among this class of scales, the K6/K10 scales appear to be the best candidate instruments for clinical practice, particularly in settings outside of psychiatric and substance abuse treatment programs. The guiding framework for creation of the K6/K10 was the theoretical and research-derived observation that persons with diverse psychiatric disorders manifest a common set of symptoms indicative of non-specific distress (Dohrenwend, Shrout, Ergi, & Mendelsohn, 1980; Kessler et al., 2002). The original goal for developing the K6/K10 scales was to include one of them in general population surveys such as, the National Survey on Drug Use and Health (NSDUH; formerly the National Household Survey on Drug Abuse [NHSDA]). These tools help states comply with the provisions of Public Law 102-321, which establishes the federal requirements for states to generate estimates of serious mental illness and to qualify for and set the amounts of block grant funding (Kessler et al., 2003). Beginning with a pool of 612 items derived from 18 existing psychological screening scales (e.g., the Beck Depression Inventory, Symptom Checklist-90), Kessler and his colleagues (Kessler et al., 2002) used analytic procedures derived from item response theory to distill a subset of 10 questions (the K10) and a completely overlapping subset of 6 questions (the K6) that identified with maximum sensitivity, individuals meeting the following two criteria: A past-year diagnosis of any DSM-IV Axis I psychiatric disorder and a Global Assessment of Functioning (GAF) score below 60 (i.e., moderate to severe impairment in psychological symptoms and functioning; see American Psychiatric Association [APA], 2002). These particular criteria were selected because they comported with the criteria used by the U.S. Substance Abuse and Mental Health Services Administration (SAMHSA) in their block grant formula for funding public mental health services to the states (see Kessler et al., 2003).

The calibration of the K6/K10 scales cut-scores was done to identify individuals above the 90th percentile in symptom severity, which is consistent with estimates that 6 percent to 10 percent of the general population need psychiatric treatment services at any given time (Kessler et al., 2002). In further validation studies, the K6/K10 scales were found to perform as well as longer screening instruments such as, the World Health Organization Disability Assessment Schedule (WHO-DAS; Rehm et al., 1999) and the CIDI-SF in identifying individuals with SMI, with the two scales performing about equally well in the U.S. and Australian general populations (Furukawa, Kessler, Slade, & Andrews, 2002; Kessler et al., 2003). Because of the near equivalent performance of the K6 and the K10, the shorter K6 was added to the NHSDA and U.S. National Health Interview Survey (NHIS) questionnaires to yield estimates of the need for psychiatric treatment in the general population. Kessler et al. (2003) noted, however, that the K10 might be more sensitive than the K6 in populations in which a larger proportion of those assessed has clinically significant emotional distress, which would likely be the case among persons admitted to drug treatment programs. Both scales are available in interviewer-administered and self-administered formats on the Internet at: http://www.hcp.med.harvard.edu/ncs/K6-K10/index.html. (The scales are available in English and German versions with versions in other languages to follow.)

In summary, the need to provide better screening for mental illness among individuals with substance-use disorders is well established given the high prevalence of psychiatric problems in this population and the complicated clinical courses among individuals with co-occurring disorders. Among the currently available screening instruments, the K6/K10 scales are excellent instruments, owing to their solid grounding in item response theory, their brevity, their ease of administration, and their established validity in large national and international general population studies. Given their continued use in general population surveys, an additional benefit of using the K6 or K10 in treatment settings is, as Kessler et al. (2003) argued, "to provide a crosswalk between community epidemiological research and clinical research by allowing a comparison of the severity distribution of non-specific distress among community vs. clinical cases" (p. 189). In the analyses that follow, we examine the 2001 NHSDA results using K6 items to calculate the rates of co-occurring substance use and psychiatric disorders and to compare the characteristics of participants with and without co-occurring psychiatric and substance-use disorders.

METHODS

Overview

The data analyzed for this study were derived from the 2001 NHSDA public-use data set. Additional details on the 2001 NHSDA sampling design, protocol, questionnaire, and construction of the public-use data set as well as the data set and codebook are available from the U.S. Department of Health and Human Services [DHHS], Substance Abuse and Mental Health Services Office Administration [SAMHSA], Office of Applied Studies [OAS] and the Inter-University Consortium for Political and Social Research at the University of Michigan [ICPSR] (DHHS, 2003). Conducted annually since 1991, the primary purpose of the NHSDA is to assess the levels of substance use, abuse, and dependence among non-institutionalized residents of the United States, 12 years of age and older. The NHSDA survey uses a multi-stage area probability sampling design with stratification and clustering to select participants. The sampling frame includes residents of non-institutional settings such as college dormitories, group homes, and military installations, but excludes residents in institutional settings such as prisons, jails, and hospitals. In 2001, to improve the validity of the self-reported information, the NHSDA survey questionnaire was self-administered by participants using audio computer-assisted interviewing (ACAI) software. The overall response rate for the 2001 NHSDA survey was 73 percent (DHHS, 2003).

Construction of the final 2001 NHSDA public-use data set included logical editing to correct for inconsistent responses and imputation of missing values that stem from errors or non-responses (DHHS, 2003). In all instances for the variables used in this study, imputed and revised values were necessary for only a small proportion (less than 2%) of cases. When available, we used the imputed, revised versions of the demographic (e.g., marital status) and substance use variables (e.g., age of first use) for our analytic models.

Participants

Juvenile participants are not assessed for SMI using the K6 questions; hence, we excluded them from the analyses. Our sample consisted of 38,132 adults, 18 years of age and older, who completed the 2001 NHSDA survey. Because our focus was on screening for co-occurring disorders, we further selected 7,089 adult participants (19% of the total unweighted sample) who, according to their K6 scores and their responses to the DSM-IV substance-use disorder questions, either had a past-year SMI warranting clinical intervention (2,590; 6.8% of the total unweighted sample), had abused or were dependent on alcohol or other drugs in the past year (3,519; 9.2%), or had a co-occurring past-year SMI and substance-use disorder (982; 2.6%). Depending on the analyses, we used different combinations of these three groups to compare participants on selected characteristics.

Measures

Co-occurring disorders. Co-occurring disorders were calculated based on the variables that measured SMI and any past-year substance abuse and dependence. The K6 items embedded in the mental health section of the 2001 NHSDA questionnaire were used to measure SMI. Participants respond to the K6 items by indicating the extent to which they experienced each of 6 symptoms of general psychological distress in the month they felt the most anxious, depressed or nervous in the preceding year. Item scores are based on 5-point Likert-type scales that range from 0 ("none of the time") to 4 ("all of the time"), yielding summary scores that range from 0 to 24. To calculate the presence of an SMI, we used a score of 13 or above, which general population studies have established as an optimal cut-point (Kessler et al., 2003).

Substance abuse and dependence were measured by questions from the section of the 2001 NHSDA questionnaire that assesses symptoms associated with drug use, and which are consistent with DSM-IV substance-use disorder criteria (APA, 2002). Responses to the sequence of questions for each substance are summarized by variables that represent past-year abuse or dependence on alcohol and on other substances that include: marijuana, cocaine, heroin, stimulants, analgesics, hallucinogens, inhalants, sedatives, and tranquilizers. Participants were assessed as abusing or dependent on a substance if they met the DSM-IV criteria for any of these drugs.

Past-year treatment history. Receipt of substance abuse and mental health treatment services in the past year was assessed through a series of questions that are specific to treatment modalities (e.g., outpatient mental health treatment, participation in AA or other self-help groups for substance use). To assess past-year treatment history of respondents, we used the variables that summarize mental health and substance use treatment across modality (e.g., any mental health treatment) as well as perceived need for treatment.

Demographic characteristics. Our multivariate statistical models included a number of demographic variables as covariates. These variables are associated with SMI and drug dependence in the research and clinical literature (e.g., Mueser, Noordsy, Drake, & Fox, 2003) and include: gender, ethnicity, age group, educational level, employment status, marital status, and the population density of the metropolitan statistical area (MSA) where the respondent resided at the time of the interview. These variables were extracted from the demographics section of the NHSDA questionnaire.

Analyses

We conducted all analyses using the survey analytic procedures included with Stata SE statistical software (Stata Corporation, 2003), which allowed us to incorporate variables representing sample weight, strata, and cluster into the bivariate and multivariate statistical models. We used these variables to estimate standard errors and variances corrected for design effects that stem from the multi-stage sampling design of the 2001 NHSDA survey. We also calculated a normalized, adjusted sample weight. The normalized sample weight was simply a linear transformation of the sample weight that maintained the observed sample size while reflecting the influence of the weight (i.e., selection probability). The normalized, adjusted weight yielded the same estimates as the sample weight without adjustment and did not inflate the sample size: Hence, we conducted all statistical tests using the normalized weight variable. To reduce the possibility of an inflated Type I error attributable to running multiple statistical tests, we adopted a more conservative alpha level of $p < .01$ instead of the conventional $p < .05$ for assessing the statistical significance of our results (Tabachnick & Fidell, 2001).

We first ran bivariate analyses to compare participants with and without a substance-use disorder on their responses to the K6 items and to the overall scale to determine if participants with substance use disorders had different response profiles on the K6 compared with persons who had no substance-use disorders. We conducted bivariate analyses to compare participants on demographic and drug use characteristics based on their co-occurring disorder status (i.e., none, SMI only, substance abuse or dependence only, co-occurring disorders). Finally, we conducted multivariate analyses using binary logistic regression models of the association between SMI and substance abuse and dependence for the most commonly used substances: alcohol, marijuana, cocaine, heroin, and analgesics. These models controlled for differences in participant demographic characteristics and examined the likelihood that participants with an SMI would report a substance-use disorder. The dependent measure in each model was substance abuse or dependence for one of the 5 most commonly used substances compared with no substance abuse or dependence.

RESULTS

Table 1 shows the K6 item results for the NHSDA adult participants by substance disorder status. The column percentages show the proportion of participants who had experienced a symptom all of the time or most of the time in their worst month of the previous year. Participants with a past-year substance use disorder, either abuse or dependence, consistently reported experiencing the symptoms of psychological distress assessed by the K6 to a greater degree than participants without a substance use disorder, with all item differences statistically significant at the p < .001 level. These findings support Kessler et al.'s (2002) conclusion that the final items selected for inclusion in the K6 all demonstrated high diagnostic sensitivity. After summing the K6 items and applying the criterion of a cut-score of 13 or higher as indicating a clinically significant SMI, more than 7% of the sample met this criterion. Participants with a past-year substance-use disorder were over three times as likely to have a past year SMI (21%) compared with participants without an SMI (6%), a difference that was also statistically significant at the p < .001 level. In terms of co-occurring disorders then, about one-fifth of the participants in this general population sample with a substance-use disorder also had a past-year co-occurring SMI.

TABLE 1. K6 Results by Past-Year Substance Abuse/Dependence Status: Percentage of Participants Reporting Symptoms All or Most of the Time

K6 Item	Any Substance Abuse or Dependence in the Past Year			
	No Abuse or Dependence	Abuse or Dependence	All Participants	
(1) Nervousness	5.3%	17.7%	6.2%	***
(2) Hopelessness	5.3	17.7	6.2	***
(3) Restless or fidgety	5.1	16.0	5.9	***
(4) So depressed nothing could cheer up	4.7	14.6	5.4	***
(5) Everything was an effort	7.7	19.6	8.6	***
(6) Worthlessness	5.5	17.6	6.4	***
Serious Mental Illness (K6 Total > = 13)	6.3	21.0	7.4	***
Mean K6 Score (0 - 24 possible)	3.7	7.4	4.0	***

Note. All figures are based on the weighted Ns and unless otherwise indicated, are percentages. The unweighted N for those with no substance abuse or dependence in the past year was 33,631 (88.2%) and was 4,501 (11.8%) for those abusing or dependent on any substance, including alcohol, in the past year. Percentage comparisons are based on a Rao-Scott conversion of the Chi-square statistic and were estimated using weighted data and variables for clustering and stratification. The mean comparison of the K6 total score is based on a t-test that assumes unequal variances.
***p < .001

Comparisons on demographic characteristics among the subsample of participants who met the criteria for SMI (N = 3,519), a substance-use disorder (N = 2,590), or co-occurring disorders (N = 982) are shown in Table 2. All statistical comparisons of participants in these three groups, except for ethnicity, were statistically significant at the p < .001 level. Participants with SMI only were much more likely to be female (67%) than participants with a past-year substance-use disorder only (28%) and those with a co-occurring disorder (48%). The profile of participants with SMI only, compared with other participants, is that they tended to be older, married, to be out of the labor force, to live in a smaller metropolitan statistical area (MSA) or not in an MSA at all, and to have a lower chance of having been arrested in the past year. On most characteristics, except gender, participants with co-occurring disorders were more similar to participants with a substance-use disorder "only" than they were to participants with SMI only. Participants with co-occurring disorders tended to be younger, single, more likely to be unemployed or employed part-time (though close to 50% reported being employed) and to have a much greater chance of having been arrested in the past year, possibly attributable to their substance use. Nearly twice as many participants with a past-year substance-use disorder or a co-occurring disorder reported an arrest in the preceding year compared with participants with SMI only.

Patterns of substance use and of mental health and substance use treatment among these same three groups of participants are presented in Table 3. In the first set of comparisons, proportions of participants reporting having ever used a particular substance, those with a past-year substance-use disorder or a co-occurring disorder were more likely to report using most of the substances listed, compared with participants with SMI only. In particular, a greater percentage of those with a substance use or co-occurring disorder reported ever using cocaine, crack, hallucinogens, tranquilizers, and analgesics. Chi-square tests of these differences were all statistically significant at the $p < .01$ or $p < .001$. Restricting the comparisons further to those with a substance use disorder, the data shown in Table 3 also reveal a pattern in which higher proportions of those with a co-occurring SMI reported having ever used a drug, compared with those without a co-occurring SMI. Statistical comparisons of the drug use reported by these two groups of participants (not shown in Table 3) yielded the following significant differences: cocaine ($F(1, 45) = 6.71$, $p < .01$), crack ($F(1, 45) = 8.93$, $p < .01$), hallucinogens ($F(1, 45) = 13.00$, $p < .001$), tranquilizers ($F(1, 45) = 27.69$, $p < $

TABLE 2. Demographics by Co-Occuring Disorder Status[a,b,c,d,e]

	Serious Mental Illness Only (N = 3,519)	Substance Use Disorder Only (N = 2,590)	Co-Occuring Disorders (N = 982)	Sig.
Gender				
Female	67.0%	28.1%	48.6%	***
Ethnicity				
White	75.2	73.9	74.8	
African-American/Black	11.1	9.2	13.0	
Hispanic	8.8	12.7	8.5	
Other	4.9	4.2	3.7	
Age Group				
18-25	19.3	36.4	39.8	***
26-34	18.7	20.5	22.9	
35+	62.0	43.0	37.3	
Marital Status				
Single (Never Married)	29.1	51.3	51.0	***
Divorced	25.3	15.8	18.5	
Married	45.7	32.9	30.5	
Education (Highest Grade)				
Less than High School	21.1	16.0	24.2	***
High School Graduate/GED	34.5	31.9	35.5	
Some College	27.2	29.1	24.9	
College Graduate	17.2	23.1	15.5	
Employment Status				
Full Trime	45.9	64.7	49.8	
Part Time	13.9	14.7	18.2	
Unemployed	3.8	4.8	8.8	
(Other, including not in labor force)	36.5	15.8	23.3	
Population Density				
MSA > 1 Million	38.6	46.2	42.9	***
MSA < 1 Million	37.2	34.4	35.3	
Not in MSA	24.3	19.5	21.8	
Arrested Past Year	20.7	42.4	40.0	***

Note. N's shown are based on the unweighted data from 2001 NHSDA participants ages 18 and older. Tests of significance are based on modified Pearsons chi-square converted to an F statistic using a second order Rao and Scott correction. Column percentages may not add to 100 due to rounding.

$**p < .01, ***p < .001$.

TABLE 3. Substance Use and Treatment History by Co-Occurring Disorder Status

	Serious Mental Illness Only	Substance Use Disorder Only	Co-Occuring Disorders	Sig.
	(N = 3,519)	(N = 2,590)	(N = 982)	
Ever Used[a]				
Alcohol	86.9%	99.3%	98.8%	
Marijuana	51.4	77.5	83.7	
Cocaine	20.2	42.0	49.6	**
Crack	5.0	13.6	20.6	**
Heroin	2.8	6.8	10.5	
Hallucinogens	19.6	43.8	54.4	***
Inhalents	12.2	29.8	32.9	
Tranquilizers	11.4	22.0	36.0	***
Sedatives	6.9	11.3	16.4	
Stimulants	13.6	23.4	34.0	***
Analgesics[d]	15.8	33.4	51.5	***
Any illicit drug execept marijuana	40.0	66.5	78.6	***
Past Year Abuse or Dependence[b]				
Alcohol	-	84.3	78.2	
Marijuana	-	16.3	25.0	***
Cocaine	-	5.7	9.2	
Heroin	-	4.5	7.7	
Hallucinogens	-	1.5	4.9	***
Inhalants	-	0.3	1.1	
Tranquilizers	-	1.0	2.6	***
Sedatives	-	.2	2.3	**
Stimulants	-	1.3	3.5	***
Analgesics[d]	-	4.0	11.5	***
Past-Year Mental Health Treatment[c]				
Inpatient	4.5	-	9.4	**
Outpatient	31.3	-	26.9	
Prescribed medication	39.8	-	38.2	
Any treatment received	46.8	-	45.3	
Needed treatment but did not receive	29.2	-	38.9	***

	Serious Mental Illness Only	Substance Use Disorder Only	Co-Occuring Disorders	
	(N = 3,519)	(N = 2,590)	(N = 982)	Sig.
Past-Year Substance Use Treatment[b]				
Alcohol Use	-	7.8	13.3	**
Drug Use	-	5.6	9.5	
Any treatment received	-	10.6	17.4	***

Note. N's shown are based on the unweighted data from 2001 NHSDA participants ages 18 and older. Tests of significance are based on modified Pearsons chi-square converted to an F statistic using a second order Rao and Scott correction. Column percentages may not add to 100 due to rounding.

[a] Statistical comparisons are for all three groups of particpants.

[b] Statistical comparisons are between participants with a past-year substance use disorder with co-occuring disorders only.

[c] Statistical comparisons are between participants with an SMI and with co-occuring disorders only.

[d] Analgesics includes illegal use of non-prescription pain relievers such as Darvon, Darvocet, Percodan, Vicodin, and Tylenol with Codeine and excludes non-prescription drugs such as aspirin and Tylenol.

**p < .01, ***p < .001.

.001), stimulants (F(1, 45) = 15.96; p < .001), and analgesics (F(1, 45) = 40.11; p < .001).

The second group of comparisons on type of drug, shown in Table 3, were also restricted to participants with a substance use disorder because, by definition, those with an SMI only did not meet the criteria for abuse or dependence on any substance. The overall pattern for these comparisons was the same as for ever using a substance; higher proportions of those with a co-occurring disorder reported abuse or dependence on the following drug classes: marijuana, hallucinogens, tranquilizers, sedatives, stimulants, and analgesics. Those with co-occurring disorders were also more likely to report abuse or dependence on a larger number of substances (.96) than those without a co-occurring disorder (.55; t = 8.67, p < .001). In terms of drug use and dependence then, those with a co-occurring SMI and substance-use disorder tend to use and to become dependent on a wider array of substances, compared with those without a co-occurring SMI.

We compared the past year mental health treatment histories of those with co-occurring disorders to those with SMI only. Two comparisons were statistically significant: those with co-occurring disorders were more likely to report inpatient mental health treatment in the past year

(9% compared with 4%; $F(1, 3,562) = 10.59$, $p < .001$) and more likely to report needing but not receiving mental health treatment in the past year (39% compared with 23%; $F(1, 3,562) = 31.11$, $p < .001$). Similarly, comparisons of those with and without a co-occurring SMI on past year treatment for substance use showed that those with a co-occurring disorder were more likely to report treatment for an alcohol use disorder (14% compared with 8%; $F(1, 4,500) = 8.93$, $p < .01$) and any past-year substance use disorder (17% compared with 11%; $F(1, 4,500) = 11.86$, $p < .001$).

In the final set of analyses, we examined the relationship between SMI and substance abuse and dependence disorders using binary logistic regression models. The results of these analyses are shown in Table 4. In the logistic regression models, past-year substance abuse or dependence for each of the 5 most commonly used substances was the dependent variable. We coded past-year abuse or dependence as 1 and no past-year use or dependence as 0. Hence, odds ratios larger than 1 signify model predicators associated with an increased chance of abusing or being dependent on a substance while odds ratios lower than 1 signify a decreased chance of abuse or dependence. Predictors in the models included all of the demographic variables shown in Table 2 as well as a variable representing past-year SMI based on the K6. Both the omnibus F-tests of all 5 models as well as the predictor representing SMI were statistically significant. In each case, having a past-year SMI was associated with an increase in the odds of having a past-year substance use disorder. Controlling for the demographic characteristics in the models, the magnitudes of these relationships were substantial, ranging from those with an SMI being more than 3 times as likely to report abuse or dependence on alcohol to 8 times more likely to report abuse or dependence on analgesics.

DISCUSSION

We believe the findings from this study demonstrate the importance of screening for SMI among substance users. Using the K6 as the screening tool for SMI, we found that 21% of those with a substance use disorder had a co-occurring SMI that likely warrants clinical attention. Conversely, (although not reported in the analyses section) we also found that 27% of those with an SMI had a co-occurring substance-use disorder. These results indicate that in a general population sample, at least one-fifth of those with a substance use disorder require treatment

TABLE 4. Binary Logistic Regression Models of Substance Use and Serious Mental Illness

	Alcohol		Marijuana		Cocaine		Heroin		Analgesics	
	OR	(SE)	OR	(SE)	OR	(SE)	OR	(SE)	OR	(SE)
Model: Abuse of Dependence compared to No Abuse or Dependance										
Gender (reference category = Males)										
Females	0.37	(.02)***	0.36	(.04)***	0.38	(.07)***	0.42	(.09)***	0.66	(1.4)
Ethnicity (reference category = Whites)										
African-American	0.69	(.07)***	0.85	(.12)	1.34	(.38)	1.49	(.47)	0.24	(.11)
Hispanic	0.92	(.09)	0.71	(.14)	1.33	(.49)	1.39	(.58)	1.03	(.34)
Other	0.57	(0.7)***	0.71	(.20)	0.81	(.53)	0.88	(.68)	1.34	(.97)
Age Group (reference category = 18-25)										
26-35 years-old	0.70	(.05)***	0.49	(.08)***	1.89	(.54)	2.29	(.75)	0.91	(.21)
36+ years	0.37	(.03)***	0.20	(.04)***	1.13	(.34)	1.61	(.53)	0.58	(.18)
Marital Status (reference category = single)										
Divorced, separated	0.86	(.09)	0.76	(.20)	0.54	(.18)	0.48	(.18)	0.71	(.27)
Married	0.43	(.03)***	0.28	(.06)***	0.29	(.10)***	0.25	(.10)***	0.65	(.20)
Education Level (reference category = < high school)										
High School/GED	0.91	(.08)	0.79	(.12)	1.03	(.26)	1.28	(.38)	0.62	(.16)
Some College	1.11	(.16)	0.51	(.08)***	0.53	(.15)	0.67	(.22)	0.51	(.16)
College Graduate	1.07	(.06)	0.31	(.07)***	0.15	(.06)***	0.16	(.08)***	0.34	(.13)**
Employment Status (reference category = full time)										
Part time	0.96	(.08)	1.18	(.16)	1.23	(.36)	1.30	(.41)	1.53	(.52)
Unemployed	1.18	(.16)	1.84	(.38)**	2.58	(.89)**	2.06	(.89)	1.51	(.26)
(Other, including not in labor force)	0.66	(.06)***	0.75	(.12)	1.04	(.26)	0.87	(.24)	0.84	(.24)
Population Density (reference category = MSA > 1 Million)										
MSA < 1 Million	0.99	(.07)	0.95	(.12)	0.63	(.15)	0.52	(.13)**	0.96	(.24)
Not in MSA	0.91	(.07)	0.81	(.11)	0.44	(.13)**	0.41	(.14)	0.97	(.24)
Serious Mental Illness (reference category = no SMI)	3.38	(.18)***	4.03	(.54)***	4.58	(.91)***	5.18	(1.16)***	8.5	(2.05)***
Omnibus F Test of Model Significance	$F_{(17,884)} =$ 79.11***		$F_{(17,884)} =$ 43.08***		$F_{(17,884)} =$ 20.50***		$F_{(17,884)} =$ 17.58***		$F_{(17,884)} =$ 22.78***	

$$**p < .01, ***p < .001$$

Note. Unweighted N for all three models = 38,132. Statatard errors are based on data weighted for sampling probabilities and controlling for design effects due to stratification and clustering. Co-efficient tests of significance are based on t-tests. Omnibus tests of significance are based on modified Pearson chi-squares converted to an F Statistic using a second order Rao and Scott correction.
[a] Analgesics includes illegal use of non-prescription pain relievers such as Darvocet, Percodan, Vicodin, and Tylenol with Codeine and excludes non-prescription drugs such as asprin and Tylenol.

129

for a psychiatric disorder. It is likely that an even higher proportion of those seeking treatment for substance use disorders need concurrent mental health treatment given the greater tendency for those with co-occurring disorders to seek treatment, compared with those without co-occurring disorders (Mueser et al., 1998; Wu, Kouzis, & Leaf, 1999). Despite the greater tendency of those with co-occurring disorders to seek treatment though, we also found that over half, as well as over half of the participants with single disorders, did not receive treatment services in the preceding year. In particular, drug treatment for all participants with substance use disorders appeared to be especially inadequate regardless of the presence of a co-occurring disorder. These findings are consistent with those of other studies, which have shown that the majority of individuals with substance use and psychiatric disorders do not get treatment (Wu et al., 1999).

With respect to the demographic and clinical characteristics of those with co-occurring disorders, our study yielded results that were also consistent with previous research. Demographically, participants with co-occurring disorders were more similar to participants with substance use disorders than they were to participants with SMIs. Participants with co-occurring disorders and substance-use disorders were more likely than participants with SMIs to be male, younger, unmarried, unemployed, and to have a criminal history (Negrete, 2003). Clinically, we found those with co-occurring disorders had more severe substance use than those without a co-occurring disorder as indicated by their tendency to report using and abusing or being dependent on a larger number of substances than those without co-occurring disorders. This finding is consistent with Negrete's (2003) description of the drug-using behavior of schizophrenics as particularly "chaotic, polymorphous, and opportunistic" (p. 17), suggesting the pattern of drug-seeking and drug use is related to the general behavioral disorganization caused by severe psychiatric disorders. Moreover, we also found that those with co-occurring disorders were more likely to report receiving treatment in an inpatient mental health facility and to have needed, but not received, mental health treatment services in the preceding year. These findings support those of other studies in which persons with co-occurring disorders had more severe psychiatric symptoms and often sought out or received psychiatric treatment in more expensive acute care inpatient facilities (Dickey & Azeni, 1996).

Our results support the use of the K6 as a practical screening measure. Although not a validation study per se, we found high consistency among the K6 items in discriminating those with SMI from those without SMI. Moreover, the proportion of participants in the total 2001 NHSDA sample with SMI, as measured by K6 criteria (7%), is consistent with the stated objective of the developers of the K6 to identify approximately the top 10% of the population in terms of symptom severity and need for clinical intervention (Kessler et al., 2002).

It is important to note, however, that when using the K6 in populations in which the base rates of psychiatric disorders and psychological distress are higher than in the general population, such as those seeking drug treatment or criminal justice populations, the K6 will likely identify more than 10% as needing clinical attention. For example, administration of the K6 to a group of adult male arrestees resulted in identification of 17% as having SMI (Swartz & Lurigio, 2004)-not because the K6 generated false positives but simply because the study used a cut-point based on general population samples. We know, however, that higher proportions of criminal justice offenders have SMIs and need psychological treatment (e.g., see Lurigio et al., 2003), which was reflected in their higher K6 scores. In these circumstances, if resources are available, the standard cut-point for the K6 can certainly be used for clinical decisions. However, recalibrating the K6 cut-point to comport with the population on which the tool will be used, is also recommended if identifying the top 10% of the population in terms of symptom severity remains the goal (see Kessler et al., 2002).

The study's primary limitation was its exclusive reliance on self-reported data to determine level of substance use and psychiatric symptoms. Because these behaviors are stigmatized, they are likely to be under-reported (e.g., Harrison, 1997), even with the methodological improvements in the 2001 NHSDA data collection protocols, such as the use of ACAI. Moreover, as we have already noted, because the NHSDA sample is derived from the general population, the prevalence rate of co-occurring substance-use and psychiatric disorders is likely lower than in clinical and institutional populations.

In conclusion, we believe that screening for co-occurring psychiatric disorders among substance abusers will become the norm and that treatment for co-occurring disorders will become more common given the prevalence of such disorders and the poor clinical outcomes that occur when they are undetected and untreated. We suggest that social workers and other clinicians who work with substance abusing populations consider incorporating the K6 scale into their routine assessment protocol. The brevity of administration time-about 2 minutes-means respondent burden is low and is more than offset by the diagnostic information obtained. The availability of the K6 in the public domain and the soon-to-be-available translations of the K6 into other languages mean that it can feasibly be used with a wide variety of populations and in a wide array of clinical settings.

REFERENCES

American Psychiatric Association [APA]. (2002). *Diagnostic and Statistical Manual of Mental Disorders, Text-Revision.* Washington, DC: Author.

Cournos, F., & McKinnon, K. (1997). HIV seroprevalence among people with severe mental illness in the United States: A critical review. *Clinical Psychology Review, 17*(3), 259-269.

Derogatis, L.R., Lipman, R. S., Covi, L. (1973). SCL-90: An outpatient psychiatric rating scale, preliminary report. *Psychopharmacology Bulletin, 9,* 13-28.

Dickey, B., & Azeni, H. (1996). Persons with dual diagnoses of substance abuse and major mental illness: Their excess costs of psychiatric care. *American Journal of Public Health, 86*(7), 973-977.

Dickey, B., Normand, S.-L. T., Weiss, R. D., Drake, R. E., & Azeni, H. (2002). Medical morbidity, mental illness, and substance-use disorders. *Psychiatric Services, 53*(7), 861-867.

Dohrenwend, B. P., Shrout, P. E., Ergi, G. E., & Mendelsohn, F. S. (1980). Measures of non-specific psychological distress and other dimensions of psychopathology in the general population. *Archives of General Psychiatry, 37,* 1229-1236.

Drake, R. E., Essock, S. M., Shaner, A., Carey, K. B., Minkoff, K., Kola, L., et al. (2001). Implementing dual diagnosis services for clients with severe mental illness. *Psychiatric Services, 52*(4), 469-476.

First, M. B., Spitzer, R. L., Gibbon, M., & Williams, J. B. W. (1997). *Structured Clinical Interview for DSM-IV Axis I Disorders, Research Version, Non-patient Edition (SCID-I/NP).* New York: Biometrics Research, New York State Psychiatric Institute.

Furukawa, T. A., Kessler, R. C., Slade, T., & Andrews, G. (2002). The performance of the K6 and K10 screening scales for psychological distress in the Australian national survey of mental health and well-being. *Psychological Medicine, 33,* 357-362.

Harrison, L. H. (1997). The validity of self-reported drug use in survey research: An overview and critique of research methods. In L. Harrison, and A. Hughes (Eds.), *The validity of self-reported drug use: Improving the accuracy of survey estimates* (DHHS Publication No. ADM 97-4147, pp. 17-36). Washington, DC: U.S. Department of Health and Human Services.

Havassy, B. E., Alvidrez, J., & Owen, K. K. (2004). Comparisons of patients with comorbid psychiatric and substance-use disorders: Implications for treatment and service delivery. *American Journal of Psychiatry, 161*(1), 139-145.

Johnson, D. L. (1997). Overview of severe mental illness. *Clinical Psychology Review, 17*(3), 247-257.

Kalichman, S. C., Kelly, J. A., Johnson, J. A., & Bulto, M. (1994). Factors associated with risk for HIV infection among chronic mentally ill adults. *American Journal of Psychiatry, 151*(2), 221-227.

Kessler, R.C., Andrews, G., Colpe, L.J., Hiripi, E., Mroczek, D.K., Normand, S.-L.T., Walters, E.E., & Zaslavsky, A. (2002). Short screening scales to monitor population prevalences and trends in nonspecific psychological distress. *Psychological Medicine. 32*(6), 959-976.

Kessler, R. C., Andrews, G., Mroczek,D., Ustun, T. B., & Wittchen, H. U. (1998). The World Health Organization Composite International Diagnostic Interview Short-Form (CIDI-SF). *International Journal of Methods in Psychiatric Research, 7*, 171-185.

Kessler, R.C., Barker, P.R., Colpe, L.J., Epstein, J.F., Gfroerer, J.C., Hiripi, E., Howes, M.J, Normand, S-L.T., Manderscheid, R.W., Walters, E.E., Zaslavsky, A.M. (2003). Screening for serious mental illness in the general population *Archives of General Psychiatry, 60*(2), 184-189.

Kessler, R. C., McGonagle, K. A., Zhao, S., Nelson, C. B., Hughes, M., Eshleman, S., Wittchen, H. U., & Kendler, K. S. (1994). Lifetime and 12-month prevalence of DSM-III-R psychiatric disorders in the United States: Results from the national comorbidity study. *Archives of General Psychiatry, 51*, 8-19.

Kessler, R. C., & Walters, E. (2002). The national comorbidity survey. In M. T. Tsuang, & M. Tohen (Eds.), *Textbook in psychiatric epidemiology* (2nd ed., pp. 343-362). New York: John Wiley & Sons.

Lacro, J. P., Dunn, L. B., Dolder, C. R., Leckband, S. G., & Jeste, D. V. (2002). Prevalence of and risk factors for medication nonadherence in patients with schizophrenia: A comprehensive review of the literature. *Journal of Clinical Psychiatry, 63*(10), 892-909.

Lurigio, A. J., Cho, Y. I., Swartz, J. A., Johnson, T.P., Graf, I., & Pickup, L. (2003). Standardized assessment of substance-related, other psychiatric, and comorbid disorders among probationers. *International Journal of Offender Therapy & Comparative Criminology, 47*(6), 630-652.

McLellan, A. T., Kushner, H., Metzger, D., Peters, R., Smith, I., Grissom, G., Pettinati, et al. (1992). The fifth edition of the Addiction Severity Index, *Journal of Substance Abuse Treatment, 9*, 199-213.

Mueser, K. T., Noordsy, D. L., Drake, R. E., & Fox, L. (2003). *Integrated treatment for dual disorders.* New York: The Guilford Press.

Mueser, K. T., Drake, R. E., & Wallach, M. A. (1998). Dual diagnosis: A review of etiological theories. *Addictive Behaviors, 23*(6), 717-734.

Murphy, J. M. (2002). Symptom scales and diagnostic schedules in adult psychiatry. In M. T. Tsuang, & M. Tohen (Eds.), *Textbook in psychiatric epidemiology* (2nd ed., pp. 273-332). New York: John Wiley & Sons.

Negrete, J. C. (2003). Clinical aspects of substance abuse in persons with schizophrenia. *Canadian Journal of Psychiatry, 48*(1), 14-21.

Overall, J. E., & Gorham, D. R. (1962). The Brief Psychiatric Rating Scale. *Psychological Report, 10*, 799-812.

Regier, D. A., Farmer, M. E., Rae, D. A., Locke, B. Z., Keith, S. J., Judd, L. L., & Goodwin, F. K. (1990). Comorbidity of mental disorders with alcohol and other drug abuse: Results from the Epidemiological Catchment Area (ECA) Study. *Journal of the American Medical Association, 264*(19), 2511-2518.

Regier, D. A., Kaelber, C. T., Rae, D. S., Farmer, M. E., Knauper, B., Kessler, R. C., & Norquist, G. S. (1998). Limitations of diagnostic criteria and assessment instruments for mental disorders. *Archives of General Psychiatry, 55*(2), 109-115.

Rehm, J., Üstün, T. B., Saxena, S., Nelson, C. B., Chatterji, S., Ivis, F. & Adlaf, E. (1999). On the development and psychometric testing of the WHO screening instrument to assess disablement in the general population. *International Journal of Methods in Psychiatric Research, 8*, 110-123.

Ries, R. K., & Comtois, K. A. (1997). Illness severity and treatment services for dually diagnosed severely mentally ill outpatients. *Schizophrenia Bulletin, 23*(2), 239-246.

Robins L.N., Helzer, J.E., Croughan J., & Ratcliff, K.S. (1981). National Institute of Mental Health Diagnostic Interview Schedule: Its history, characteristics, and validity. *Archives of General Psychiatry, 38*, 381-389.

Robins, L. N., Wing, J., Wittchen, H. U., Helzer, J. E., Babor, T. F., Burke, J., Farmer, A., Jablenski, A., Pickens, R., Regier, D. A., Sartorius, N., & Towle, L. H. (1988). The Composite International Diagnostic Interview. *Archives of General Psychiatry, 45*, 1069-1077.

Sheehan, D. V., Lecrubier, Y., Sheehan, K. H., Amorim, P., Janavs, J., Weiller, E., Hergueta, T., Baker, R., & Dunbar, G. C. (1998). The Mini-International Neuropsychiatric Interview (MINI): The development and validation of a structured diagnostic psychiatric interview for the DSM-IV and ICD-10. *Journal of Clinical Psychiatry, 59*, 22-33.

Slade, T. B., & Andrews, G. (2002). Empirical impact of DSM-IV diagnostic criteria for clinical significance. *The Journal of Nervous & Mental Disease. 190*(5), 334-337.

Soyka, M. (2000). Substance misuse, psychiatric disorder, and violent and disturbed behavior. *British Journal of Psychiatry, 176*, 345-350.

Stata Corporation (2003). Stata SE (Version 8.1). [Computer software]. College Station, TX: Author.

Stiffman, A. R., Stiley, C. W., Horvath, V., Hadley-Ives, E., Polgar, M., Elze, D. et al. (2001). Organizational context and provider perception as determinants of mental health service use. *The Journal of Behavioral Health Services & Research, 28*(2), 188-204.

Substance Abuse and Mental Health Services Administration [SAMHSA] (2002). *Report to Congress on the prevention and treatment of co-occurring substance abuse disorders and mental disorders.* Rockville, MD: SAMHSA. Retrieved March 13, 2003 from: http://www.samhsa.gov/publications/publications.html.

Swartz, J. A., & Lurigio, A. J. (2004). *Use of the K6/K10 scales for screening for serious mental illness among criminal offenders.* Manuscript in preparation.

Swartz, M. S., Swanson, J. W., Hiday, V. A., Borum, R., Wagner, H. R., & Burns, B. J. (1998). Violence and severe mental illness: The effects of substance abuse and nonadherence to medication. *American Journal of Psychiatry, 155*(2), 226-231.

Tabachnick, B. G., & Fidell, L. S. (2001). *Multivariate statistics, Fourth edition.* Needham Heights, MA: Allyn & Bacon.

Teplin, L., & Swartz, J. (1989). Screening for severe mental disorder in jails: The development of the referral decision scale. *Law and Human Behavior, 13*(1), 1-18.

U.S. Dept. of Health and Human Services, Substance Abuse and Mental Health Services Administration, Office of Applied Studies. (2003). National Household Survey on Drug Abuse, 2001 [Computer file]. ICPSR version. Research Triangle Park, NC: Research Triangle Institute [producer], 2002. Ann Arbor, MI: Inter-University Consortium for Political and Social Research [distributor], 2003.

Wood, J. M., Garb, H. N., Lilienfeld, S. O., & Nezworski, M. T. (2002). Clinical assessment. *Annual Review of Psychology, 53*, 519-543.

Wu, L-T., Kouzis, A. C., & Leaf, P. J. (1999). Influence on comorbid alcohol and psychiatric disorders on utilization of mental health services in the national comorbidity survey. *American Journal of Psychiatry, 156*(8), 1230-1236.

Evaluating Rapid Assessment Instruments' Psychometric Error in a Practice Setting: Use of Receiver Operating Characteristics Analysis

Timothy B. Conley, PhD

SUMMARY. *Objective:* This paper presents a clear methodological example for practitioners' evaluation of rapid assessment instruments' psychometric error. *Participants:* One hundred and twenty nine incarcerated multiple offender drunk drivers were administered 3 rapid assessment instruments. The average age was 39, males comprised 83% and 81% were white. Thirty percent were married; 45% had never married. *Method:* Receiver Operating Characteristics analysis compared instrument scores to a criterion diagnosis. False positive and false negative rates were graphed, tabled and examined. *Findings:* All three instruments were reliable (alpha > .85) but subject to false positive and/or false

Timothy B. Conley is affiliated with the Department of Social Work, University of Montana, Missoula, MT 59812.

[Haworth co-indexing entry note]: "Evaluating Rapid Assessment Instruments' Psychometric Error in a Practice Setting: Use of Receiver Operating Characteristics Analysis." Conley, Timothy B. Co-published simultaneously in *Journal of Evidence-Based Social Work* (The Haworth Social Work Practice Press, an imprint of The Haworth Press, Inc.) Vol. 2, No. 1/2, 2005, pp. 137-154; and: *Addiction, Assessment, and Treatment with Adolescents, Adults, and Families* (ed: Carolyn Hilarski) The Haworth Social Work Practice Press, an imprint of The Haworth Press, Inc., 2005, pp. 137-154. Single or multiple copies of this article are available for a fee from The Haworth Document Delivery Service [1-800-HAWORTH, 9:00 a.m. - 5:00 p.m. (EST). E-mail address: docdelivery@haworthpress.com].

http://www.haworthpress.com/web/JEBSW
Digital Object Identifier: 10.1300/J394v02n01_08

negative diagnostic rates in excess of 14%. *Conclusion:* Receiver Operating Characteristics analysis is an effective practical methodology for evaluating the performance of rapid assessment instruments in clinical settings allowing practitioners to knowingly manage psychometric error. *[Article copies available for a fee from The Haworth Document Delivery Service: 1-800-HAWORTH. E-mail address: <docdelivery@haworthpress.com> Website: <http://www.HaworthPress.com> © 2005 by The Haworth Press, Inc. All rights reserved.]*

KEYWORDS. Assessment, psychometric error, receiver operating analysis, measurement error

The use of brief written measurement instruments for the rapid assessment of a client's situation has long been part of social work's practice base (Fischer & Corcoran, 2000; Hudson, 1982). Social workers' use of rapid assessment instruments is increasingly common in court clinics, child welfare offices and other social service settings (Cherpitel, 1995, 1997; Conigrave, Hall, & Saunders, 1995; Springer, Abell, & Hudson, 2002). McMurtry, Rose, and Cisler (2003) presented a workshop at the Society for Social work and Research's 7th annual conference entitled "Identifying and Administering the Most-Used Rapid Assessment Instruments in Research" which advocated their use. Psychometric measurement error is an inevitable component of any instrument; Fischer and Corcoran (2000) caution that since no measure in the behavioral and social sciences is completely reliable and valid, practitioners simply must strive for the best they can get.

It is the responsibility of the practitioner to insure that the validity of cut-points for Rapid assessment instruments is managed practically and responsibly. The cut-point is the test score at which a condition is presumed met: Those over the cut-point have it and all those under do not. For example, The MAST was originally designed to screen for alcoholism among hospitalized psychiatric patients (Selzer, 1971), and cut-points (or scores) of > 5 indicated a diagnosis of alcoholism. When assessment instruments like this are created, their reliability and validity are tested on a specific sample. The cut-points established for that sample are generally assumed to be accurate. However, the psychometric properties of any index or test-like factor structure and internal consistency reliability-may differ across specific practice samples. The same is true for cut-points and responsible practitioners must take these differences (measurement errors) into consideration. This requires examining an instrument's behavior in specific practice settings.

This study worked with multiple offender drunk drivers and presents the procedures for establishing sample specific cut-points for three rapid assessment instruments: The Severity of Alcohol Dependence Questionnaire (SAD-Q) (Stockwell, Murphy, & Hodgeson, 1983), the Alcohol Use Disorders Identification Test (AUDIT) (Saunders, Aasland, Babor, De La Fuente, & Grant, 1993) and the Michigan Alcoholism Screening Test (MAST) (Selzer, 1971). The study uses Receiver Operating Characteristics (ROC) analysis (Murphy et al., 1988) to determine the cut-point at which each instrument's score most accurately converges with a diagnoses of alcohol dependence as established by DSM-IV based interviewing (American Psychiatric Association, 1994). It informs practitioners on how to manage the over-diagnosis or under-diagnosis of substance abuse/dependence problems in this practice sample by examining the most effective cutoff scores for the three tests, taking into account the impact of psychometric measurement error on practice. Through this example, practitioners in other settings are encouraged to engage in a similar process of population specific instrument validation.

METHOD

Sample

Study participants were 129 consecutively admitted clients in a court ordered multiple-offender 14 day residential drunk driver program: This included all clients admitted over the 8 weeks allowed by the program for the study. The sample was 83% male, with an average age of 39. Race was reported as White by 81% of the sample, Unknown or no answer by 11%, Black by 3.4% and the remainder were Hispanic, Asian, and Alaskan Native. Forty-five percent were never married, 30% were currently married, and the rest either divorced, widowed, or separated. The average level of education was 12.37 years.

Measures

The Severity of Alcohol Dependence Questionnaire, Alcohol Use Disorders Identification Test, and the Michigan Alcoholism Screening

Test are all alcohol use related rapid assessment instruments currently in use with program participants.

Severity of Alcohol Dependence Questionnaire (SAD-Q)

The SAD-Q was designed by Stockwell et al. (1979) specifically to operationalize the concepts of the alcohol dependence syndrome (Edwards & Gross, 1976) and is mostly concerned with tolerance and withdrawal. This is a 20-item questionnaire consisting of five sub-scales with four items in each. It is used by the program primarily for the purpose of identifying individuals with physiological dependence and assumes that there is a parallel development of severity and frequency of morning symptoms of withdrawal, quantity of alcohol consumed on a typical heavy drinking day, and frequency of relief drinking. Thus, avoidance of withdrawal as a learned behavioral response is a key concept. The test items themselves are designed to cover a range of severity of symptomotology and they measure frequency of experience on four point scales of: (0) almost never, (1) sometimes, (2) often, and (3) nearly always. When measuring the reinstatement of symptoms on the mornings after two days of heavy drinking, preceded by a few weeks of abstinence, the items measure symptoms as: (0) not all, (1) slightly, (2) moderately, or (3) quite lot. Thus the total minimum score for the questionnaire is 0 and the maximum is 60.

A SAD-Q cut-point of 35 suggests severe dependence. However, Stockwell et al. (1979) were appropriately concerned with psycho- metric error and wisely cautioned that cut-points should be interpreted cautiously and examined for sample specific applicability, that is, context validity. In a 1985 study, Meehan, Webb, and Unwin, researchers in Ireland, validated the SAD-Q using un-structured clinical interview ratings as criteria for a group of 102 patients admitted to a general psychiatric hospital. There was a 75% concordance between the clinical ratings and SAD-Q when a cut-point of 30 was used to indicate severe dependence.

The SAD-Q has exhibited excellent internal consistency reliability (alpha > .90) across a series of studies (Stockwell, Murphy, & Hodgeson, 1983). Stockwell, Sitharthan, McGrath, and Lang (1994) reported Chronbach's alphas ranging from .86 to .98 in their samples drawn from both the general population and from attendants of a controlled drinking clinic (both in Australia). Given that the SAD-Q shares a common theoretical base with DSM-IV diagnostic criteria for alcohol dependency, the alcohol dependence syndrome (Edwards & Gross, 1976), it was anticipated for this study that relative to the other instruments, the SAD-Q would more effectively converge with the interview diagnosis.

The Alcohol Use Disorders Identification Test (AUDIT)

The AUDIT instrument was developed by the World Health Organization to identify persons whose alcohol consumption has become hazardous or harmful to their health. It consists of 10 items ostensibly measuring three conceptual domains: Harmful drinking, dependence, and hazardous drinking. Scores on this test range from 0 to 40. In its brief history it has generated a very large body of research literature (Allen, Litten, Fertig, & Babor, 1997). Using an exceptionally thorough and complex set of assessments as a criteria, Saunders et al. (1993) employed Receiver Operating Characteristic analysis on the AUDIT and suggested a cut-point of 8 as being most accurate for identifying alcohol use disorders in general samples across cultures. Skipsey, Burlson, and Kranzler (1997) report that this rapid assessment instrument exhibits good internal consistency (alpha = .94). With data from a sample of 82 persons diagnosed with DSM-III-R drug dependence they used ROC analysis to evaluate psychometric error; they found the instrument most accurate at a cut-point of 8.

Volke, Steinbauer, Cantor, and Holzer (1997) also used ROC analysis to evaluate AUDIT scores from 1,333 primary care patients at a family practice representing a broad socioeconomic range, a mixture of insured and uninsured patients, White, African-American, and Mexican American males and females. They found that the test positively predicted between 89% and 95% of alcohol dependent patients who met an ICD-10 diagnosis of alcohol dependence and that its predictive value is unaffected by patient background.

The Michigan Alcoholism Screening Test (MAST)

The MAST is a 25-item pencil and paper questionnaire. It is a reliable (alpha generally > .90) self report instrument designed to diagnose alcoholism and is considered a valuable diagnostic instrument with a long clinical and research history (Gibbs, 1983; Lapham et al., 1995; Mischke & Venneri, 1987; Ross, Gavin, & Skinner, 1990). The total MAST score can range from 0 to 53, with item weights that range from zero to five. The MAST's items highlight various problems clinically assumed to be associated with alcohol use, including medical, interpersonal, and legal consequences (Selzer, 1971). The author originally recommended a cutoff score of 5 for a diagnosis of alcoholism. However, he later suggested that to reduce the number of false positives, the following cut-points be used: 0-4, not alcoholic; 5-6, may be alcoholic; 7 or more, alcoholic (Selzer, Vinokur, & Rooijen, 1975).

Ross, Gavin, and Skinner (1990) conducted a study into the diagnostic validity of the MAST and Alcohol Dependence Scale (Horn, Skinner, Wanburg, & Foster, 1984) in the assessment of DSM-III-R classified alcohol disorders with voluntary inpatient chemical dependency treatment unit participants. They employed the NIMH Diagnostic Interview Schedule (Robins, Helzer, Croughan, & Ratcliff, 1981) as their criterion for diagnosing alcohol disorders and used ROC analysis to determine that the optimal cut-point for the MAST was 12/13 for this specific sample.

Rapid assessment instruments used by the Driving Under the Influence of Liquor (DUIL) program share the qualities of being brief, easily administered by para-professional staff, hand scored, and relatively easy to interpret. Each test's score ranges on a continuum from 0 to a maximum by summing responses to items and higher scores ostensibly indicate a higher likelihood of assessing positive for an alcohol related condition.

Criterion

The criterion chosen for this study is a DSM-IV specific subset of items from the Alcohol Use Disorders and Associated Disabilities Interview Schedule (AUDADIS), (Grant & Hassin, 1992; Grant & Towle, 1990). Ustun et al. (1997) conducted research into the reliability and validity of this interview schedule and concluded, as did Grant et al. (1995) that it is a reliable and valid method of interviewing for alcohol dependence in various samples. Other criterion considered for this study included the Structured Clinical Interview for Dependence, the Composite International Diagnostic Interview and the Schedules for Clinical Assessment in Neuropsychiatry (all reviewed by Grant & Towle, 1990). The Alcohol Use Disorders and Associated Disabilities Interview Schedule was chosen for its advantages of being brief, easily administered, easily scored for diagnostic purposes and cost free, as it is in the public domain (see Appendix). Moreover, the program where the study was conducted was clinically oriented towards DSM-IV and this interview schedule effectively operationalizes those diagnostic criteria.

The Alcohol Use Disorders and Associated Disabilities Interview Schedule's items are employed in this study as a semi-structured interview administered by an experienced clinician, as this most closely reflects the actual clinical assessment practice at the program where the study was conducted. In this way the implications for practice are more readily acceptable to the program's clinicians, an important point to honor when seeking to advance research based practice at the clinic level. There are 7 DSM-IV criteria for chemical dependency and the summed number of criteria met (0 through 7) may then be used as a ratio level scale, as was done by Grant et al. (1994). If 3 or more criteria are met, clients are considered positive for a diagnosis of alcohol dependence. The Alcohol Use Disorders and Associated Disabilities Interview Schedules' results provide a powerful and generalizable criterion measure for ROC analysis.

Data Collection

The SAD-Q, AUDIT, and MAST were administered by the principal investigator in that order to participants in groups of thirty or more in a classroom setting as pencil and paper tests on the morning of the first day after admission to the program. Four consecutive admission groups were studied over the course of eight weeks. A standardized administration protocol insured consistency of test administration with regards to sequence, instruction and responses to participant questions. Despite the potential threat posed by response bias issues (Babor, Stephens, & Marlat, 1987), participants were required to list their name and date of birth. The tests are an integral part of the program's assessment regimen and this information is required on all other written tasks performed by clients. It allowed for a 'real world' examination of the instruments' performance while they are actually being used at the program. At test time, the participants were each given an appointment card to see the principal investigator, an MSW clinician specializing in addictions, within three days of test taking. When seen individually, the participants were invited to participate in a study concerning the tests' validity. For those that agreed, informed consent (approved by a College Institutional Review Board) was signed and witnessed. Those that did not agree were offered the benefit of a confidential professional evaluation of their drinking behavior anyway. Only one client declined to participate. All participants received the Alcohol Use Disorders and Associated Disabilities Interview Schedule interview with results recorded on copies of the Appendix, and each received a DSM-IV diagnosis based on this interview. A sign up list was kept for all participants who wished to receive a copy of the final study, and the principal investigator furnished an e-mail address, a mailbox address and a telephone number for contact purposes.

DATA ANALYSIS RESULTS AND DISCUSSION

All test and interview results were entered into SPSS 10.0 (SPSS, 2001) item by item, and portrayed as a graph and tables. True positive, true negative, false positive and false negative rates were given for each instrument at all possible cut-points, allowing for graphic and tabular presentation of results. As a statistical procedure, ROC (Murphy et al., 1988; Hsaio, Bartko, & Potter, 1989) is fairly new in its application to social science research and a thorough description of its statistical theory and mathematical equations may be found in a comprehensive book by Swets (1996), though the 1988 article by Murphy et al. is more practical. ROC was included in SPSS software version 10.0 as a graphing procedure (SPSS, 2001).

For this study, participants exhibiting 3 or more DSM-IV criteria (the diagnostic threshold according to DSM-IV) are considered to meet the condition of alcohol dependence. Those with 2 or less are not. By designating 1 = condition met and 0 = condition not met as a criterion, this sets a 'true' standard against which each instruments' scores may be compared. For example, for any given study participant a MAST score may be compared to the criterion. A participant may score 15 on the MAST (well above the standard cut-point of 7) and yet their interview diagnosis could indicate that they met only 2 DSM-IV criteria (condition not met) and are thus not considered alcohol dependent. In this case the ROC procedure would identify a false positive finding by the test. Moreover, a participant may score 2 on the MAST yet be positive according to the criteria in which case the test results in a false negative. By examining all data on all tests, ROC analysis creates a visual representation of each test instrument's true positive rate plotted against false positive rate *across the complete range of possible test scores.*

ROC analysis also allows the researcher/practitioner to determine the optimal instrument cut-point for identifying alcohol use problems in individuals in the specific sample, that is, *the cut-point at which the test will result in the lowest possible overall number of mis-classifications.* This statistical procedure has previously been used successfully to evaluate alcoholism screening instruments in other clinical settings (Cherpitel, 1995, 1997; Conigrave, Hall, & Saunders, 1995; Skipsey, Burlson, & Kranzler, 1997; Volke, Steinbauer, Cantor, & Holzer, 1997).

If the ability of a test instrument to discriminate between those who meet the condition and those who do not is no better than chance (.50), the resulting ROC graphic curve will be a diagonal line. If the test shows better than chance the line will be above the diagonal-the further above, the more accurate the test. A perfect test (1.0) will completely follow the left and top line of the graphing box. The Area Under the Curve-but above the diagonal-and its variance may be measured as it will fall between (.50) for an instrument whose ability to discriminate is no better than chance, to (1.0) for an instrument which discriminates perfectly (Ross, Gavin, & Skinner, 1990). The Area Under the Curve may itself be statistically analyzed for strength and significance (including confidence interval) as was done by Cherpitel (1995). For this current study an ROC curve was plotted for all possible cut-points for each test instrument and the Area Under the Curve analyzed for strength and significance.

The Area Under the Curve statistic challenges the hypothesis that the test is doing better than chance at predicting the condition. Table 1, *Area Under the Curve*, demonstrates that each test was significant. Therefore the null hypothesis is rejected; the instruments tests are able to predict the condition. Each test fell within its confidence interval (p. < .001).

By graphing the full range of pairs of *sensitivity* and 1-specificity (false positive) for all three tests, the ROC curves offer a rich picture of the potential information content of the tests throughout the range of possible cut-points. A graph of the three curves which plots sensitivity on the vertical axis (Y) by 1-*specificity* on the horizontal axis (X) is illustrated in Figure 1.

TABLE 1. Area Under the Receiver Operating Curve for the SAD-Q, MAST, and AUDIT

	AUC (SE)	Asymptotic Sig. (a)	C.I. (p. < .05)
SAD-Q	.797 (.047)	.000	(.705) (.889)
MAST	.816 (.042)	.000	(.733) (.889)
AUDIT	.838 (.040)	.000	(.760) (916)

(a) null hx: true area = 0.50
N = 129

FIGURE 1. Receiver Operating Curve

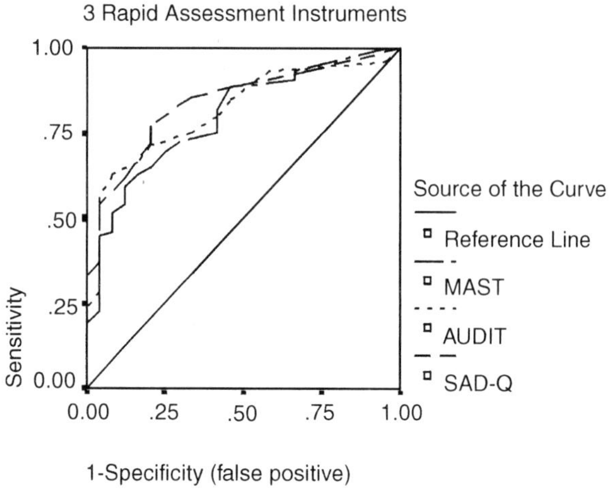

3 Rapid Assessment Instruments

Table 2 was designed to examine each instrument's *sensitivity* (the proportion of the persons who actually meet the condition and are classified as meeting it-true positive) and *specificity* (the proportion of persons who do not actually meet the condition and are classified as not meeting it-true negative). False positive and false negative rates for each cut-point presented were added for clarity, as these are of most interest to practitioners. Only a partial range of relevant scores is represented by the table in the interest of space. Choosing a lower cut-point for practice use generally results in higher sensitivity and lower specificity. The optimal cut-point then will be the best balance between the two. Of salient concern in a treatment program such as Driving Under the Influence of Liquor, is sensitivity (true positive) and 1-specificity (false positive). The important clinical question becomes: to what degree is the program willing to tolerate classifying somebody as not having an alcohol related condition, when in fact they are diagnosable (false negative)?

The SAD-Q exhibited very strong internal consistency reliability with this sample (Alpha = .91). For the SAD-Q the suggested cut-point is 1-2, the point at which 85.7% of those with a DSM-IV diagnosis are identified as having the diagnosis and 77.7% of those without the diagnosis are classified as not having the diagnosis. While at this cut-point the test will falsely identify 33.3 % of those who do not have the condi-

TABLE 2. Sensitivity and Specificity for the SAD-Q, MAST, and AUDIT at Select Cut-Points

	Cut-point	Sensitivity	Specificity	False Positive	False Negative
SAD-Q	1/2	.857	.777	.223	.143
	2/3	.771	.792	.208	.229
	3/4	.724	.792	.208	.276
	4/5	.619	.875	.125	.381
MAST	7/8	.933	.667	.333	.067
	10/11	.819	.583	.417	.181
	11/12	.752	.583	.417	.248
	12/13	.724	.708	.292	.276
	13/14	.695	.750	.250	.305
	14/15	.648	.792	.208	.352
	15/16	.629	.833	.167	.371
AUDIT	4/5	.848	.542	.458	.152
	5/6	.800	.583	.417	.200
	6/7	.752	.667	.333	.248
	7/8	.714	.792	.208	.286
	8/9	.667	.833	.167	.333
	9/10	.669	.917	.083	.371

Cutoff values are the averages of two consecutive ordered observed test values.
N = 129

tion as having it, it is of more importance that the program would only initially perceive 14.3 % of those who do have the condition as not having it. It is hazardous to indicate to a multiple offender drunk driver they do not have an alcohol dependency problem when in fact they do. This finding indicates an optimal cut-point for the test dramatically lower than that found by either Stockwell et al. (1979) or Meehan, Webb, and Unwin (1985) with their different client samples and much lower than that in use by the program. The finding highlights the importance of establishing sample specific cut-points for rapid assessment instruments and raises the question of what cut-point would be most useful with other groups such as adolescents, elderly, outpatients, persons with disabilities, etc. Only when the questionnaire's cut-point is validated against an interview based criterion with these samples will this be known.

It is also possible that the low optimal cut-point for this sample of persons convicted of driving under the influence is related to the criterion itself, the Alcohol Use Disorders and Associated Disabilities Interview Schedule. Weiczorek, Miller, and Nochajski (1991) outlined several gaps in the research literature with regards to screening drunk drivers, finding it a major problem that currently available screening instruments have not been standardized for use with this specific population. Moreover, they were appropriately critical of research processes whereby newer assessment instruments are validated using an older instrument as a criterion-with neither instrument compared to a more widely accepted standard such as DSM-IV criteria. Both they and Conley (2001) advocate specifically for the use of DSM-IV standards in evaluating both drunk drivers and the instruments used to evaluate them and this study supports that recommendation.

The MAST exhibited strong internal consistency reliability with this sample (Alpha = .87). The cut-point of 10-11 will correctly identify 81.9% of the participants who meet the diagnosis, but to achieve this the test will only correctly identify 58.3% of those who do not have the condition. Put another way, the false positive rate-those that do not have the condition that the test indicates do-would be one minus specificity or about 41.7%. This is unacceptably high. The optimal cut-point suggested for this test then is 13-14, which will correctly identify 69.5% of this sample's alcohol dependent clients and 75.0% of those who do not, while falsely diagnosing as negative 30.5 % of the cases who do in fact meet the condition. This is nearly twice the cut-point of 7 in use at the program now which, according to this study of 129 participants, would identify 33.3% of those who do not have the condition as having it. Clearly the program has been erring on the side of caution by only classifying 6.7% of those meeting the criteria not meeting it. Given the level of social impairment which drinking has caused this population there has been an understandably high level of skepticism among program personnel with regards to clients who appear to not be alcohol dependent.

The cut-point for the MAST suggested here is the one which would meet the specific needs of this program with this clientele; it is the most appropriate for this particular program. By knowing the error rate and where it lies, the error may be consciously managed in a way that is understandable and acceptable to the program's practitioners and useful to the clients.

The AUDIT also exhibited good internal consistency reliability with this sample (Alpha = .85). At a cut-point of 4-5 the AUDIT will correctly identify 84.8 % of those who truly meet the diagnosis but at the expense of diagnosing 45.8% of those who don't have the condition as having it (one minus specificity, false positive). The optimal cut-point suggested for this test then is 7-8, where 71.4% who truly have the condition are diagnosed as having it and only 20.8% of those who do not have the condition are diagnosed as having it. At this cut-point, 28.6% of those with the condition *met* would be diagnosed as *not met*. The AUDIT was the most difficult test to find a balanced cut-point for. This may be due to conceptual and theoretical differences in the background of the instrument and the criterion. The AUDIT seeks to identify harmful/hazardous drinking while DSM-IV criteria are grounded more in the alcohol dependence syndrome theory (Edwards & Gross, 1976). Nonetheless, the research practice of comparing the test to a criterion and examining the cut-points using ROC highlights for the practitioner the test's strengths and shortcomings.

Establishing the context specific validity of any rapid assessment instrument is not immediate but develops experientially over time as data accumulates. More important than simply asking if a test is valid, is to ask what interpretation one can draw from the responses to items on a particular scale (Davidson, 1987). Fischer and Corcoran (2000) detail several advantages and disadvantages of rapid assessment instruments which are supported by this study. They caution that instrument reliability and validity are only estimates derived from norming on particular groups, leaving it open to question whether or not particular instruments are reliable and valid for particular individual clients and client groups. For the Driving Under the Influence of Liquor program, discontinued use of the AUDIT is advised. This is not a general critique of the test, which has proven very valid and reliable with a variety of clientele-it is just not a particularly good fit for this one. Moreover, once aware of the psychometric error they could expect from the SAD-Q and MAST the program's counselors were more comfortable with their use, despite the error rates.

ROC analysis is an effective method for determining sample specific optimal cut-points for rapid assessment instruments when screening for substance dependence disorders in a practice setting. Understanding the risks for false positives and false negatives allows practitioners to interpret tests responsibly and to knowingly manage the information provided. There may be clinical settings where any false negative rate is unacceptable for a particular rapid assessment instrument and only thorough face to face interviewing (not infallible itself) should be used. Rapid assessment instruments should be used for screening, not diagnosis, and the ROC analysis process could bolster confidence in their use and allow clinics to make more judicious use of their resources when further specialized assessment/diagnosis seems to be in order. The

DUIL program specifically is advised to minimize the extent they rely on any test information which, even at its best, misclassifies a high percent of participants. Brief, semi-structured clinical interviewing based on the Alcohol Use Disorders and Associated Disabilities Interview Schedule criteria, (which is suggested for reasons outlined earlier) is advised to insure higher rates of diagnostic accuracy. Moreover, support is provided for Fischer and Corcoran's (2000) suggestion that multiple instruments be used in conjunction with clinical interviewing. It is best not to over-rely on any psychometric instrument, as assessment is an imprecise science.

This study was limited by the size (129) and homogeneity of its sample, hampering its generalizability. Moreover, the use of a single criterion for diagnosing an alcohol related problem, while common in clinical practice, fails to lend strength to the findings. Further research could look at a larger sample taken over a longer period of time; it may be that the Driving Under the Influence of Liquor program participant characteristics differ by season as do rates of arrest and conviction. Moreover, it could be useful to over-sample women and minorities over time to examine how the instruments behave for these clients and which cut-points are most effective at identifying alcohol problems for them.

The Alcohol Use Disorders and Associated Disabilities Interview Schedule criterion was chosen for its brevity, relative ease of administration and scoring, being cost free, and being acceptable to a program which already employs DSM-IV criteria. For research purposes however, other criteria such as those reviewed by Grant and Towle (1990) could be used and may portray a different performance by the instruments-findings which would further bolster the program's ability to understand and manage measurement error.

Gathering and analyzing data from rapid assessment instruments and criterion interviews is a fairly complex process, one that requires a program to take a quantitative approach. Its practicality may be somewhat limited depending on the research skills of the practitioners, but its use presents an opportunity for social work researchers and practitioners to work together, advancing empirically based and valid assessment of client problems.

REFERENCES

Allen, J.P., Litten, R.Z., Fertig, J.B., & Babor, T. (1997). A review of research on the Alcohol Use Disorders Identification Test. *Alcoholism: Clinical and Experimental Research, 21* (4), 613-619.

American Psychiatric Association. (1994). *Diagnostic and statistical manual of mental disorders, 4th ed.* Washington DC: American Psychiatric Association.

Babor, T.F., Stephens, R.S., and Marlatt, G.A. (1987). Verbal report methods and clinical research on alcoholism: Response bias and its minimization. *Journal of Studies on Alcohol, 48,* 410-14.

Cherpitel, C.J. (1995). Analysis of cut points for screening instruments for alcohol problems in the emergency room. *Journal of Studies of Alcohol 56,* 695-700.

Cherpitel, C.J. (1997). Brief Screening Instruments for Alcoholism. *Alcohol Health and Research World, 21* (4), 348-351.

Conigrave, K.M., Hall, W.D., & Saunders, J.B. (1995). The AUDIT questionnaire: Choosing a cut-off score. *Research Report. Addiction, 90,* 1349-1356.

Conley, T.B. (2001) Construct Validity of the MAST and AUDIT with multiple offender drunk drivers. *Journal of Substance Abuse Treatment, 20,* 287-295.

Davidson, R. (1987). Assessment of the alcohol dependence syndrome: A review of self-report screening questionnaires. *British Journal of Clinical Psychology, 26,* 243-255.

Edwards, G., & Gross, M. (1976). Alcohol dependence: Provisional description of a clinical syndrome. *British Medical Journal, 1,* 1058-1061.

Fischer, J., & Corcoran, K. (2000). *Measures for clinical practice: A source book* (3rd ed.). NY: The Free Press.

Gibbs, L.E. (1983). Validity and reliability of the Michigan Alcoholism Screening Test: A review. *Drug and Alcohol Dependence, 12,* 279-285.

Grant, B.F., & Hasin, D.S. (1992). *The Alcohol Use Disorder and Associated Disabilities Interview Schedule.* Rockville, MD: National Institute of Alcohol Abuse and Alcoholism.

Grant, B.F., Harford, T.C., Dawson, D.A., Chou, P., Dufor, M., & Pickering, R. (1994). Prevalence of DSM-IV alcohol abuse and dependence: United States, 1992. *Alcohol Health and Research World, 18* (3), 243-248 (NIAAA's Epidemiologic Bulletin # 35).

Grant, B.F., Harford, T.C., Dawson, D.A., Chou, P., & Pickering, R. (1995). The Alcohol Use Disorder and Associated Disabilities Interview Schedule (AUDADIS): Reliability of alcohol and drug modules in a general population sample. *Drug and Alcohol Dependence, 39,* 37-44.

Grant, B.F., & Towle, L. (1990). Standardized diagnostic interviews for alcohol research. *Alcohol Health & Research World, 14* (4), 340-348.

Horn, J.L. Skinner, H.A., Wanburg, K.W., & Foster, F.M. (1984). *The Alcohol Dependence Scale (ADS).* Toronto: Addiction Research Foundation.

Hsaio, J.K., Bartko, J.M., & Potter, W.Z. (1989). Diagnosing diagnosis: Receiver operating characteristic methods and psychiatry. *Archives of General Psychiatry, 46,* 664-667.

Hudson, W. W. (1982). *The Clinical Measurement Package: A Field Manual.* Tallahassee, FL: WALMYR Publishing Co.

Lapham, S.C., Skipper, B.J., Owen, J.P., Kleyboecker, K., Teaf, D., Thompson, B., & Simpson, G. (1995). Alcohol abuse screening instruments: Normative test data collected from a first DWI offender screening program. *Journal of Studies on Alcohol, 56,* 51-59.

McMurtry, S.L., Rose S.J., & Cisler, R.A. (2003) Identifying and administering the most-used rapid assessment instruments in research. Workshop presented at the Society for Social Work and Research 7th annual conference, Washington DC, 2003. Abstract retrieved on-line 12-21-03 at: *http://www.sswr.org/papers2003/618.htm*

Meehan, J.P., Webb, M., & Unwin, A. (1985). The Severity of Alcohol Dependence Questionnaire (SAD-Q) in a sample of Irish problem drinkers. *British Journal of Addictions, 80* (1), 57-64.

Mischke, H.D., & Venneri, R. (1987). Reliability and validity of the MAST, Mortimer-Filkins Questionnaire and CAGE in DWI assessment. *Journal of Studies on Alcohol, 48* (5), 492-501.

Murphy, J.M., Berwick, D.M., Weinstein, M.C., Borus, J.F., Budman, S.H., & Klerman, G.L. (1988). Performance of screening and diagnostic tests: Application of receiver operating characteristic analysis. *Archives of General Psychiatry, 44*, 550-555.

Robins, L.N., Helzer, J.E., Croughan, J., & Ratcliff, K.S. (1981). National Institute of Mental Health Diagnostic Interview Schedule: Its history, characteristics, and validity. *Archives of General Psychiatry, 38*, 381-389.

Ross, H.E., Gavin, D.R., & Skinner, H.A. (1990). Diagnostic validity of the MAST and the Alcohol Dependence Scale in the assessment of DSM-III alcohol disorders. *Journal of Studies on Alcohol, 51* (6), 506-513.

Saunders, J.B., Aasland, O.G., Babor, T.F., De La Fuente, J.R., & Grant, M. (1993). Development of the AUDIT: WHO collaborative project on early detection of persons with harmful alcohol consumption-II. *Addiction 88*, 791-804.

Selzer, M.L. (1971). The Michigan Alcoholism Screening Test: The quest for a new diagnostic instrument. *American Journal of Psychiatry, 127*, 1653-1658.

Selzer, M.L., Vinokur, A., & Rooijen, L. (1975). A self-administered short Michigan Alcoholism Screening Test (SMAST). *Journal of Studies on Alcohol, 36*, 117-126.

Skipsey, K., Burleson, J.A., & Kranzler, H.R. (1997). Utility of the AUDIT for identification of hazardous and harmful drinking in drug dependent patients. *Drug and Alcohol Dependence, 45* (3),157-63.

Springer, D.W., Abell, N., & Hudson, W.W. (2002). Creating and validating rapid assessment instruments for practice and research part 1. *Research on Social Work Practice, 12* (3), 408-439.

SPSS (2001). Version 10.0 for P.C. *http://www.spss.com*

Stockwell, T., Hodgson, R., Edwards, G., Taylor, C., & Rankin, H. (1979). The development of a questionnaire to measure severity of alcohol dependence. *British Journal of Addiction 74*, 79-87.

Stockwell, T., Murphy, D., & Hodgson, R. (1983). The Severity of Alcohol Dependence Questionnaire: Its use, reliability and validity. *British Journal of Addiction, 78*, 145-155.

Stockwell, T., Sitharthan, T., McGrath, D., & Lang, E. (1994). The measurement of alcohol dependence and impaired control in community samples. *Addiction, 89*, 167-174.

Swets, J.A. (1996). *Signal detection theory and ROC analysis in psychology and diagnostics: Collected papers.* Mahawa, NJ: Lawrence Erlbaum Associates.

Ustun, B., Compton, W., Mager, D., Babor, T., Baiyewu, O., Chatterji, S., Cottler, L., Gogus, A., Mavreas, V., Peters, L., Pull, C., Saunders, J., Smeets, R., Stipec, M.-R., Vrasti, R., Hasin, D.S., Room, R., Van den Brink, W. Regier, D., Blaine, J., Grant,

B.F., & Sartorius, N. (1997). WHO study on the reliability and validity of the alcohol and drug use disorders instruments: Overview of methods and results. *Drug and Alcohol Dependence, 47*, 161-169.

Volke, R.J., Steinbauer, J.R., Cantor, S.B., & Holzer, C.E. (1997). The Alcohol Use Disorders Identification Test (AUDIT) as a screen for at risk drinking in primary care patients of different racial/ethnic backgrounds. *Addiction, 92*, 197-206.

Weiczorek, W.F., Miller, B.A., & Nochajski, T.H. (1991). *Screening of DWI offenders: Needs and prospects.* The Problem Drinker-Driver Project: New York State Division of Alcohol Abuse and Alcoholism: Research note 91-4, July 1991. ISSN # 1049-1813.

APPENDIX

0 = not met
1 = met

Alcohol Use Disorders and Associated Disabilities Interview Schedule
(AUDADIS)   _____

Adapted From: 1992 National Longitudinal Alcohol Epidemiologic Survey:
DSM-IV Alcohol Dependence Diagnostic Criteria and Associated Questionnaire
Items-Public Domain

Diagnostic Criteria for Alcohol Dependence

0 = met
1 = not met

Diagnostic Criterion: Tolerance (DSM-IV 1)

Questionnaire Items: **dsmd1**_____

A)_____ Find that your usual number of drinks had much less effect on you that
it once did.
B)_____ Find that you had to drink much more than you once did to get the
effect you wanted.

(Tolerance need only to have occurred once during the past year for the criterion to be
positive.)

Diagnostic Criterion: Withdrawal syndrome of withdrawal relief/avoidance   **dsmd2**_____
(DSM-IV 2)

Questionnaire Items:

Have any of the following experiences happened to you when the effects of
alcohol were wearing off, several hours after drinking, or the morning after
drinking?

A)_____   For example did you ever:
_____a) Have trouble falling asleep or staying awake.
_____b) Find yourself shaking when the effects of alcohol wear off.
_____c) Feel depressed, irritable, or nervous.
_____d) Feel sick to your stomach or vomit when the effects of alcohol were
wearing off.
_____e) Have a very bad headache.
_____ f) Find yourself sweating or your heart beating fast when the effects of
alcohol were wearing off.
_____g) See, feel, or hear things there were not really there.
_____h) Have fits or seizures when the effects of alcohol were wearing off.

APPENDIX (continued)

B)_____ Take a drink to get over any of the bad after effects of drinking.
C)_____ Take a drug other than aspirin, Tylenol, (tm), or Advil (tm) to keep from having a hangover or to get over the bad after-effects of drinking.
D)_____ Take a drink to keep from having a hangover or to make yourself feel better when you had one.

(Two or more symptoms of withdrawal must have occurred at least twice during the past year for the criterion to be positive.)

Diagnostic Criterion: Drinking larger amounts over a longer period of time than intended (DSM-IV 3).
Questionnaire Items: **dsmd3**_____

A)_____Start drinking even though you decided not to or promised yourself you would not.
B)_____End up drinking more than you meant to.
C)_____Keep on drinking for a much longer period of time that you had intended to.

Diagnostic Criterion: Persistant desire or unsuccessful efforts to cut down or control drinking (DSM-IV 4).
Questionnaire Items: **dsmd4**_____

A)_____Want to stop or cut down on your drinking.
B)_____Try to stop or cut down on your drinking but found you could not do it.

Diagnostic Criterion: Great deal of time spent in activities to obtain alcohol, to drink, or to recover from its effects (DSM-IV 5).
Questionnaire Items: **dsmd5**_____

A)_____Spend so much time drinking that you had little time for anything else.
B)_____Spend a lot of time being sick or with a hangover from drinking.
C)_____Spend a lot of time making sure that you always had alcohol available.

Diagnostic Criterion: Important social, occupational, or recreational activities given up or reduced in favor of drinking (DSM-IV 6).
Questionnaire Items: **dsmd6**_____

A)_____Give up or cut down on activities that were important to you in order to drink-like work, school, or associating with friends or relatives.
B)_____Give up or cut down on activities that you were interested in or that gave you pleasure in order to drink.

Diagnostic Criterion: Continued to drink despite knowledge of having a persistent or re-current physical or psychological problem caused or exacerbated by drinking (DSM-IV 7).
Questionnaire Items: **dsmd7**_____

A)_____Continued to drink even though you knew it was making you feel depressed, uninterested in things, or suspicious or distrustful of other people.
B)_____Continued to drink even though you know it was causing you a health problem or making a health problem worse.

Substance Use in a State Population of Incarcerated Juvenile Offenders

Michael G. Vaughn, MA, MALS
Matthew O. Howard, PhD
Kirk A. Foster, MDiv, MSW
Michael K. Dayton, BA
Jonathan L. Zelner, BA

SUMMARY. This study examined the prevalence and patterns of illicit drug use among a state population of 723 incarcerated juvenile offenders. In addition to alcohol and marijuana, results indicated high rates of illicit substance use involving a wide range of substances including amphetamines, opiate drugs, prescription drugs, and solvents. Further, significant gender and ethnic differences were observed with regard to

Michael G. Vaughn is affiliated with the Comorbidity and Addictions Center, George Warren Brown School of Social Work Washington University, St. Louis, MO.

Matthew O. Howard is affiliated with the School of Social Work and Department of Psychiatry, University of Michigan, Ann Arbor, MI.

Kirk A. Foster, Michael K. Dayton, and Jonathan L. Zelner are affiliated with the George Warren Brown School of Social Work, Washington University, St. Louis, MO.

Address correspondence to: Michael G. Vaughn, MA, MALS, Doctoral student, Comorbidity and Addictions Center, George Warren Brown School of Social Work, Washington University, St. Louis, MO 63130-4899 (E-mail: mvaughn@wustl.edu).

This project was supported by Grant # 1 RO3 DA015556-01 (Matthew O. Howard, PhD, PI).

[Haworth co-indexing entry note]: "Substance Use in a State Population of Incarcerated Juvenile Offenders." Vaughn, Michael G. et al. Co-published simultaneously in *Journal of Evidence-Based Social Work* (The Haworth Social Work Practice Press, an imprint of The Haworth Press, Inc.) Vol. 2, No. 1/2, 2005, pp. 155-173; and: *Addiction, Assessment, and Treatment with Adolescents, Adults, and Families* (ed: Carolyn Hilarski) The Haworth Social Work Practice Press, an imprint of The Haworth Press, Inc., 2005. pp. 155-173. Single or multiple copies of this article are available for a fee from The Haworth Document Delivery Service [1-800-HAWORTH, 9:00 a.m. - 5:00 p.m. (EST). E-mail address: docdelivery@haworthpress.com].

Digital Object Identifier: 10.1300/J394v02n01_09

alcohol and drug related problems, suicidal ideation, and age of substance use initiation. *[Article copies available for a fee from The Haworth Document Delivery Service: 1-800-HAWORTH. E-mail address: <docdelivery@ haworthpress.com> Website: <http://www.HaworthPress.com> © 2005 by The Haworth Press, Inc. All rights reserved.]*

KEYWORDS. Substance abuse, juvenile offenders, incarcerated youth, adolescent substance use, juvenile justice

Research on the use of psychoactive substances among incarcerated juvenile offenders, though still in its infancy, is beginning to document lifetime prevalence of drug use and abuse at pronounced levels. This state of affairs is not only overwhelming to juvenile justice systems with limited screening and treatment resources, but also portends negative outcomes for youth in their post-incarceration transition phase. Indeed, this is significant given that in the most recent census of juveniles in corrections, 134,011 youth resided in nearly 3,000 facilities in the U.S. (Sickmund, 2004). Although large, this figure represents just a snapshot of youth who are incarcerated at any one time.

Most studies of substance use among juveniles in corrections have examined detained youth not yet adjudicated to state systems of incarceration (Abram, Teplin, McClelland, & Dulcan, 2003; Dembo, Williams, Fagan, & Schmeidler, 1993; Hando, Howard, & Zibert, 1997; Potter & Jenson, 2003; Teplin, 1990; Teplin, 1994; Teplin, Abram, McClelland, Dulcan, & Mericle, 2002). At present, limited research is available on the substance use, abuse and dependence patterns of youth in state systems of juvenile justice residential care. Further few, if any, of these investigations have examined state populations of incarcerated youth utilizing instruments capable of detailed assessment of past and current illicit drug use. Nonetheless, these studies provide data that are useful in understanding the epidemiology of illicit drug use in juvenile justice samples. In what is perhaps the most important of these studies, Teplin and colleagues (2002) found in a randomly drawn sample 1,829 detained Cook County youth that approximately half of representative males and females had a diagnosable substance use disorder.

Examining these and other studies of substance use among juveniles in corrections reveals several themes important for both researchers and practitioners alike. First, the genesis of delinquent behavior and substance use are linked (Elliott, Huizinga, & Menard, 1989; Hawkins,

Catalano, & Miller, 1992; Huizinga, Loeber, Thornberry, & Cothern, 2000; Stice, Myers, & Brown, 1998: Zhang, Wieczorek, & Welte, 1997). Thus, indicating similar etiologies. Second, juvenile offenders initiate their substance use career earlier than non-delinquents (Dembo, Pacheco, Schmiedler, Fisher, & Cooper, 1997; Dembo, Williams, Fagan, & Schmiedler, 1993; Van Kammen, Loeber, & Stouthamer, 1991) and court-referred youth use and abuse substances at rates higher than non-referred youth (Huizinga & Jakob-Chien, 1998; Rounds-Bryant, Kristiansen, Fairbank, & Hubbard, 1998). Further, illicit substance abuse heightens the risk for future referrals (Cottle, Lee, & Heilbrun, 2001). Finally, substance use disorders do not exist in isolation as the majority of juvenile offenders also possess a comorbid mental health disorder, including ADHD, anxiety, and depression (Thompson, Riggs, Mukilich, & Crowley, 1996; Teplin et al., 2002; Wasserman, McReynolds, Lucas, Fisher, & Santos, 2002). Taken together, these studies lend support to the notion of delinquency and substance use being part of a problem behavior spectrum (Huizinga, Loeber, Thornberry, & Cothern, 2000).

Current findings with youth in residential juvenile justice care provide little information pertaining to cognitive impairments stemming from the use of illicit drugs, psychosocial problems relating to family and peers, or specific data regarding the varieties of substances commonly used such as inhalants, club drugs and prescription drugs. Most studies have found that the preferred drug of use among juvenile offenders is marijuana (Potter & Jenson, 2003; Teplin et al., 2002; Vaughn, Howard, & Curtis, in press). Further evidence of the ubiquity of marijuana use among juvenile offenders is derived from Arrestee Drug Abuse Monitoring (ADAM) data. ADAM utilizes urinalysis detection methods in 23 major sites and findings since 1991 reveal dramatic increases in positive marijuana screens among youthful adult arrestees ages 18 to 20 (Golub & Johnson, 2001).

The purpose of the present paper is to characterize the substance use patterns of adolescents in a state population of incarcerated juvenile offenders. Primary research questions were as follows. (1) How prevalent is lifetime illicit drug use among incarcerated juvenile offenders in residential treatment? (2) What are the patterns of substance use and abuse by gender, ethnic group and geographic region? (3) What is the mean age of initiation for various illicit drugs? (4) What is the prevalence of substance related problems, mental health diagnoses, suicidal ideation, and trauma? Answers to the aforementioned questions will inform practitioners and policy-makers about the treatment needs of youth in a relatively large system of juvenile justice. In addition, this data can illuminate areas of research where key hypotheses can be formulated and tested as well as stimulate further research.

METHODS

Data

This paper reports findings from analyses of survey data obtained from a statewide population of juvenile offenders in Missouri State Division of Youth Services (DYS) custody. Study team members conducted face-to-face structured interviews with all respondents. Interviewing commenced in January 2004 and was completed in July 2004. Research team members were trained to administer the structured interview and to respond to potential problems arising during the interview process. Data security, coding, entry, and cleaning were maintained and executed by trained research associates under the guidance of the study's principal investigator. Formal written consent was obtained by DYS and all study protocols were approved by the Washington University Internal Review Board (IRB).

The study is a population-based investigation consisting of all youth incarcerated at 32 DYS residential treatment centers in Missouri. Most DYS youth commitments involve youth who are new to DYS (greater than 90%). Thus, only a small percentage of youth in DYS care are serving second or third commitments. Youth are mandated to residential care for a variety of transgressions including major and minor felonies, misdemeanors, and status offenses. For example, in year 2000 evaluation, 12.1% were committed for class A/B felonies, 40.2% for less serious felonies, and 32.4% for misdemeanor offenses. The average time served by youths is typically between 4-8 months and 7.5 months in the present survey. In total, 728 interviews were conducted. Of these, 4 were stopped when interviewers determined that youth were too functionally impaired to complete the interview, and 1 youth elected not to complete the interview. These 5 interviews are not included in the dataset. Further, 2 youth were transferred to other facilities while interviewers were in the facility and as such were not available for interviewing. Finally, 10 youth who were listed on facility rosters when interviewers arrived were on furlough and could not be interviewed. In sum, of a total of 740 youth eligible to participate, 728 were available for interview, of which all began the interview and 723 completed it. This translates into a 97.7% response rate.

Measures

In addition to demographic data, this report presents data derived from a range of substance use measures. Data pertaining to the lifetime prevalence and frequency of use of 22 substances including alcohol, heroin, cocaine, amphetamines, marijuana, inhalants, and hallucinogens were obtained from a comprehensive substance use assessment. Additionally, three subscales were used from the seven-scale Massachusetts Youth Screening Instrument-Second Version (MAYSI-2) (Grisso, Barnum, Fletcher, Cauffman, & Peuschold, 2001): Substance-related problems, suicidal ideation, and trauma experiences. These subscales consist of a series of items arranged in a "yes" or "no" dichotomous response format. The total number of affirmative item responses is then summed to provide an overall scale score. These total scores are subsequently used to identify youth at cautionary or exceptionally high symptom levels in order for these particular youth to receive priority in treatment and service allocation. Studies utilizing the MAYSI-2 in incarcerated youth samples have found it to be reliable (Grisso & Barnum, 2000). Current mental health diagnosis and prior "blackout" experiences were based on self-report.

Variables

Demographic variables: These variables consisted of age, gender, ethnicity, level of education, geographic region of residence, and family receipt of public assistance (an SES proxy).

Substance use variables: The primary substance use variable for this research is "lifetime history" of a particular substance including the self-reported estimate of frequency of use and age of initiation. Frequency of use variables were measured for each substance by asking whether they had used the drug fewer than five, five to ten, 11 to 99, or 100 plus times. In addition, the eight item MAYSI-2 Alcohol and Drug problems subscale was included. For example, a sample question is "Have you gotten in trouble when you've been high or have been drinking?"

Mental health diagnosis and problems: These variables included self-report of mental health diagnosis, blackout experiences lasting greater than twenty minutes derived from a head injury, current prescribed medication, MAYSI-2 suicidal ideation (6 items) and traumatic experiences (5 items) subscales.

Analysis

The data analysis strategy for the present study was primarily descriptive in nature. The goal was to detail elemental patterns of substance use and related mental health conditions in an accessible manner for scholars, policy-makers, and practitioners alike. Analysis and presentation of data proceeded as follows. Frequencies and measures of central tendency for the aforementioned variables were tabled where appropriate. Reliability analyses utilizing Cronbach's alpha were computed for each MAYSI-2 subscale used. Analysis of Variance (ANOVA) techniques with Scheffe Post Hoc analysis and t-tests to assess statistically significant mean differences between groups were executed. Magnitudes in the difference between binary groups, such as gender, were delineated by effect size calculations using Cohen's *d*. Effect size magnitude was interpreted as .20 (small), .50 (medium), and .80 (large) as suggested by Cohen (1988).

RESULTS

Population Characteristics

Characteristics of study participants are presented in Table 1. Not unexpectedly, most youth were male (87%). In terms of ethnicity, the population was predominately White (55.3%) and African-American (32.9%), followed by Latino/Latina (3.9%), Multiethnic or Biracial (6.2%), and other (1.5%). The mean age was 15.5 (*SD* = 1.23) with a range from 11 to 20. The mean grade completed was 9.3 (*SD* = 1.31). In terms of geographic region, the majority of youth reported their home residence as either urban (39.1%) or small town (39.6%), followed next by suburban area (13.8%) and rural/country area (7.5%). Approximately 40% of youth reported coming from a home that received public assistance (i.e., food stamps, AFDC). The mean time spent in the custody was 7.5 months, yet this was highly variable as shown by a standard deviation of 8.5 months. The majority of youth (84%) reported being in detention prior to adjudication to their current DYS residence.

TABLE 1. Characteristics of Youth Incarcerated in State of Missouri DYS Facilities (N = 723)

	N (%)	M (SD)
Sex		
Male	629(87.0)	
Female	94(13.0)	
Ethnicity		
African-American	238(32.9)	
White	400(55.3)	
Latino/Latina	28(3.9)	
Multiethnic	45(6.2)	
Other*	11(1.5)	
Age		15.5(1.23)
11-yr.-old	3(0.4)	
12-yr.-old	6(0.8)	
13-yr.-old	41(5.7)	
14-yr.-old	78(10.8)	
15-yr.-old	194(26.8)	
16-yr.-old	277(38.3)	
17-yr.-old	109(15.1)	
18-yr.-old	5(0.7)	
19-yr.-old	3(0.4)	
20-yr.-old	5(0.7)	
Grade Level		9.3(1.31)
Region		
Urban	283(39.1)	
Suburban	100(13.8)	
Small town	286(39.6)	
Rural or country area	54(7.5)	
Public Assistance		
Yes	288(40.0)	
No	425(59.0)	
Time in Custody (months)		7.5(8.47)
In Detention prior to Adjudication		
Yes	607(84.0)	
No	116(16.0)	

*Includes Native American and Asian

Mental Health Disorders and Related Conditions

Table 2 reports current prevalence of mental health diagnosis and related conditions. Approximately one-half of youth had received a mental health diagnosis excluding any substance use disorder (51.4%). By far the most common mental health disorder found was Attention Deficit Hyperactivity Disorder (ADHD) followed by Bipolar Disorder. One

TABLE 2. Prevalence of Mental Health Disorders and Related Conditions in 723 Youth Incarcerated in State of Missouri DYS Facilities

	N (%)	M (SD)
Current Mental Health Diagnosis[1]		
Yes	370 (51.4)	
No	350 (48.6)	
Hearing Voices not Actually There		
Yes	106 (14.7)	
No	617 (85.3)	
Blackout Experience due to Head Injury		
Yes	132 (18.3)	
No	588 (81.7)	
Receiving Medication		
Yes	419 (58.0)	
No	304 (42.0)	
Alcohol and Drug Problem Index (MAYSI-2)		
Total		3.86 (2.36)
Gender		
Male		3.93 (4.58)
Female		4.40 (2.36)
Ethnicity*		
African-American		3.08 (2.14)
White		4.22 (2.45)
Latino/Latina		5.00 (2.96)
Multiethnic		3.76 (2.53)
Other		4.91 (2.16)
Suicide Ideation Index (MAYSI-2)		
Total		2.22 (2.37)
Gender**		
Male		2.01 (2.30)
Female		3.50 (2.38)
Ethnicity**		
African-American		1.13 (1.81)
White		2.69 (2.44)
Latino/Latina		2.50 (2.49)
Multiethnic		3.13 (2.26)
Other		3.82 (2.09)
Traumatic Experiences Index (MAYSI-2)		
Total		2.96 (1.61)
Gender		
Male		2.94 (1.60)
Female		3.12 (1.68)
Ethnicity		
African-American		3.01 (1.58)
White		2.85 (1.64)
Latino/Latina		3.47 (1.58)
Multiethnic		3.24 (1.48)
Other		3.45 (1.75)

[1] Does not include a substance use disorder.
Significant differences between groups (t-tests and ANOVA) at *$p < .005$, **$p < .001$.

hundred and six (14.7%) youth reported "having heard voices that were not actually there." The number of youth experiencing a period of unconsciousness (20 minutes or more) due to head injury was 132 (18.3%). A substantial percentage of youth were currently receiving prescribed medication for a diagnosed condition (58%).

Scores from the MAYSI-2 Alcohol and Drug Problems, Suicidal Ideation, and Traumatic Experiences subscales are also presented in Table 2. The total population mean score on the Alcohol and Drug Problems Index (Coefficient alpha = .83) was 3.86 (SD = 2.36). Males scored lower than females, (M = 3.93, SD = 4.58) versus (M = 4.40, SD = 2.36). This difference was not statistically significant and the effect size magnitude difference was small ($d = -.14$). There were significant differences between ethnic groups ($F = 4.36$, $p < .005$) with African-Americans being the lowest scoring group ($M = 3.08$, $SD = 2.14$) and Latino/Latinas the highest ($M = 5.0$, $SD = 2.96$). Post Hoc tests (Scheffe) reveals that a significant mean difference between Whites and African-Americans ($p = .005$) with African-Americans scoring 1.9 less than whites. The Suicidal Ideation Index (Coefficient alpha = .91) revealed a population mean of 2.22 (SD = 2.37). Significant differences between gender ($t = 39.2$, $p < .001$) and ethnic groups ($F = 21.97$, $p < .001$) were observed. There was a moderate-to-large effect size difference between males and females ($d = .64$), with females displaying higher scores. Also, as was the case with the Alcohol and Drug Problems subscale, African-Americans were the lowest scoring group ($M = 1.12$, $SD = 1.81$) with the Biracial/Multiethnic and other (included Asians and Native-Americans) categories attaining the highest scores ($M = 3.13$, $SD = 2.26$; $M = 3.82$, $SD = 2.09$) respectively. Post Hoc testing shows statistically significant mean differences between African-Americans and Whites ($p < .001$), Multiethnic groups ($p < .001$). The Traumatic Experiences subscale (Coefficient alpha = .77 for females and .68 for males) revealed a population mean of 2.96 ($SD = 1.61$). No significant differences were found between gender and ethnic groups. White youth displayed the lowest scores ($M = 2.86$, $SD = 1.64$), while the Latino/Latina group had the highest scores ($M = 3.47$, $SD = 1.58$).

Lifetime Prevalence and Frequency of Use of Major Substances of Abuse

Table 3 presents lifetime prevalence rates and frequency of lifetime use of major drugs of abuse (i.e., alcohol, marijuana) for various psychoactive substances. Prior alcohol, cigarette and marijuana use was nearly universal. Further, these drugs were characterized by a heavy fre-

TABLE 3. Lifetime Prevalence and Frequency of Major Substances of Abuse Among 723 Youth Incarcerated in State of Missouri DYS Facilities[1]

	N (%)
Alcohol (excludes malt liquor)	
Lifetime Prevalence	613 (84.8)
Frequency of use	
Fewer than 5 times	112 (15.5)
5-10 times	90 (12.4)
11-99 times	193 (26.7)
100+ times	218 (30.2)
Amphetamines	
Lifetime Prevalence	233 (32.2)
Frequency of use	
Fewer than 5 times	62 (8.6)
5-10 times	41 (5.7)
11-99 times	61 (8.4)
100+ times	75 (10.4)
Cigarettes	
Lifetime Prevalence	618 (85.5)
Frequency of use	
Fewer than 5 times	46 (6.4)
6-10 times	34 (4.7)
11-99 times	63 (8.7)
100+ times	473 (65.4)
Cocaine (including crack)	
Lifetime Prevalence	
Frequency of use	169 (23.4)
Fewer than 5 times	
5-10 times	67 (9.3)
11-99 times	49 (6.8)
100+ times	47 (6.5)
	52 (7.2)
Ecstacy (MDMA)	
Lifetime Prevalence	143 (19.8)
Frequency of use	
Fewer than 5 time	71 (9.8)
5-10 times	34 (4.7)
11-99 times	25 (3.5)
100+ times	13 (1.8)
Hallucinogens	
Lifetime Prevalence	167 (23.1)
Frequency of use	
Fewer than 5 times	77 (10.7)
5-10 times	30 (4.1)
11-99 times	39 (5.4)
100+ times	19 (2.6)
Marijuana	
Lifetime Prevalence	626 (86.6)
Frequency of use	
Fewer than 5 times	59 (8.2)
5-10 times	31 (4.3)
11-99 times	98 (13.6)
100+ times	436 (60.6)

	N (%)
Opiates (not heroin)	
Lifetime Prevalence	233(32.2)
Frequency of use	
Fewer than 5 times	85(11.8)
5-10 times	49 (6.8)
11-99 times	47 (6.5)
100+ times	52 (7.2)
Prescription drugs (without a prescription)	
Lifetime Prevalence	154 (21.3)
Frequency of use	
Fewer than 5 times	42 (5.8)
5-10 times	35 (4.8)
11-99 times	45 (6.2)
100+ times	31 (4.3)
Tranquilizers	
Lifetime Prevalence	229 (31.7)
Frequency of use	
Fewer than 5 times	65 (9.0)
5-10 times	41 (5.7)
11-99 times	62 (8.6)
100+ times	61 (8.4)
Barbiturates	
Lifetime Prevalence	80 (11.1)
Frequency of use	
Fewer than 5 times	19 (2.6)
5-10 times	18 (2.5)
11-99 times	23 (3.2)
100+ times	21 (2.9)
Cough Syrup (not prescribed)	
Lifetime Prevalence	124 (17.2)
Frequency of use	
Fewer than 5 times	51 (7.0)
5-10 times	32 (4.4)
11-99 times	28 (3.9)
100+ times	12 (1.7)
GHB	
Lifetime Prevalence	13 (1.8)
Frequency of use	
Fewer than 5 times	9 (1.2)
5-10 times	1 (0.1)
11-99 times	3 (0.4)
100+ times	0 (0.0)
Heroin	
Lifetime Prevalence	47 (6.5)
Frequency of use	
Fewer than 5 times	23 (3.1)
5-10 times	12 (1.7)
11-99 times	7 (1.0)
100+ times	5 (0.7)
Inhalants	
Lifetime Prevalence	281 (38.9)
Specific Inhalant	
Air freshener	58 (8.0)

TABLE 3 (continued)

	N (%)
Butane	50 (6.9)
CO_2	65 (9.0)
Freon	44 (6.1)
Gasoline	159 (22.0)
Nail polish	61 (8.4)
Nitrous oxide	45 (6.2)
Paint	60 (8.3)
PC duster	106 (14.6)
Permanent marker	106 (14.6)
Spray paint	83 (11.5)
Whippets	44 (6.1)
White out	52 (7.2)
Ketamine	
Lifetime Prevalence	26 (3.6)
Frequency of use	
Fewer than 5 times	16 (2.2)
5-10 times	4 (0.5)
11-99 times	3 (0.4)
100+ times	4 (0.5)
Malt Liquor	
Lifetime Prevalence	359 (49.7)
Frequency of use	
Fewer than 5 times	69 (9.5)
5-10 times	66 (9.1)
11-99 times	117 (16.2)
100+ times	107 (14.8)
PCP	
Lifetime Prevalence	154 (21.3)
Frequency of use	
Fewer than 5 times	81 (11.2)
5-10 times	24 (3.3)
11-99 times	31 (4.3)
100+ times	17 (2.3)
Steroids	
Lifetime Prevalence	20 (2.8)
Frequency of use	
Fewer than 5 times	11 (1.5)
5-10 times	4 (0.5)
11-99 times	4 (0.5)
100+ times	1 (0.1)

[1] Note: Percentages displayed are for the total population, not the sub-sample that used each drug.

quency of use. For example, 436 (60.3%) youth reported using marijuana on more than 100 occasions in their lives. A wide variety of substances had lifetime prevalence rates between twenty and thirty percent (i.e., amphetamines, cocaine, ecstasy, hallucinogens, opiates, PCP prescription drugs without a prescription and tranquilizers).

Lifetime prevalence of inhalant use showed a concerning use pattern characterized by a wide variety of solvents use, particularly gasoline 159 (22%), "PC duster" 106 (14.6%), and permanent marker use 106 (14.6%). The lifetime prevalence of cough syrup to get high was a striking 124 (17.2%). The rates of barbiturate (11.1%) and heroin use (6.5%) were also concerning given the age of this population and the long-term addiction potential associated with these agents. When compared to national surveys such as the Monitoring the Future Study the rates found in this study are considerably higher than those reported by youth in the general population.

Age of First Use by Substance, Gender and Ethnicity

As shown in Table 4, the mean age for initiating use of cigarettes (10.6), marijuana (11.3), and alcohol (11.6) preceded the use of amphetamines, cocaine, opiates, prescription drugs and tranquilizers by approximately two years. The mean age for substance use initiation for males and females was similar (10.6 for males, 10.8 for females), non-statistically significant and negligible-to-small in magnitude ($d = .08$). In terms of ethnicity, the multi-ethnic/bi-racial and "other" categories initiated use of substances the earliest. African-Americans were the latest substance use initiating group ($M = 11.7$, $SD = 2.17$). Whites and Latinos/Latinas were similar at ages 10.1 and 10.0, respectively.

Lifetime Prevalence Rates by Geographic Region

Table 5 presents data on the geographic region of residence of the population of incarcerated youth. Youth from urban areas reported high rates of marijuana use and PCP (Phencyclidine) use. Overall, suburban youth reported the highest rates of substance use. For example, prevalence rates for suburban youth were the highest in the alcohol, amphetamine, cocaine, marijuana, opiates, and prescription drug categories. Youth from small towns reported the highest rate of tranquilizer use. Compared to suburban and small town youth, rural adolescents and urban youth reported the lowest rates of substance use. Perhaps reflecting availability of certain substances in geographic locals, significant be-

TABLE 4. Mean Age of First Use by Illicit Substance, Gender, and Ethnicity (N =723)

	M % (SD)
Substance	10.6 (2.62)
Cigarettes	11.3 (2.23)
Marijuana	11.6 (2.71)
Alcohol	13.4 (1.80)
Tranquilizers	13.5 (1.70)
Amphetamines	13.5 (1.58)
Opiates	13.6 (1.97)
Cocaine/Crack	13.6 (1.63)
Prescription drugs	14.3 (1.30)
Ecstacy	
Gender	10.6 (2.64)
Male	10.8 (2.53)
Female	
Ethnicity	11.7 (2.17)
African-American	10.1 (2.49)
White	10.0 (2.58)
Latino/Latina	9.95 (2.26)
Biracial or Multiethnic	9.36 (1.63)
Other	

tween group differences were found for amphetamines ($F = 6.38$, $p < .001$), ecstasy ($F = 6.02$, $p < .001$), marijuana ($F = 7.40$, $p < .001$), opiates ($F = 5.20$, $p < .001$), PCP ($F = 5.68$, $p < .001$) and tranquilizers ($F = 3.50$, $p < .05$). Analysis of Post Hoc tests reveals statistically significant mean differences between urban youth and small town youth with urban youth reporting less use of Opiates ($p = .005$), Tranquilizers ($p = .02$), and Amphetamines ($p = .001$). Ecstasy and PCP use, however, were higher for urban youth. There were also statistically significant differences between suburban and urban youth with respect to Amphetamines ($p = .02$), with suburban youth reporting greater prevalence of lifetime use. Finally, youth from rural or country areas reported significantly less mean lifetime use of Marijuana when compared to urban ($p = .001$) or suburban ($p = .001$) adolescents.

DISCUSSION AND IMPLICATIONS FOR POLICY AND PRACTICE

Lifetime prevalence of multiple forms of illicit substance use was extensive in the current study population. Further, significant differences

TABLE 5. Mean Lifetime Prevalence of Drug Use by Geographic Region[1]

	Mean % (SD)
Alcohol	
Total	(84.8) (.36)
Urban	(82.3) (.38)
Suburban	(92.0) (.27)
Small town	(85.3) (.35)
Rural or country area	(81.5) (.39)
Amphetamines*	
Total	(32.3) (.47)
Urban	(23.0) (.42)
Suburban	(40.0) (.49)
Small town	(38.5) (.49)
Rural or country area	(33.3) (.48)
Cigarettes	
Total	(85.5) (.35)
Urban	(84.1) (.37)
Suburban	(87.0) (.34)
Small town	(86.0) (.35)
Rural or country area	(87.0) (.34)
Cocaine or Crack Cocaine	
Total	(23.4) (.42)
Urban	(18.7) (.39)
Suburban	(31.0) (.46)
Small town	(25.2) (.43)
Rural or country area	(24.1) (.43)
Ecstasy*	
Total	(19.8) (.40)
Urban	(26.1) (.44)
Suburban	(24.0) (.43)
Small town	(13.6) (.34)
Rural or country area	(11.1) (.32)
Hallucinogens	
Total	(23.1) (.42)
Urban	(18.8) (.39)
Suburban	(31.0) (.46)
Small town	(24.1) (.43)
Rural or county area	(25.9) (.44)
Marijuana*	
Total	(86.6) (.34)
Urban	(90.5) (.29)
Suburban	(93.0) (.26)
Small town	(83.6) (.37)
Rural or country area	(70.4) (.46)
Opiates*	
Total	(32.2) (.47)
Urban	(24.0) (.43)
Suburban	(39.0) (.49)
Small town	(38.1) (.49)
Rural or country area	(31.5) (.47)

TABLE 5 (continued)

	Mean % (SD)
PCP***	
Total	(21.3) (.41)
Urban	(27.6) (.45)
Suburban	(25.0) (.44)
Small town	(16.1) (.37)
Rural or country area	(9.3) (.29)
Prescription Drugs	
Total	(21.3) (.41)
Urban	(17.3) (.38)
Suburban	(25.0) (.44)
Small town	(24.1) (.43)
Rural or country area	(20.4) (.41)
Tranquilizers*	
Total	(31.7) (.47)
Urban	(25.4) (.44)
Suburban	(30.0) (.46)
Small town	(37.8) (.49)
Rural or country area	(35.2) (.48)

[1] Includes major drugs of abuse.
Significant difference between groups (ANOVA) at $^*p < .05$, $^{**}p < .01$, $^{***}p < .001$.

were found by gender, ethnicity and geographic region. The co-occurrence of illegal behavior, drug use, and mental health disorders should raise serious concerns, both at social policy and practitioner levels, about the nature and treatment of multi-problem youth. These survey findings build on previous research on youth in jails and detention centers and provide compelling documentation that could prove useful to programmers and practitioners in the juvenile justice system.

These findings, however, are limited by a lack of multivariate tests as well as detailed information on the social contexts from which study youth emerged. For example, we have not examined these relationships between substance use and demographic factors while controlling for relevant covariates. Also, investigations that contain extensive family, peer, and neighborhood information would further clarify the relationships between patterns of substance use, mental health status and anti-social behavior. Future studies should also seek to follow youth at earlier points in time in order to examine the developmental sequences that influence the initiation and subsequent changes in substance use.

It appears that practitioners in juvenile justice settings can fruitfully apply screening measures and diagnostic testing to enhance substance abuse treatment. One way to do this is to employ screening measures such as the MAYSI-2 at intake and then assess youth who score above threshold levels with the self-administered computerized Diagnostic Interview Schedule for Children (DISC) for diagnostics (e.g., Wasserman et al., 2002). This type of approach is relatively both quick and inexpensive and may improve the overall efficiency of services to incarcerated youth. There is also evidence that assessment instruments can be usefully employed for incarcerated youth for the purpose of transitional planning into the community (Trupin, Turner, Stewart, & Wood, 2004). In addition, recent research has documented several interventions that can be useful for up to a year for adolescent substance abusers (Vaughn & Howard, 2004). Thus, there are evidence-based approaches that can potentially improve the lives of referred youth and improve the general service delivery to youth in need. It should be noted that these approaches should not take precedence over, but be delivered in tandem with, preventive interventions that can be employed at a much earlier juncture in time.

REFERENCES

Abram, K. M., Teplin, L. A., McClelland, G. M., & Dulcan, M. K. (2003). Comorbid psychiatric disorders in youth in juvenile detention. *Archives of General Psychiatry*, *60*, 1097-1108.

Cohen, J. (1988). *Statistical power for the behavioral sciences.* (2nd ed.) Hillsdale, NJ: L. Erlbaum Associates.

Cottle, C.C., Lee, R.J., & Heilbrun, K. (2001). The prediction of criminal recidivism in juveniles: A meta-analysis. *Criminal Justice and Behavior*, *29*, 367-394.

Dembo, R., Pacheco, K., Schmeidler, J., Fisher, L., & Cooper, S. (1997). Drug use and delinquent behavior among high risk youths. *Journal of Adolescent Substance Abuse*, *6*, 1-25.

Dembo, R., Williams, l., Fagan, J., & Schmeidler, J. (1993). The relationships of substance abuse and other delinquency over time in a sample of juvenile detainees. *Criminal Behaviour and Mental Health*, *3*, 158-179.

Derogatis, L.R. (1993). *Brief symptom inventory: Administration, scoring, and procedures manual.* Minneapolis, MN: National Computer Systems, Inc.

Derogatis, L. R., & Savitz, K. L. (2000). The SCL-90-R and brief symptom inventory (BSI) in primary care. In Maruish, M. E. (Ed.), *Handbook of Psychological Assessment in Primary Care Settings*, pp. 297-334, Mahwah, NJ: Lawrence Erlbaum Associates.

Elliott, D.S., Huizinga, D., & Menard, S. (1989). *Multiple problem youth: Delinquency, substance use, and mental health problems.* New York: Springer-Verlag.

Golub, A., & Johnson, B. D. (2001). *The rise of marijuana as the drug of choice among youthful adult arrestees.* Research in Brief. Washington DC: U.S. Department of Justice, National Institute of Justice.

Grisso, T., Barnum, R. (2000). *Massachusetts Youth Screening Instrumen-2: User's Manual and Technical Report.* Worcester MA: University of Massachusetts Medical School.

Grisso, T., Barnum, R., Fletcher, K. E., Cauffman, E., & peuschold, D. (2001). Massachusetts youth screening instrument for mental health needs of juvenile justice youths. *Journal of the American Academy of Child & Adolescent Psychiatry, 40,* 409-418.

Hando, J., Howard, J., & Zibert, E. (1997). Risky drug practices and treatment needs of youth detained in New South Wales juvenile justice centres. *Drug and Alcohol Review, 16,* 137-145.

Hawkins, J.D., Catalano, R.F., & Miller, J.Y. (1992). Risk and protective factors for alcohol and other drug problems in adolescence and early childhood: Implications for substance abuse prevention. *Psychological Bulletin, 112,* 64-105.

Huizinga, D., & Jakob-Chien, C. (19980. The contemporaneous co-occurrence of serious and violent juvenile offending and other problem behaviors. In R. Loeber, & D.P. Farrington (Eds.), *Serious and violent juvenile offenders: Risk factors and successful interventions.* (pp. 47-67). Thousand Oaks CA: Sage.

Huizinga, D., Loeber, R., Thornberry, T.P., & Cothern, L. (2000). Co-occurrence of delinquency and other problem behaviors. *Juvenile Justice Bulletin,* November. Washington DC: U.S. Department of Justice, Office of Justice Programs. Office of Juvenile Justice and delinquency Prevention.

Potter, C. C., & Jenson, J. M. (2003). Cluster profiles of multiple problem youth: Mental health problem symptoms, substance use, and delinquent conduct. *Criminal Justice and Behavior, 30,* 230-250.

Rounds-Bryant, J.L., Kristiansen, P.L., Fairbank, J.A., & Hubbard, R.L. (1998). Substance use, mental disorders, abuse, and crime: Gender comparisons among a national sample of adolescent drug treatment clients. *Journal of Child & Adolescent Substance Abuse, 7,* 19-34.

Sickmund, M. (2004). Juveniles in corrections. *Juvenile Offenders and Victims National report Series Bulletin.* Washington DC: U.S. Department of Justice, National Institute of Justice.

Stice, E., Myers, M.G., & Brown, S.A. (1998). Relations of delinquency to adolescent substance use and problem use: A prospective study. *Psychology of Addictive Behaviors, 12,* 136-146.

Teplin, L. (1990). The prevalence of severe mental disorder among male urban jail detainees: Comparison with the Epidemiological Catchment Area Program. *American Journal of Public Health, 80,* 663-669.

Teplin, L. (1994). Psychiatric and substance abuse disorders among male urban jail detainees. *American Journal of Public Health, 84,* 290-293.

Teplin, L.A., Abram, K.M., McClelland, G.M., Dulcan, M.K., & Mericle, A.A. (2002). Psychiatric disorders in youth in juvenile detention. *Archives of General Psychiatry, 59,* 1133-1143.

Thompson, L., Riggs, P., Mukilich, S., & Crowley, T. (1996). Contribution of ADHD symptoms to substance problems and delinquency in conduct disordered adolescents. *Journal of Abnormal Child Psychology, 24.* 325-347.

Trupin, E. W., Turner, A. P., Stewart, D., & Wood, P. (2004). Transition planning and recidivism among mentally ill juvenile offenders. *Behavioral Sciences and the Law, 22,* 599-610.

Van Kammen, W.B., Loeber, R., & Stouthamer-Loeber, M. (1991). Substance use and its relationship to conduct problems and delinquency in young boys. *Journal of Youth & Adolescence, 20,* 399-413.

Vaughn, M. G., & Howard, M. O. (2004). Adolescent substance abuse treatment: A synthesis of controlled evaluations. *Research on Social Work Practice, 14,* 325-335.

Vaughn, M. G., & Howard, M. O., & Curtis, M. P. (in press). Is ecstasy (MDMA) use associated with symptoms of anxiety or depression among incarcerated juvenile offenders? *Journal of Evidence-Based Social Work.*

Wasserman, G. A., McReynolds, L. S., Lucas, C. P., Fisher, P., Santos, L. (2002). The voice DISC-IV with incarcerated male youths: Prevalence of disorder. *Journal of the American Academy of Child & Adolescent Psychiatry, 41,* 314-318.

Zhang, L., Wieczorek, W.F., & Welte, J.W. (1997). The impact of age of onset of substance use on delinquency. *Journal of research on Crime & Delinquency, 34,* 253-268.

Primary Caregiver and Child Attachment: An Important Assessment Issue for Substance Use in African American and Hispanic Youth

Carolyn Hilarski, PhD

SUMMARY. This descriptive pilot study examined the relationship between African American and Hispanic youth's reported substance use and their perceived attachment with their primary caregiver. Thirty ($N = 30$) African American and Hispanic adolescents, age 14 through 17, were divided into two groups, those who reported using alcohol and/or drugs (n = 15) and those who did not (n = 15) The two groups were matched on race, age, gender, violence exposure, and community. Utilizing SPSS to conduct intercorelational and t-test analyses, the results showed that the African American and Hispanic youth who reported alcohol and/or drug use were significantly more likely to self-report greater problems in their primary caregiver relationships than those who did not. These findings suggest that assessment of family process is es-

Carolyn Hilarski is Assistant Professor, Social Work Department, College of Liberal Arts, Rochester Institute of Technology, 18 Lomb Memorial Drive, Rochester, NY 14623-5604 (E-mail: cxhgsw@rit.edu).

[Haworth co-indexing entry note]: "Primary Caregiver and Child Attachment: An Important Assessment Issue for Substance Use in African American and Hispanic Youth." Hilarski, Carolyn. Co-published simultaneously in *Journal of Evidence-Based Social Work* (The Haworth Social Work Practice Press, an imprint of The Haworth Press, Inc.) Vol. 2, No. 1/2, 2005, pp. 175-189; and: *Addiction, Assessment, and Treatment with Adolescents, Adults, and Families* (ed: Carolyn Hilarski) The Haworth Social Work Practice Press, an imprint of The Haworth Press, Inc., 2005, pp. 175-189. Single or multiple copies of this article are available for a fee from The Haworth Document Delivery Service [1-800-HAWORTH, 9:00 a.m. - 5:00 p.m. (EST). E-mail address: docdelivery@haworthpress.com].

Digital Object Identifier: 10.1300/J394v02n01_10

sential when a youth presents with substance use. Moreover, a universal prevention effort might entail incorporating healthy family process education as part of a preschool curriculum. *[Article copies available for a fee from The Haworth Document Delivery Service: 1-800-HAWORTH. E-mail address: <docdelivery@haworthpress.com> Website: <http://www.HaworthPress.com> © 2005 by The Haworth Press, Inc. All rights reserved.]*

KEYWORDS. Attachment, substance abuse, African American, Hispanic, adolescents

INTRODUCTION AND LITERATURE REVIEW

The yearly cost of substance use and abuse is estimated at two hundred fifty billion dollars to which alcohol issues consume a major portion. This appalling sum pays for prevention and social welfare efforts, health care costs, reduced productivity, and drug related crime (Martin, 2001).

For adolescents, alcohol continues to be the most popular mood altering substance used inside the United States, with 25% of thirteen-year-olds reporting alcohol use in the previous thirty days. This is a serious circumstance, since adolescents who begin drinking before the age of 15 are at great risk for an alcohol diagnosis sometime in their lifetime (Grant & Dawson, 1997).

The issue of illegal drug use among adolescents is relatively unchanged, as a significant portion of twelfth graders report using drugs each year (Johnston, O'Malley, & Backman, 2000a). To illustrate, marijuana continues to be a popular drug among teens, and although amphetamine, hallucinogen, and heroin use has remained steady, the use of ecstasy and steroids is increasing.

Substance use and abuse can have acute and chronic effects for adolescents. Most obvious is the development of addiction, which prevents optimal emotional, educational, physical, and social maturation. Although addiction may not be the universal outcome of adolescent alcohol or drug (AOD) use, for some, any use may have profound consequences, particularly, on the still developing body and mind (Battjes, Gordon, O'Grady, Kinlock, & Carswell, 2003).

Alcohol and/or drug use is one of the most common presenting issues in mental health services for children and adolescents (Santisteban, Perez-Vidal, Schwartz, & LaPerriere, 2003). Yet, there is no current empirical understanding of why this is so. One consistently emerging factor is the caregiver and child relationship (Brook, Richter, & Whiteman, 2000; Hadley, Holloway, & Mallinckrodt, 1993; Santisteban et al., 2003). Research finds that an essential element to healthy child development is a caregiver who is physically and emotionally available, from birth through adolescence (Brook, Whiteman, Balka, & Hamburg, 1992).

A connected relationship forms between the child and the primary caregiver during early infancy. The nature of this connection influences the child's self-concept, worldview, personality, and life-long relationships (Brook et al., 1992; Hadley et al., 1993). The youths' successful progress through the challenges of the life-span stages depends upon the child's perception of the caregiver and child bond or attachment. For example, Brook et al. (1992) found that a positive parent-child attachment was the basis for the child's development of traditional values. These values influence the youth's choices regarding the use of drugs and alcohol. Hoffman's (1993) research concurred finding that *attachment to the family* had both direct and indirect controls on the child's life path.

Attachment Theory

In the early twentieth century, researchers began to observe the effects of maternal deprivation on child development. They focused on the effects of prolonged institutional care, whether it was in hospital or in child-care institutions, and on frequent changes in primary caregivers during the early years of life. Two major views become apparent.

The first, drive theory, proposed that a stimulus pushes the individual to satisfy an instinctual need. Thus, a child's primary life sustaining need for food draws him/her to the primary caregiver, who additionally satisfies a secondary need for personal relationships. According to Freud's drive theory, infants and children love their primary caregiver because they have internalized them as the satisfiers of their basic needs (Taylor, 1956). In the United States, drive theory took the form of behaviorism or learning theory. This theory maintains that the association between the child's hunger, a primary need, and its satisfaction with food, the reinforcer, influences the relationship with the caregiver (Bowlby, 1958).

Bowlby (1956) observed that children separated from their caregivers developed what he called affectionless personalities. Moreover, a subgroup of these infants suffered from failure to thrive even though their basic biological needs were met. His conclusion was that the caregiver and child relationship was as important as the satisfaction of the basic needs of nutrition, clothing, and housing. From these observations, attachment theory was born.

Attachment theory proposes that individuals engage in biologically based behaviors meant to maintain or restore safety (Bowlby, 1958). From birth, a person is instinctively drawn to develop relationships with others in order to obtain protection, comfort, and support. These attachment relationships, depending upon the quality of the responsiveness of the attachment figure, influence the child's development, whether it is healthy or unhealthy. To illustrate, when the child's innate attachment seeking behavior is triggered by the experience of, for example, a threat, the primary caregiver's response is critical. A common perception of a threat would be hunger, discomfort because of temperature or pain, or an unfamiliar person or situation. If the caregiver's response to the infant's distress is sensitive, comforting, and helpful, the infant's anguish will reduce. If this is a consistent outcome, the child learns to trust the caregiver. When the child perceives that the caregiver is emotionally available to comfort, reassure, and intervene when necessary, the child has the confidence to engage in necessary self-esteem building exploratory activities. Thus, the caregiver serves as a secure base from which the child may investigate the world independently. This encourages interaction and trust building with others, which promotes differentiation and health (Cicchetti, Rogosch, & Toth, 1998).

When a youth is faced with an insensitive or rejecting primary caregiver, the child's internal working model of safety is distorted and emotional regulation is difficult and at times overwhelming (Cicchetti & Toth, 1998). Alcohol or drug use may be perceived as helpful with modifying these unwanted thoughts and emotions. Indeed, drug use may become a defense mechanism to reduce the anxiety associated with the thoughts related to fear of being out of control. Drugs literally take the place of the nurturing attachment by briefly altering the negative feelings related to the child's perception of the unworthy and unlovable self (Hadley et al., 1993).

Adolescent Alcohol and Drug Use and Attachment

There appears to be no single etiological factor for mood altering substance use or abuse. Some theoretical agreement focuses on the interacting influences of biology, psychology, and social variables (Marlatt, 1985). Yet, central to many human psychological disease theories is the mother and child relationship. The basic premise is that childhood experiences are associated with an understanding of the self and the environment, and this understanding influences the individual's developmental path. For example, agitated caregiver and child interactions that are perceived by the child as traumatic result in poor affect tolerance, self-regulation, and impoverished interpersonal relations, that, in due course, places the child at risk for substance abuse (Khantzian, 1980). Moreover, the caregiver and child relationship appears even more influential with Hispanic youth (Frauenglass, Routh, Pantin, & Mason, 1997). Although, Hispanic youth report drug use that is comparable to Caucasian youth, the influence of the caregiver and child relationship is greater with Hispanic youth (R.H. Coombs, Paulson, & Richardson, 1990).

Summary

A subgroup of children negotiate adolescence successfully. Others navigate this crucial developmental stage with great difficulty. The successful and not successful do not cluster around monetary, intellectual, social, or cultural lines. There are no unfailing predictors of how an adolescent will complete the journey to adulthood. However, attachment theory provides a persuasive explanation. Youth who do not feel bonded with their primary caregiver possess distorted internal working models, associated with low self-esteem. They also present with little adaptive functioning and poor impulse control, which influences their problem solving and mood regulating abilities in addition to affecting peer relationships (Grossmann, 1999). Youth not satisfactorily connected to a primary caregiver may perceive this circumstance as traumatic rejection and problem solve the issue by self-medicating with mood altering substances.

PURPOSE AND HYPOTHESES

This descriptive pilot study was interested in assessing, in an African American and Hispanic non-clinical convenience sample, if a relationship existed between the youth's alcohol and/or drug use and their perceived attachment with their primary caregiver.

The hypotheses were:

1. African American and Hispanic youths' attitude towards their primary caregiver is significantly associated with self-reported substance use.
2. African American and Hispanic youth who report substance use are significantly more likely to self-report greater problems with their primary caregiver relationship than those who do not.

It is vital to study factors associated with substance use in special populations. Especially in populations where substance use is highly associated with cultural and environmental stressors. Substance abuse has not been studied in a minority population with attachment theory as a guiding principle. The outcome will influence prevention intervention efforts. Additionally, the level of violence exposure found in these youth will add to previous findings.

METHODS

Participants

A convenience sample of 30 youth residing in an urban environment in upstate New York fulfilled this preliminary descriptive study. The participants ranged in age from 14 to 17 ($M = 15.93$, $SD = 1.11$). The sample included 16 females (53.3%) and 14 males (46.7%). The youth self identified as 80% African American, 10% Black-Hispanic, 3.3% Hispanic/White, 3.3% Puerto Rican, and 3.3% American Hispanic.

Instruments

Each participant completed, individually, a paper and pencil questionnaire that included a measure of satisfaction with their primary caregiver, alcohol and drug use, exposure to violence and loss, and demographic information. The survey took about 45 minutes.

The Child's Attitude Toward Mother (CAM) (Hudson, 1982) is a twenty-five item survey designed to measure the child's perception of satisfaction with his/her mother (primary caregiver) relationship. The survey offered seven responses, from 1 = none of the time to 7 = all of the time, with higher scores indicating greater relationship problems. Questions included "my mother gets on my nerves" and "I think my mother is terrific." The CAM has demonstrated discriminant validity by distinguishing between children with and without primary caregiver relationship problems. The one-week test-retest reliabilities ranged from .95 to .96 (Hudson, 1982, p. 1019). This study collapsed the responses to 1 = none of the time to a little of the time and 0 = some of the time to all of the time. Time and attention issues were a guiding force for this decision. The participants were also offered, "do not know" as a neutral response, which was calculated as zero. Summed scores offered continuous data.

Substance use was measured with the questions "Have you ever used alcohol?" and "Have you ever used drugs?" The responses offered were 'yes' = 1 or 'no' = 2, dichotomous data.

The Community Violence Survey (CVS) (Richters, 1993) examined the youth participants' exposure to neighborhood violence. This survey asked the participants to rate the frequency with which they experienced, witnessed, or heard about different violent acts in their neighborhood. An example question was, "Have you been shot by a gun?" yes = 1 or no = 0. Further questions included exposure to shootings, stabbings, sexual assault, muggings, drug deals, arrests by the police, murders, and suicides. Summed scores offered continuous data. This measure has been used with school-aged children residing in violent neighborhoods. A one-week test-retest reliability factor was estimated at .84 (Richters, 1993).

Procedures

A grass roots urban group intent on changing their neighborhood decided to begin their quest with assessing the thoughts and feelings of the local youth regarding their community. A pre-law college student and member of the community group, volunteered to do a field survey of two seventh grade classes from the local middle school. Permission was obtained from the school administrator and a teacher volunteered two of her classes for the dialogue. One of the questions posed to the class members was, *"What are some of your concerns about your neighborhood?"* The students' verbal responses were unanimous *"Drugs and violence."* The interviewer then asked *"What about drugs and violence?"* and the students' responses were, *"There are too many gangs and drive by shootings,"* *"No one cares,"* *"Everyone is doing drugs,"* in addition to several concerns that *"Family and friends will be hurt in some way because of the drugs and violence."*

The outcome of this limited field survey was a sense that adolescents in this community were feeling afraid and anxious. Moreover, the youth were thinking that it was normal to use drugs. Further, the youth were exposed to significant loss and violence and feeling that no one cared. The community group decided to obtain more information.

Two neighborhood youth and members of the grass roots organization volunteered to continue surveying the community youth. The volunteer adolescent surveyors (age 18 and 19) engaged in a 4-hour training process given by a local college professor trained in social science research. The surveyor training included role-play regarding how to respond to participant/parent questions about consent forms, what to expect regarding the survey, and potential participant questions during the survey. Additionally, education regarding all documentation, such as informed consent provided by parent and teen participants and how to complete the debriefing process and exit appraisal. Surveyors were provided with the telephone numbers of both a mental health practitioner and the youth participant's primary caregiver in case of an emergency. Moreover, youth surveyors were in weekly supervision contact with the university professor.

The surveyors canvassed the neighborhood for voluntary adolescent participants, living with one biological parent, over the course of three months in late 2003. Each potential participant was given a letter describing the study and the data collection procedures along with two copies of parent and youth informed consent forms. Adolescents (ages 14 through 17) with signed parental and youth informed consent forms were selected as participants. All of those youth contacted agreed to participate. The selected youth completed surveys, individually, during school hours at the middle school library. Participants were paid $10 for their time. All completed surveys were kept in a locked file cupboard in the school library. The university professor collected the surveys weekly during the supervision sessions.

Analysis

Descriptive analyses of the participants' demographic and characteristic data were completed (see Table 1). Each response to the substance use question went into one of two groups: Substance use and no substance use. The summed CAM and CVS scores were placed consecutively.

Pearson product correlation examined hypothesis one and an independent t test evaluated hypothesis two. Analysis was completed using the Statistical Package for the Social Sciences (SPSS) 11.5.

TABLE 1. Demographic and Descriptive Data (N = 30)

Age
14-15 years	23%
16-17 years	77%

Gender
Males	47%
Females	53%

Major Life Events (deaths, divorce, marriages, moves)
1-3 Events	63%
4	37%

Attend After School Program
Yes	37%
No	63%

Sent to Principal (in past year)
Never	67%
Sometimes	17%
Often	17%

Absent from School (in past year)
Never	40%
Sometimes	47%
Often	13%

Violence Exposures (ever)
1-15 events	53%
16+	47%

Gone to the Hospital (past year)
None	60%
1 or more times	40%

Youth Resided with:
Mother	100%

RESULTS

This descriptive pilot study investigated the relationship between African American and Hispanic adolescents' perceptions of their relationship problems with their primary caregiver and their reported substance use behavior.

Hypothesis 1 stated that the participant's attitude towards their relationship with their primary caregiver would be significantly associated with their self-reported substance use. Results of the correlational analyses presented in Table 2 showed that one of the six correlations was statistically significant supporting hypothesis one. Thus, it appeared that, in this small sample, there was a statistically significant relationship between reported substance use and perceived problem issues with the primary caregiver. Violence exposure was not significantly associated with substance abuse or child's relationship with primary caregiver.

From the surveys collected, two groups (see Table 3) were formed, a substance use group (n = 15) and no substance use group (n = 15). A follow up independent-samples t test evaluated if any significant differences in violence exposure existed between those youth who reported using alcohol or drugs (group one) and those who did not (group two). The test was not significant, $t(28) = -.591, p = .560$, meaning that both group one ($M = 14.33, SD = 5.72$) and group two ($M = 15.67, SD = 6.62$) reported, on average, similar community violence experiences.

A two-way contingency analysis was conducted to evaluate if demographic differences existed between groups one and two. The variables were race with two levels (African American = 1 and Hispanic = 2), gender with two levels (male = 1 and female = 2), and substance use with two levels (yes = 1 and no = 2). There were no significant differ-

TABLE 2. Intercorrelations Between Substance Use, CVS, and CAM Scores (N = 30)

Scales	1	2	3
(1) Substance Use	-		
(2) CVS	-.111	-	
(3) CAM	.458*	.123	-

*Correlation is significant at the .05 level (2-tailed)
Note. (CAM) Child's Attitude Toward Mother; (CVS) Community Violence Survey

TABLE 3. Group Demographics

	Group 1 (AOD use)	Group 2 (No AOD use)
Age		
14-15 years	(2) 13%	(5) 33%
16-17 years	(13) 73%	(10) 67%
Race		
African American	(15) 100%	(12) 80%
Hispanic		(3) 20%
Gender		(6) 40%
Male	(8) 53%	
Female	(7) 47%	(9) 60%

ences between group one and group two regarding race X^2 $(1, N = 30) =$ .536, $p = .464$ or gender X^2 $(1, N = 30) = 3.33, p = .07$.

A paired samples t-test was used to evaluate if there were differences between the two groups regarding age. The results indicated that the mean age in group one ($M = 16.00$, $SD = .925$) was not significantly different from the mean age in group two ($M = 15.87$, $SD = 1.30$), (t (28) = .323, $p = .749$. Thus, both groups were not significantly different regarding age, race, or gender variables. All of the participants lived in the same community.

The results of an independent-samples t test to evaluate hypothesis two that African American and Hispanic youth who reported alcohol and/or drug use were significantly more likely to self-report greater problems in their primary caregiver relationships than those who did not was significant, t (28) = 2.73, $p = .011$. The mean CAM score in group one ($M = 14.27$, $SD = 2.02$) was greater that the mean CAM score in group two ($M = 12.00$, $SD = 2.51$).

DISCUSSION

The main findings of this descriptive pilot study support previous research (Bell, Forthun, & Sun, 2000; Brennan & Shaver, 1995; Brook et al., 2000) that the primary caregiver and youth relationship is an influencing factor in whether the youth chooses to use alcohol or drugs. Adolescents who described their primary caregiver as trustworthy, patient, and understanding were significantly less likely to report mood-altering substance use in comparison to youth who described their primary caregiver as unresponsive, critical, or over or under protective. The youth's preferences regarding their caregiver relate to attachment theory, which guided and is supported by this research.

Limitations

There were several limitations in this pilot study. First, there was a selection threat to internal validity as the participants were volunteers. Second, the use of self-report instruments increased the possibility that questioned events or experiences were over or underestimated or imprecise through recall or gender influences. Third, the small sample size decreased the reliability of the outcome. Additionally, the sample was primarily African American and living in an urban environment. Thus, the results are not generalizable to other racial and ethnic groups or other types of environments. Finally, there was a social interaction threat. Data collection took place over a three-month period leaving the opportunity for participants and potential participants to talk to one another about the survey and their responses to the survey.

Implications for Practice

These findings and confirmation in future studies will have important clinical implications. Since the primary caregiver and child relationship heavily influences the child's personality and the child's personality and relationship with the primary caregiver is associated with substance use, early family assessment is essential. If a family disturbance is found, an early prevention effort that includes restructuring of the family dynamics is essential. However, a family intervention is helpful at any place along the continuum when substance use and family disruption is present (Santisteban et al., 2003).

A brief strategic/structural family therapy (BSFT) model is effective, especially with African American and Hispanic youths, although, researchers believe it is a helpful model for all ethnic groups (Santisteban et al., 1997). In Hispanic families where caregiver influence appears to be strong, research revealed that Hispanic participants who reported satisfying relationships with their caregivers were less involved with mood-altering substance use and less influenced by substance using peers (Coombs, Paulson, & Richardson, 1991).

The BSFT model conceptualizes a family as a complex system of interdependent members who mutually influence the behaviors of one another through interactions. Within the family system, interdependent interactions tend to recur and create repetitive patterns that actually define the 'structure' of the family (Santisteban et al., 2003). These repetitive interactive patterns are essential in the developmental adjustment of family members and basic to the etiology and maintenance of pathology in the system (Frauenglass et al., 1997). BSFT focuses on helping the family members to first recognize problematic behavior, then, to problem solve the issue through 'win-win' negotiations. The earlier the intervention is implemented in families with unhelpful structures and processes, the better the outcome (Santisteban et al., 2003).

In changing family interactions, the BSFT therapist will work in the 'here and now' and focus on observable family exchanges. Restructuring is one element of this model and entails working with boundaries and alliances in order to establish the caregiver as the leader of the family and discourage inappropriate alliances that may exist between care-giver and child.

Further therapeutic work involves *individual healing*, with an object relations underpinning. This prevention effort may coexist with family therapy. The goals of this intervention relate to changing the youth's un-helpful internal scheme. The adolescent is encouraged to integrate the inner identification of the self with a more realistic frame. In addition, the work of differentiating from the *object* is necessary for ego building. This will support the youth for the demands of the family work (Hadley et al., 1993).

Future Research

The preliminary findings in this study suggest that further research is essential with sample sizes large enough to sustain conclusions. Additionally, all of the youth in this study reported significant exposure to loss and community violence, yet chose to deal with their trauma differently. This study suggests that this 'difference' is related to the primary caregiver and child relationship. Perhaps this is due to gener- ational transmission, as the primary caregiver's perception of the *self and world* is conveyed to the child (Cicchetti & Aber, 1998; Figley, 1989). In any case, future studies might engage in an in-depth examination of the family structure and process. This would be helpful in furthering our understanding of why youth choose different paths. It would also help to fine tune and empirically evaluate a family prevention effort. Additionally, future research may want to compare peer group prevention with family prevention efforts, as, in some instances, peer groups appear to increase dysfunctional behavior in youth (Dishion, McCord, & Poulin, 1999).

REFERENCES

Battjes, R. J., Gordon, M. S., O'Grady, K. E., Kinlock, T. W., & Carswell, M. A. (2003). Factors that predict adolescent motivation for substance abuse treatment. *Journal of Substance Abuse Treatment, 24*(3), 221-232.

Bell, N. J., Forthun, L. F., & Sun, S. W. (2000). Attachment, adolescent competencies, and substance use: Developmental considerations in the study of risk behaviors. *Substance Use & Misuse, 35*(9), 1177-1206.

Bowlby, J. (1958). The nature of the child's tie to his mother. *International Journal of Psychoanalysis, 39*(Sept/Oct), 350-373.

Bowlby, J. (1978). Attachment theory and its therapeutic implications. *Adolescent Psychiatry, 6*(5-33).

Brennan, K. A., & Shaver, P. R. (1995). Dimensions of adult attachment, affect regulation, and romantic relationship functioning. *Personality and Social Psychology Bulletin, 21*(3), 267-283.

Brook, J. S., Richter, L., & Whiteman, M. (2000). Effects of parent personality, upbringing, and marijuana use on the parent-child attachment relationship. *Journal of American Academy of Child Adolescent Psychiatry, 39*(2), 240-248.

Brook, J. S., Whiteman, M., Balka, E. B., & Hamburg, B. A. (1992). African American and Peurto Rican drug use: Personality, familial, and other environmental risk factors. *Genetic, Social, and General Psychology Monographs, 118*(4), 47-438.

Cicchetti, D., & Aber, J. L. (1998). Contextualism and developmental psychopathology [editorial]. *Developmental Psychopathology, 10*(2), 137-141.

Cicchetti, D., Rogosch, F. A., & Toth, S. L. (1998). Maternal depressive disorder and contextual risk: Contributions to the development of attachment insecurity and behavior problems in toddlerhood. *Developemental Psychopathology, 10*(2), 283-300.

Cicchetti, D., & Toth, S. L. (1998). The development of depression in children and adolescents. *American Psychology, 53*(2), 221-241.

Constantino, J. N. (1995). Early relationships and the development of aggression in children. *Harvard Review Psychiatry, 2*(5), 259-273.

Coombs, R. H., Paulson, M. J., & Richardson, M. A. (1990). Peer vs. parental influence in substance use among Hispanic and Anglo children and adolescents. *Journal of Youth & Adolescence, 20*(1), 73-88.

Coombs, R. H., Paulson, M. J., & Richardson, M. A. (1991). Peers vs. parental influences in substance use among Hispanic and Anglo children and adolescents. *Journal of Youth & Adolescence, 20*(1), 73-88.

Dishion, T. J., McCord, J., & Poulin, F. (1999). When interventions harm: Peer groups and problem behavior. *American Psychologist, 54*, 755-764.

Figley, C. R. (1989). *Helping traumatized families.* San Francisco, CA, U.S.: Jossey-Bass Inc, Publishers.

Frauenglass, S., Routh, D. K., Pantin, H. M., & Mason, C. A. (1997). Family support decreases influence of deviant peers on Hispanic adolescents' substance use. *Journal of Clinical & Child Psychology, 26*(1), 15-23.

Grant, B. F., & Dawson, D. A. (1997). Age at onset of alcohol use and its association with DSM-IV alcohol abuse and dependence: Results from the National Longitudinal Alcohol Epidemiologic Survey. *Journal of Substance Abuse, 9*, 103-110.

Grossmann, K. E. (1999). Old and new internal working models of attachment: The organization of feelings and language. *Attach Human Developement, 1*(3), 253-269.

Hadley, J. A., Holloway, E. L., & Mallinckrodt, B. (1993). Common aspects of object relations and self-representations in offspring from disparate dysfunctional families. *Journal of Counseling Psychology, 40*(3), 348-356.

Hudson, W. W. (1982). A measurement package for clinical social workers. *Journal of Applied Behavioral Science, 18*(2), 229-238.

Johnston, L. D., O'Malley, P. M., & Backman, J. G. (2000a). *National survey results on drug use from the monitoring the future study, 1975-1999.* Rockville, MD: U.S. Department of Health and Human Services.

Khantzian, E. J. (1980). An ego/self theory of substance dependence: A contemporary psychoanalytic perspective. *NIDA Res Monogr, 30*, 29-33.

Marlatt, G. A. (1985). *Relapse prevention: Theoretical rational and overview of the model.* New York: Guilford Press.

Martin, S. E. (2001). The links between alcohol, crime and the criminal justice system: explanations, evidence and interventions. *American Journal of Addiction, 10*(2), 136-158.

Richters, J. E. (1993). Community violence and children's development: Toward a research agenda for the 1990s. *Psychiatry, 56*(1), 3-6.

Santisteban, D. A., Coatsworth, D. J., Perez-Vidal, A., Mitrani, V., Jean-Gilles, M., & Szapocznik, J. (1997). Brief structural/strategic family therapy with African and Hispanic high risk youth. *Journal of Community Psychology, 25*(5), 453-472.

Santisteban, D. A., Perez-Vidal, A., Schwartz, S. J., & LaPerriere, A. (2003). Efficacy of brief strategic family therapy in modifying Hispanic adolescent behavior problems and substance abuse. *Journal of Family Psychology, 17*(1), 121-134.

Taylor, J. A. (1956). Drive theory and manifest anxiety. *Psychol Bull, 53*(4), 303-320.

Zeanah, C. H. (1996). Beyond insecurity: A reconceptualization of attachment disorders of infancy. *Journal of Consult Clinical Psychology, 64*(1), 42-52.

Defining Relapse
from a Harm Reduction Perspective

Katie Witkiewitz, MA, PhC

SUMMARY. In the treatment of addictions, engaging in any substance use following treatment is often viewed as a treatment failure. This paper provides theoretical and empirical support for a harm reduction approach to the evaluation of treatment outcomes. Such an approach focuses on consequences associated with the post-treatment drinking, without using rigid definitions of "success" or "failure." Harm reduction approaches to alcohol treatment are introduced and recommendations for future research and social work practice are provided. *[Article copies available for a fee from The Haworth Document Delivery Service: 1-800-HAWORTH. E-mail address: <docdelivery@haworthpress.com> Website: <http://www. HaworthPress.com> © 2005 by The Haworth Press, Inc. All rights reserved.]*

KEYWORDS. Relapse, alcohol treatment, harm reduction, relapse prevention, treatment outcomes

Katie Witkiewitz is affiliated with the Addictive Behaviors Research Center, University of Washington, Department of Psychology, Seattle, WA 98195 (E-mail: kate19@ u.washington.edu).

This research was supported by National Institute of Alcohol Abuse and Alcoholism Grant R21 AA013942-01.

[Haworth co-indexing entry note]: "Defining Relapse from a Harm Reduction Perspective." Witkiewitz, Katie. Co-published simultaneously in *Journal of Evidence-Based Social Work* (The Haworth Social Work Practice Press, an imprint of The Haworth Press, Inc.) Vol. 2, No. 1/2, 2005, pp. 191-206; and: *Addiction, Assessment, and Treatment with Adolescents, Adults, and Families* (ed: Carolyn Hilarski) The Haworth Social Work Practice Press, an imprint of The Haworth Press, Inc., 2005, pp. 191-206. Single or multiple copies of this article are available for a fee from The Haworth Document Delivery Service [1-800-HAWORTH, 9:00 a.m. - 5:00 p.m. (EST). E-mail address: docdelivery@haworthpress.com].

The average yearly expenditure on alcohol treatment in the United States is roughly $5.5 billion, and the overall economic cost of alcohol abuse and dependence is estimated to be greater than $184.6 billion (Harwood, 2000). Approximately 2.2 million Americans receive alcohol treatment each year (National Institute of Alcohol Abuse and Alcoholism, NIAAA, 1998) and it is estimated that 17.6 million Americans meet criteria for alcohol abuse or dependence (Grant, Dawson, Stinson, Chou, Dufour, & Pickering, 2004). Based on these estimates if the United States government spent the same amount (approximately $2,500 per person) for all individuals actually needing treatment (approximately 17 million) then the average expenditure would be $42.5 billion dollars. These staggering estimates have sparked the development of alternative, less expensive, forms of alcohol treatment (e.g., Fleming, Barry, Manwell, Johnson, & London, 1997), but engaging individuals in treatment remains a greater problem.

Alcohol dependent individuals may resist treatment for any number of reasons (e.g., financial, time-commitment, treatment access), but the most often cited reasons include the self-perception that their drinking is not a problem, the stigma and embarrassment of being called an "alcoholic," and negative attitudes toward treatment (Cunningham, Sobell, Sobell, Agrawal, & Toneatto, 1993; Sobell, Sobell, Toneatto, & Leo, 1993). Not wanting to quit drinking and resistance to abstinence based treatments may also present a barrier to individuals who otherwise would seek treatment for their problem drinking (Humphreys & Klaw, 2001).

Considering most individuals who need alcohol treatment do not receive services and many who do receive treatment do not maintain treatment goals, it is imperative that addiction practitioners, educators, policy makers, and program administrators work towards the goal of improving treatment engagement, retention, and outcomes. The current article provides an overview of relapse following alcohol treatment and how harm reduction approaches may help the addiction field move closer to this goal. First, data is presented on relapse rates and treatment outcomes, highlighting the importance of defining treatment outcomes from a harm reduction perspective. Second, relapse prevention, as a harm reduction approach to alcohol treatment, is introduced. Third, a conceptualization of relapse as a dynamic process is presented. Finally, recommendations for future research and social work practice are provided.

RELAPSE AND DEFINITION OF TREATMENT OUTCOMES

One of the major problems with treatment for addictive behaviors is the high rates of relapse to substance use (Hunt, Barnett, & Branch, 1971). Relapse has been defined as the process in which an individual who is attempting to change a behavior experiences a set-back leading to the resumption of the target behavior (Marlatt, 1985; Witkiewitz & Marlatt, 2004). Within the relapse process, a lapse is defined as an initial setback (e.g., a discrete drinking episode) and a prolapse is defined as the return to the goal behavior (abstinence or moderate drinking) following an episode of drinking. A finding that has been consistently identified in both the research and clinical literature is that lapses are the modal outcome for patients with alcohol dependence (Connors, Maisto, & Zywiak, 1996).

Litman (1986) described alcoholism as a "relapsing condition," and the empirical research supports this conception. Investigations conducted within the last decade have found relapse rates ranging from 28% to 86% (Cooney, Litt, Morse, Bauer, & Guapp, 1997; Greenfield, Hufford, Vagge, Muenz, Costello, & Weiss, 1998; Hall, Havassy, & Wasserman, 1990; Rychtarik, Prue, Rapp, & King, 1992; Solomon & Annis, 1990). The wide discrepancy in relapse rates across studies has been attributed to operational definitions of "relapse," ranging from "any drinking" to "heavy drinking" to "alcohol related consequences" (Maisto, Pollock, Cornelius, Lynch, & Martin, 2003). These definitions of relapse impact treatment goals, the likelihood of success, and predictive validity. Maisto and colleagues (2003) found that the "any drinking" definition of relapse at 6 months following treatment was less predictive of 12-month outcomes (drinking quantity and frequency) than were less stringent definitions of relapse (e.g., heavy drinking or drinking related consequences). Based on the "any drinking" definition the majority of the sample (74%) relapsed and the time to relapse was the shortest (median = 26 days) as compared to the other definitions of relapse. Therefore, this investigation demonstrated that using the "any drinking" definition provides a dismal view of treatment outcome and ignores important variability in drinking quantity, frequency, and consequences.

The relationship between treatment goals and relapse definitions is inherently intertwined. If a treatment program is abstinence-based, then any transgression may be viewed negatively, which may actually lead to an increase in the problematic behavior. This phenomenon, called the abstinence violation effect (Marlatt, 1985), is the negative attribution associated with the violation of self-imposed rules. Oftentimes individuals who attempt to change a target behavior set unrealistically high goals and when they are unable to achieve such standards tend to give-up on any change in the targeted direction (Polivy & Herman, 2002).

Abstinence as the sole indicator of treatment success limits the ability of professionals and their clients to accurately assess treatment gains in the direction of abstinence. Furthermore, in some populations (e.g., adolescents) the chances of achieving an abstinence goal are very slim (Maisto et al., 2003). Based on a stages of change model (Prochaska & DiClemente, 1984), individuals who are not prepared to quit drinking are not likely to engage in or experience success in abstinence-based treatments.

Nonetheless, many treatment programs and the Alcoholics Anonymous literature require abstinence goals and tend to be focused on the notion that having one drink following a period of abstention is indicative of failure. Making this assumption, the Alcoholics Anonymous website, states: "So far as can be determined, no one who has become an alcoholic has ever ceased to be an alcoholic. The mere fact of abstaining from alcohol for months or even years has never qualified an alcoholic to drink "normally" or socially . . . For the alcoholic, one drink of alcohol in any form is likely to be too much" (http://www.alcoholics-anonymous.org, last accessed April 27th, 2004).

The hypothesis that "one drink makes a drunk" was recently empirically tested using data from a large sample (n = 563) of alcohol dependent individuals who received a variety of community-based treatments (data obtained from the National Institute of Alcohol Abuse and Alcoholism-Relapse Replication and Extension Project; Lowman, Allen, Stout, & Relapse Research Group, 1996). Self-reported drinking behavior was assessed monthly for twelve months following completion of treatment. Using these data Witkiewitz (2004) investigated the individual variation in drinking quantity and frequency by modeling the within-and between-person drinking trajectories over time. Figure 1 provides a visual representation of the individual changes in drinking over the 12-month follow-up, with each line representing a person in the dataset. The Y-axis is the frequency of drinking at each time-point, as measured by percentage of days abstinent (with 100% indicating the person never drank and 0% indicating the person drank every day in the month). As shown in Figure 1, the drinking trajectories were highly variable between individuals at each time-point and within individuals across time.

Latent growth mixture modeling, a longitudinal modeling technique that combines continuous and discrete latent variables (see Muthen, 2001; Muthen & Shedden, 1999), was used to model the individual variation in post-lapse drinking trajectories. Essentially, latent growth mixture modeling can be used to cluster individuals with similar drinking into "latent classes" of drinking trajectories. In this study the heterogeneity in drinking trajectories could be summarized using four common drinking trajectories. As shown in Figure 2, each line represents the identified latent class trajectories, and the percentages indicate the number of individuals classified into that trajectory class. The four classes could be described as: (1) a small group (11%) of continuously heavy drinkers; (2) a small group (12%) of drinkers who initially drank heavily and then returned to abstinence or light drinking; (3) a small

FIGURE 1. Individual drinking trajectories for the first 12 months following treatment.

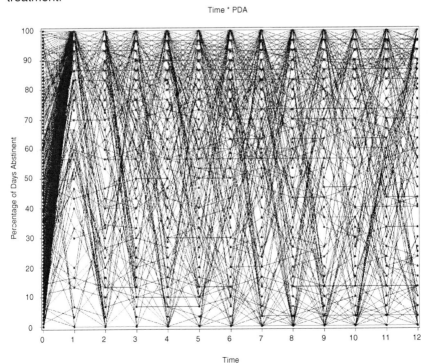

group (13%) of moderate to moderately-heavy drinkers; and (4) a large group (64%) of light drinkers and abstainers.

Contradicting the historical view of relapse and the assumption of Alcoholics Anonymous, the return to heavy drinking was not the most common outcome. Rather, the findings demonstrated initial lapses followed by a return to abstinence (prolapse) was the rule, not the exception.

Based on Witkiewitz (2004), it is not accurate to assume that a return to heavy drinking is the most common outcome following treatment for an alcohol use disorder. Rather, for the majority of individuals "one drink does not necessarily make a drunk" and a variety of drinking goals (including light and moderate drinking) are achievable. Many of the individuals in the Relapse Replication and Extension Project experienced a significant decrease in drinking related consequences and most were capable of either abstinence or light and moderate drinking.

FIGURE 2. Four trajectory classes for percentage of days abstinent.

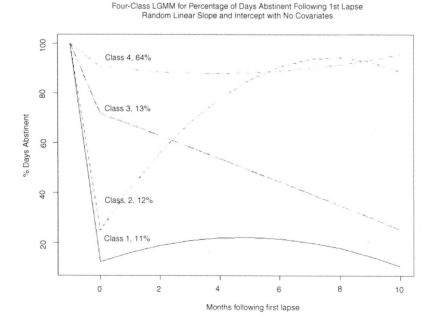

APPROACHES TO ALCOHOL TREATMENT

Considering alternatives to abstinence goals and letting clients select their own drinking goals may be threatening for some practitioners, as it may seem that supporting a non-abstinent goal encourages drinking. On the contrary, the data suggests that when provided the opportunity to self-select treatment goals an individual is likely to choose abstinence goals or move from moderation to abstinence goals during the course of treatment (Hodgins, Leigh, Milne, & Gerrish, 1997). Further, non-confrontational, client-focused approaches to alcohol treatment have demonstrated efficacy in controlled trials, particularly when delivered as a brief intervention (Miller & Wilbourne, 2002). A series of meta-analyses conducted by Miller and colleagues (Miller, Andrews, Wilbourne, & Bennett, 1998; Miller & Wilbourne, 2002) identified cognitive, behavioral, and motivational approaches as the most effective treatments; whereas mandatory Alcoholics Anonymous attendance, confrontational approaches, and milieu therapy were identified as the least effective treatments. In addition, these treatments tend to be the least desirable options among individuals with alcohol use disorders.

From the perspective of client preference, harm reduction approaches tend to be preferred over mandatory and/or confrontational treatments (Marlatt & Witkiewitz, 2002). Harm reduction is solely designed to meet an individual "where he/she is at" and develop treatment strategies based on the motivation, strengths and limitations of each client. For example consider an individual who is drinking heavily four nights a week, not willing to quit drinking, and most concerned about hangovers resulting in poor performance at work. From a harm reduction perspective the practitioner might work with the client toward a goal of not drinking on work nights. This is not to say that abstinence is ruled out for this particular client, rather it is not identified as a primary treatment goal. Further, the definition of treatment outcome would be based on the client's frequency of drinking on work nights, hangovers, and subsequent performance at work. If the individual is successful at meeting this goal then other consequences or patterns of use could become the focus of treatment. Ideally clients will change their drinking behavior in such a way as to reduce and eliminate all drinking-related consequences.

One specific harm reduction approach, relapse prevention, has received considerable empirical support in the treatment of addictive and non-addictive behaviors (Carroll, 1996; Irvin, Bowers, Dunn, & Wang,

1999; Witkiewitz & Marlatt, 2004). Originally developed as an aftercare approach to help clients maintain treatment goals and manage lapses following treatment for an alcohol use disorders (Marlatt & Gordon, 1985), relapse prevention has become a popular adjunct to many empirically-supported treatments. The primary focus of relapse prevention is to classify high risk situations, which can include any situation that increases an individual's likelihood of engaging in the identified problem behavior (e.g., heavy drinking), and then provide a number of cognitive and behavior strategies for reducing a person's susceptibility to relapse in those situations (Marlatt & Gordon, 1985). Either abstinence or moderation goals are encouraged and supported, but they are not the main focus of the intervention.

Using relapse prevention techniques for the client described in the example provided above, the practitioner and client would work collaboratively to determine what situations precede heavy drinking on work nights. The client may identify several specific situations (e.g., sporting events, social engagements, stressful day at work) and/or general situations (e.g., depressed mood, being alone, feeling anxious). Each individual's high-risk situations may differ; but there are some commonly identified situations that are risky for most individuals trying to abstain from alcohol. Marlatt and Gordon (1985) developed a detailed taxonomy of high-risk situations based on eight subcategories of relapse determinants that were identified by recovering alcoholics who experienced a relapse following treatment. These relapse determinants included: coping with negative emotional states, coping with negative physical-psychological states, enhancement of positive-emotional states, testing personal control, giving in to temptations and urges, coping with interpersonal conflict, social pressure, and enhancement of positive emotional states.

Recently, Witkiewitz, and Marlatt (2004) have re-conceptualized these relapse determinants into a dynamic model of the relapse process. Shown in Figure 3, it is proposed that lapses occur within a system of interacting risk factors.

Tonic and phasic processes (the circles) operate during a high-risk situation. Tonic processes include those factors that a person carries wherever he/she goes: These factors are present at the start of treatment and they are present at the end of treatment. Some examples of factors operating within a tonic process include: family history of alcoholism (e.g., genetic factors), age at the time of the first drink, and number of years the person was dependent on alcohol prior to treatment. Phasic processes include precipitating factors that can be highly dynamic and

FIGURE 3. Dynamic model of relapse.

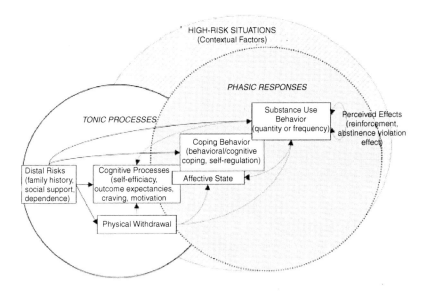

unpredictable, such as coping skills, affective states, motivation, craving, and perceived effects of using alcohol. Factors operating within a phasic process are often amenable to change and provide important targets for treatment.

Putting it all together, it is proposed that several interacting and compounding factors are operating within high-risk situations, creating a complex system of risk factors and behavioral responses where small changes in risk correspond to large changes in drinking behavior. Following from the example above, if the client has a stressful day at work and then attends a dinner party with his/her coworkers (a high-risk situation), the increase in stress may trigger a reduction in coping efficacy. The person then uses an ineffective coping response (e.g., going to the bar to get away from co-workers in the dining room), which increases his/her probability of drinking (Rabois & Haaga, 2003).

As made clear by this example, relapse is complex. Working with the client to identify high-risk situations and teaching skills for dealing with those situations will decrease the probability of lapses and may reduce the severity of a lapse, when a lapse does occur. If the client described above recognized that sitting at the bar was an ineffective coping response either before or after his/her first drink, then the likelihood of a major drinking episode followed by a hangover is decreased. However, if the client is only prepared to "not drink," then being in the bar to get away from co-workers may actually increase the client's level of stress by decreasing abstinence self-efficacy (the individual's belief in their ability abstain). If the client does have a drink and experiences the abstinence violation effect, then he/she is more likely to continue drinking heavily, which will be followed by a hangover and poor performance at work. Poor performance may cause the client to have a stressful day at work, and the cycle of relapse proneness begins again.

Recent work by our lab provides empirical support for a complex systems approach to understanding post-treatment drinking behavior (Hufford, Witkiewitz, Shields, Kodya, & Caruso, 2003; Witkiewitz, 2004; Witkiewitz & Marlatt, in press). Using statistical methods derived from catastrophe theory (Thom, 1975), a subset of nonlinear dynamical systems theory that attempts to model the discontinuous changes in behavior resulting from continuous changes in the parameters controlling the system, we have been able to quantify small, continuous differences in risk level that correspond to large, discontinuous differences in the quantity and frequency of post-treatment drinking.

Consider the following example, an individual who scores a 15 (on a 20-point depression scale) reports drinking 8 drinks per night, a second person who scores a 15 reports drinking only 1 drink per night, a third person who scores a 14 reports drinking 3 drinks per night, whereas a fourth individual who scores a 12 reports drinking 12 drinks per night. The relationship between depression scores and drinking is discontinuous: The same level of depression corresponds with large differences in drinking for the four individuals. Catastrophe theory is uniquely suited for these data, because the model seeks to identify discontinuous relationships between variables. Several risk factors (i.e., coping, negative affect, self-efficacy, abstinence violation effect, distal risk, outcome expectancies) from the dynamic model of relapse (Figure 3), have been shown to predict discontinuous drinking behavior in individuals who have received treatment for their alcohol use disorder (Witkiewitz, 2004; Witkiewitz & Marlatt, in press). Together these studies provide empirical evidence for a conceptualization of relapse as a complex process.

DEFINITIONS OF RELAPSE:
IMPLICATIONS FOR PRACTICE

Provided the definition of relapse as a complex system and given the range of drinking trajectories following alcohol treatment, it seems impractical to assume a single treatment goal (e.g., abstinence) will be appropriate for all individuals. Instead, practitioners are encouraged to consider individualized definitions of relapse that incorporate a harm reduction perspective and that account for the myriad of problems operating for each client. From this world view, reductions in drinking frequency and quantity or increasing skills for avoiding risky drinking behaviors are possible ways of defining successful treatment outcomes. Abstinence is still considered as a possible treatment goal and clinicians should encourage abstinence goals for clients who have a long history of heavy drinking, severe alcohol dependence, and/or numerous failed treatment attempts. Also, clients who are pregnant or have a health condition (e.g., Korsakoff's syndrome or chronic liver disease) that makes drinking harmful should be directed toward abstinence goals.

Realistically, individuals are struggling with dynamic and powerful instigators to drink. As treatment providers, it is possible that the best service we can offer is a supportive, pragmatic, and compassionate approach to reducing consequences associated with problem drinking. To this end, researchers and practitioners should remain open to various definitions of treatment outcomes and be prepared to work within the world view of each client. Within this flexible approach clients are encouraged to select treatment goals based on their own strengths, limitations, and motivational readiness (Miller & Rollnick, 2002).

Case example: A recent client described a period of her life in which she was successful at moderate drinking (reducing her alcohol consumption to 12 drinks per week). When I started seeing this client she was drinking four glasses of wine every night and she was unemployed. She presented to treatment with the initial goal of drinking no more than 12 drinks, but after the first week she decided to pursue a completely sober lifestyle. Every week we started the session with her describing how she was "so good" for the first few days, but then failed and drank again. After several failed attempts at abstinence we worked with her initial goal of drinking less than 12 drinks per week. Tapping into her motivation for reducing her drinking in order to obtain permanent employment, we identified high-risk situations that lead to drinking more than 12 drinks per week. We worked on drink refusal skills and I provided the client with meditation exercises she could use to reconnect herself with her goal of obtaining employment (e.g., imagining she is sitting in her new office looking out the window). After two months the client was employed part-time and drinking 6 glasses of wine per week on weekend evenings and abstaining during the work week. If we had defined relapse as "any drinking" then this client might have continued to be unsuccessful throughout the two months of treatment, or even worse, dropped out of treatment all together.

Harm reduction, a pragmatic and humanistic approach to alcohol treatment, is becoming increasingly popular in the field of social work (Brocato & Wagner, 2003; MacMaster, 2004; Seiger, 2003). By definition, as care professionals devoted to facilitating positive social changes and promoting well-being, social workers are more likely to embrace harm reduction approaches than other alcohol treatment professionals. The National Association of Social Workers (NASW) has endorsed harm reduction in many areas, including drug and alcohol treatment, needle exchange programs, and comprehensive HIV programs for IV drug users (NASW, 2000). Further, harm reduction practices are consistent with the basic values, ethical principles, and ethical standards of social workers (NASW, 1999). According to the Self-Determination ethical standard:

> Social workers respect and promote the right of clients to self-determination and assist clients in their efforts to identify and clarify their goals. Social workers may limit clients' right to self-determination when, in the social workers' professional judgment, clients' actions or potential actions pose a serious, foreseeable, and imminent risk to themselves or others. (NASW, 2000, p. 7)

This standard addresses several needs and concerns of the alcohol dependent client. The client is encouraged to choose treatment goals and work towards achieving those goals with the respect and assistance of the social worker. The code of ethics also highlights the social worker's ability to intervene with a client who is using alcohol in a self-destructive manner. In the end, the goal is to reduce the amount of personal and/or societal harm directly or indirectly caused by alcohol. Social workers are uniquely suited to pursue and achieve this goal.

Several resources for harm reduction approaches to the treatment of alcohol problems, including relapse prevention, can be found online and in print.

ONLINE RESOURCES

http://www.harmreduction.org-Harm Reduction Coalition
http://www.ihra.net/-International Harm Reduction Association
http://www.strategy.gov.uk-Alcohol Harm Reduction Strategy for England
http://www.icap.org-International Center for Alcohol Policy
http://www.bhrm.org/guidelines/RPT%20guideline.pdf-Clinical Guidelines

PRINT RESOURCES

Barber, J. G. (1994). Social work with addictions. N.Y.: New York University Press.
Daley, D. C., & Raskin, M. S. (Eds.). (1991). *Treating the chemically dependent and their families.* Newbury Park, CA: Sage.
Denning, P. et al. (2000). *Practicing Harm Reduction Psychotherapy: An Alternative Approach to Addiction.* Guilford Press.
Denning, P. et al. (2004). *Over the Influence: The Harm Reduction Guide for Managing Drugs and Alcohol.* Guilford Press.
Marlatt, G. A. (1998). *Harm Reduction.* Guilford.
Marlatt, G. A. & Gordon, J. (1985). *Relapse Prevention.* Guilford.
Peele, S. (2004). *7 Tools to Beat Addiction.* Three Rivers Press.
Tatarsky, A. (2002). *Harm Reduction Psychotherapy.* Jason Aronson.

REFERENCES

Brocato, J., & Wagner, E. F. (2003). Harm reduction: A social work practice model and social justice agenda. *Health and Social Work, 28,* 117-125.
Carroll, K. M. (1996). Relapse prevention as a psychosocial treatment: A review of controlled clinical trials. *Experimental and Clinical Psychopharmacology, 4,* 46-54.
Connors, G. F., Maisto, S. A., & Zywiak, W. H. (1996). Understanding relapse in the broader context of post-treatment functioning. *Addiction, 91* (Suppl.), 173-190.
Cooney, N. L., Litt, M. D., Morse, P. A., Bauer, L. O., & Gaupp, L. (1997). Alcohol cue reactivity, negative-mood reactivity, and relapse in treated alcoholic men. *Journal of Abnormal Psychology, 106,* 243
Cunningham, J. A., Sobell, L. C., Sobell, M. B., Agrawal, S., & Toneatto, T. (1993). Barriers to treatment: Why alcohol and drug abusers delay or never seek treatment. *Addictive Behaviors, 18* (3), 347-354.
Fleming, M. F., Barry, K. L., Manwell, L. B., Johnson, K., & London, R. (1997). Brief physician advice for problem alcohol drinkers: A randomized controlled trial in community-based primary care practices. *JAMA, 277*(13), 1039-1045.
Grant, B. F., Dawson, D. A., Stinson, F. S., Chou, S. P., Dufour, M. C., & Pickering, R. P. (2004). The 12-month prevalence and trends in DSM-IV alcohol abuse and dependence: United States, 1991-1992 and 2001-2002. *Drug and Alcohol Dependence, 74,* 223-234.

Greenfield, S. F., Hufford, M. H., Vagge, L. M., Muenz, L. R., Costello, M. E., & Weiss, R. D. (2000). The relationship of self-efficacy expectancies to relapse among alcohol dependent men and women: A prospective study. *Journal of Studies on Alcohol, 61*, 345-351.

Hall, S. M., Havassy, B. E., & Wasserman, D. A. (1991). Effects of commitment to abstinence, positive moods, stress, and coping on relapse to cocaine use. *Journal of Consulting & Clinical Psychology, 59*, 526-532.

Harwood, H. (2000). *Updating Estimates of the Economic Costs of Alcohol Abuse in the United States: Estimates, Update Methods, and Data*. Report prepared by The Lewin Group for the National Institute on Alcohol Abuse and Alcoholism, 2000. Based on estimates, analyses, and data reported in Harwood, H., Fountain, D., and Livermore, G. *The Economic Costs of Alcohol and Drug Abuse in the United States 1992*. Report prepared for the National Institute on Drug Abuse and the National Institute on Alcohol Abuse and Alcoholism, National Institutes of Health, Department of Health and Human Services. NIH Publication No. 98-4327. Rockville, MD: National Institutes of Health, 1998.

Harwood, H., Fountain, D., and Livermore, G. (1998). *The Economic Costs of Alcohol and Drug Abuse in the United States 1992*. Report prepared for the National Institute on Drug Abuse and the National Institute on Alcohol Abuse and Alcoholism, National Institutes of Health, Department of Health and Human Services. NIH Publication No. 98-4327. Rockville, MD: National Institutes of Health, 1998.

Hodgins, D. C., Leigh, G., Milne, R., & Gerrish, R. (1997). Drinking goal selection in behavioral self-management treatment of chronic alcoholics. *Addictive Behaviors, 22*, 247-255.

Hufford, M. H., Witkiewitz, K., Shields, A. L., Kodya, S., & Caruso, J. C. (2003). Applying nonlinear dynamics to the prediction of alcohol use disorder treatment outcomes. *Journal of Abnormal Psychology, 112*, 219-227.

Humphreys, K., & Klaw, E. (2001). Can targeting non-dependent problem drinkers and providing Internet-based services expand access to assistance for alcohol problems? A study of the Moderation Management self-help/mutual aid organization. *Journal of Studies on Alcohol, 62*, 528-532.

Hunt, W. A., Barnett, L. W., & Branch, L. G. (1971). Relapse rates in addiction programs. *Journal of Clinical Psychology, 27*, 455-456.

Irvin, J. E., Bowers, C. A., Dunn, M. E., & Wang, M. C. (1999). Efficacy of relapse prevention: A meta-analytic review. *Journal of Consulting & Clinical Psychology, 67* (4), 563-570.

Litman, G. K. (1986). Alcoholism survival: The prevention of relapse. In W. R. Miller, & N. Heather (Eds.), *Treating addictive behaviors: Processes of change* (pp. 391-405). New York: Plenum Press.

Lowman, C., Allen, J., Stout, R. L., & the Relapse Research Group (1996). Replication and extension of Marlatt's taxonomy of relapse precipitants: Overview of procedures and results. *Addiction, 91* (Suppl.), 51-71.

MacMaster, S. A. (2004). Harm reduction: A new perspective on substance abuse services. *Social Work, 49*, 356-363.

Maisto S.A., Pollock N.K., Cornelius J.R., Lynch K.G., & Martin C.S. (2003). Alcohol relapse as a function of relapse definition in a clinical sample of adolescents. *Addictive Behaviors, 28* (3), 449-459.

Marlatt, G. A. (1985). Relapse prevention: Theoretical rationale and overview of the model. In G. A. Marlatt, & J. R. Gordon (Eds.), *Relapse Prevention* (pp. 280-250). New York: The Guilford Press.

Marlatt, G. A., & Gordon, J. R. (1985). *Relapse prevention: Maintenance strategies in the treatment of addictive behaviors.* New York: The Guilford Press.

Marlatt, G. A., & Witkiewitz, K. (2002). Harm reduction approaches to alcohol use: Health promotion, prevention, and treatment. *Addictive Behaviors, 27*, 867-886.

Miller, W. R., Andrews, N. R., Wilbourne, P., & Bennett, M. E. (1998). A wealth of alternatives: Effective treatments for alcohol problems. In W. R. Miller, & N. Heather (Eds.), *Treating addictive behaviors: Processes of change* (2nd ed., pp. 203-216). New York: Plenum Press.

Miller, W.R., & Rollnick, S. (2002). *Motivational interviewing: Preparing people to change. 2nd edition.* New York: The Guilford Press.

Miller, W. R., & Wilbourne, P. L. (2002). Mesa Grande: A methodological analysis of clinical trials of treatments for alcohol use disorders. *Addiction, 97*, 265-277.

Muthén, B. (2001). Second-generation structural equation modeling with a combination of categorical and continuous latent variables: New opportunities for latent class-latent growth modeling. In L. M. Collins, & A. G. Sayer (Eds.), *New methods for the analysis of change* (pp. 289-322). Washington, DC: American Psychological Association.

Muthén, B., & Shedden, K. (1999). Finite mixture modeling with mixture outcomes using the EM algorithm. *Biometrics, 55*, 463-469.

National Association of Social Workers. (1999). *Code of ethics of the National Association of Social Workers.* Washington, DC: Author.

National Association of Social Workers, Practice Research Network. (2000). *Informing research and policy through social work practice.* Washington, DC: Author.

National Institute of Alcohol Abuse and Alcoholism. (1998). Drinking in the United States: Main Findings from the 1992 National Longitudinal Alcohol Epidemiologic Survey; SAMHSA (2002) National Household Survey on Drug Abuse. Washington, DC: Department of Health and Human Services.

Polivy, J., & Herman, P. (2002). If at first you don't succeed: False hopes of self-change. *American Psychologist, 57*, 677-689.

Prochaska, J. O., & DiClemente, C. C. (1984). *The transtheoretical approach: Crossing the traditional boundaries of therapy.* Malabar, FL: Krieger.

Rabois, D., & Haaga, D. A. (2003). The influence of cognitive coping and mood on smokers' self-efficacy and temptation. *Addictive Behaviors, 28*, 561-573.

Rychtarik, R. G., Prue, D. M., Rapp, S. R., & King, A. C. (1992). Self-efficacy, aftercare and relapse in a treatment program for alcoholics. *Journal of Studies on Alcohol, 53* (5), 435-440.

Sieger, B. H. (2003). Harm reduction: Is it for you? *Journal of Social Work Practice in the Addictions, 3*, 119-121.

Sobell, L. C., Sobell, M. B., Toneatto, T., & Leo, G. I. (1993). What triggers the resolution of alcohol problems without treatment. *Alcoholism: Clinical and Experimental Research, 17*, 217-224.

Solomon, K. E., & Annis, H. M. (1990). Outcome and efficacy expectancy in the prediction of post-treatment drinking behavior. *British Journal of Addiction, 85* (5), 659-665.

Thom, R. (1975). *Stabilité structurelle et morphogenèse* (Structural stability and morphogenesis). (H. Fowler, Trans.). Reading: Benjamin.

Witkiewitz, K. (2004). *Predicting Alcohol Relapse Using Nonlinear Dynamics and Growth Mixture Modeling*. Doctoral Dissertation, University of Washington.

Witkiewitz, K., & Marlatt, G. A. (2004). Relapse prevention for alcohol and drug problems: That was Zen, this is Tao. *American Psychologist, 59*(4), 224-235.

Witkiewitz, K., & Marlatt, G. A. (in press). Modeling the complexity of post-treatment drinking: It's a rocky road to relapse. *Clinical Psychology Review*.

Family-Based Treatment Models Targeting Substance Use and High-Risk Behaviors Among Adolescents: A Review

Sanna J. Thompson, PhD
Elizabeth C. Pomeroy, PhD
Kelly Gober, MSSW

SUMMARY. Recent reviews of services for families with youths coping with a wide variety of problems have strongly urged inclusion of families in all services. This manuscript will review family-based intervention models that have considerable empirical support for treating adolescent substance abuse and have demonstrated success in preventing substance use. Major interventions reviewed include: Multisystemic Family Therapy, Strengthening Families Program, Brief Strategic Family Therapy,

---

Sanna J. Thompson, Elizabeth C. Pomeroy, and Kelly Gober are affiliated with the University of Texas at Austin School of Social Work.

Address correspondence to: Sanna Thompson, PhD, University of Texas at Austin School of Social Work, Substance Abuse Research Development Program, 1717 West 6th Street, Suite 335, Campus Box R5000 Austin, TX 78703 (E-mail: SannaThompson@mail.utexas.edu).

[Haworth co-indexing entry note]: "Family-Based Treatment Models Targeting Substance Use and High-Risk Behaviors Among Adolescents: A Review." Thompson, Sanna J., Elizabeth C. Pomeroy, and Kelly Gober. Co-published simultaneously in *Journal of Evidence-Based Social Work* (The Haworth Social Work Practice Press, an imprint of The Haworth Press, Inc.) Vol. 2, No. 1/2, 2005, pp. 207-233; and: *Addiction, Assessment, and Treatment with Adolescents, Adults, and Families* (ed: Carolyn Hilarski) The Haworth Social Work Practice Press, an imprint of The Haworth Press, Inc., 2005, pp. 207-233. Single or multiple copies of this article are available for a fee from The Haworth Document Delivery Service [1-800-HAWORTH, 9:00 a.m. - 5:00 p.m. (EST). E-mail address: docdelivery@haworthpress.com].

http://www.haworthpress.com/web/JEBSW
Digital Object Identifier: 10.1300/J394v02n01_12

Multidimensional Family Therapy, and Integrated Behavioral Family Therapy. *[Article copies available for a fee from The Haworth Document Delivery Service: 1-800-HAWORTH. E-mail address: <docdelivery@haworthpress.com> Website: <http://www.HaworthPress.com> © 2005 by The Haworth Press, Inc. All rights reserved.]*

KEYWORDS. Family, treatment, adolescents, substance use, risky behaviors

FAMILIES AND HIGH-RISK YOUTH

Some have argued that families are central to the process of youth developing emotional and behavioral problems (Paradise, Cauce, Ginzler et al., 2001). Researchers contend that the relationship between vulnerability and risk becomes cemented early in life through a series of negative interactions between parent and child. The resulting difficulties in family relationships persist throughout childhood and adolescence. Poor family management, lack of positive parenting skills, and dysfunctional caregiving have been strongly related to substance use and delinquency of youth (Formoso, Gonzales, & Aiken, 2000). Conversely, family support has been shown to predict positive adjustment in childhood and adolescence; indirect evidence suggests that family support is a protective factor for adolescent substance use and conduct problems (Cauce, Reid, Landesman, & Gonzales, 1990; Wills & McNamara, 1992).

Given the family's fundamental influence on a child's life, research has consistently suggested potential benefits for including families in treatment of high-risk youth. Prevention efforts with delinquent and drug-abusing youth suggest that the single most effective form of prevention involves working with the total family system (Kumpfer, Alexander, McDonald, & Olds, 1998). Identification of situations where families may be engaged in services is a potentially beneficial method for addressing problems experienced by youth.

SUBSTANCE USE AND ADOLESCENTS

Rates of substance use among adolescent populations have become an increasing problem as the rates of substance use and abuse among American high school and college students is the highest in the industrialized world (Johnston, O'Malley, & Bachman, 2002). In 1997, ra substance use among youth 12 to 17-years of age rose to 11.7% aɪᵤ ɪɪ-licit drug use among 12-13 year-olds increased from 2.2% to 3.8% during this time period (Winters, 1999). It appears that substance use is occurring at earlier ages; some report that by age 16, half of male and female adolescents use alcohol regularly and one-quarter use marijuana (Huizinga, Loeber, & Thornberry, 1994).

Data from Monitoring the Future study (Johnston et al., 2002) suggest that adolescent drug users are often found in the juvenile justice and educational systems. Adolescents with alcohol/drug problems are often identified as delinquent, having histories of child abuse and neglect, and suffering from comorbid psychiatric conditions, especially depression and suicidality (Hawkins, Catalano, & Miller, 1992; Rahdert, & Czechowicz, 1995). Adolescents with family histories of alcoholism also report greater positive expectancies related to using substances, such as sexual enhancement and feelings of power/aggression, than do youth without family histories of alcohol abuse (Lundahl, Davis, Adesso, & Lukas, 1997).

FAMILY-BASED INTERVENTIONS

Recent reviews of services for families with youths coping with a wide variety of problems have strongly urged inclusion of families in all services (Burns, & Weisz, 2000). Many studies (e.g., Liddle, Dakof, Parker et al., 2001; Kumpfer, 1998; Henggeler, Borduim, Melton et al., 1991; Szapocznik & Williams, 2000) have demonstrated that family-oriented interventions are critical in reducing risk factors associated with substance use and these intervention models have considerable empirical support for demonstrated success in preventing adolescent substance use. Family therapies have developed from two foundational therapies that originated in the early 1970s. Structural Family Therapy, developed by Salvador Minuchin, and Strategic Family Therapy, developed by Jay Haley, are built on the assumptions that (1) families are rule-governed systems that can best be understood in context, (2) the presenting problem serves a function within the family, and (3) the concepts of boundaries, coalitions, hierarchy, power, metaphor, family life cycle development and triangles are basic to the development of a "stuck" family (Minuchin, 1974; Haley, 1973; Nichols & Schwartz, 1995). These therapeutic models are the core theories from which later models developed.

Currently, research studies have been initiated that evaluate various treatment modalities targeting adolescent substance use. Many of these studies include testing structured and manualized family interventions developed during the past two decades. For example, multi-systemic therapy (MST), strengthening family program (SFP), brief strategic family therapy (BSFT), multidimensional family therapy (MDFT), and integrated behavioral family therapy (IBFT). This manuscript reviews the empirical studies of these family-based interventions that have an emphasis on adolescent substance use. See Table 1 for a brief description of these studies.

MULTISYSTEMIC THERAPY

Multisystemic therapy (MST) treatment views individuals in terms of the complex systems in which they are embedded (Letourneau, Cunningham, & Henggeler, 2002). Individuals restructure their environments while simultaneously being influenced by them. Behavior is best understood when viewed within broader contexts, such as school, family, peers, neighborhood, services, and community institutions (Henggeler, Schoenwald, Borduin et al., 1998).

MST has been extensively evaluated, and suggests that antisocial behavior in youth is determined by a variety of correlates (Henggeler et al., 1998). These factors, along with other antisocial behaviors, such as conduct disorder and delinquency, are relevant for substance abuse (Hawkins et al., 1992; Kumpfer, DeMarsh, & Child, 1989); MST lends itself to these complex issues. The number of individual therapy sessions varies depending on the problems within the system; however, parent training typically occurs in 10 sessions (Henggeler et al., 1998).

Growing evidence supports the effectiveness of MST for substance-using adolescents. Stanton and Shadish (1997) conducted a meta-analysis of family-based treatments for drug use and found that MST effect sizes were among the highest of those reviewed. An early MST outcome study (Henggeler, 1986) used a quasi-experimental design to study youth and their families in a delinquency diversion program. Findings showed the MST was more effective than usual community services in terms of client behaviors and family relationships. Subsequently, MST has been substantiated as an evidenced- based treatment for adolescents and their families in randomized clinical trials. It has been effective in reducing out-of-home placements, delinquent behavior, substance use, and psychiatric disorders (Sheidow & Woodford, 2003).

TABLE 1. Studies of family-based treatment with focus on adolescent substance use.

Reference	Design	Sample	Outcome Variables
Multi-Systemic Therapy			
Henggeler, 1986	Quasi-Experimental; pre- and post-treatment assessments	n = 57-family ecological n = 23-alternative n = 44-control Youth and families in a delinquency diversion program	Personality Inventory Family relations Behavior Problems: conduct problems, anxious-withdrawn behaviors, immaturity, and association with delinquent peers
Henggeler, Melton, & Smith, 1992; Henggeler et al., 1991	MSFT vs. standard juvenile justice services	n = 84 juvenile offenders Random assignment	Alcohol and marijuana use Incarceration/recidivism Violence Criminal Activity
Henggeler et al., 1993	MST vs. standard juvenile justice services follow-up	n = 84 juvenile offenders Random assignment	Alcohol and marijuana use Incarceration/recidivism Aggression with peers Criminal activity Family cohesion
Borduin et al., 1995; Henggeler et al., 1991	MST vs. individual therapy	n = 200 violent juvenile offenders and families Random assignment	Arrest types: Substance use/violent crimes Arrest recidivism
Henggeler, Pickrel, & Brondino, 1996	Home-based MST vs. usual community services	n = 118 substance abusing or dependent juvenile delinquents and families Random assignment	Retention rates
Schoenwald, Ward, & Henggeler, 1996	Home-based MST vs. usual community services	n = 118 substance abusing or dependent juvenile delinquents and families Random assignment	Costs of treatment
Henggeler, Melton, Brondino, Scherer, & Hanley, 1997	MST vs. standard juvenile justice services follow-up	n = 155 adolescents Random assignment	Adherence to MST Arrests/recidivism Incarceration/recidivism
Brown, Henggeler, & Schoenwald, 1999	MST vs. standard community-based service	n = 118 substance abusing or dependent juvenile delinquents with co-morbid psychiatric disorders and families Random assignment	School attendance Mental health Adherence to MST Arrests/recidivism Incarceration/recidivism

TABLE 1 (continued)

Reference	Design	Sample	Outcome Variables
Multi-Systemic Therapy			
Henggeler, Pickrel, & Brondino, 1999	MST vs. standard juvenile justice services follow-up	n = 118 substance abusing or dependent juvenile delinquents and their families	Alcohol and marijuana use Psychiatric Symptoms Arrest/incarceration/ recidivism
Henggeler, Pickrel, & Brondino, 1999	MST vs. standard juvenile justice services follow-up	n = 118 substance abusing or dependent juvenile delinquents and their families	Alcohol and marijuana use Psychiatric Symptoms Arrest/incarceration/ recidivism
Henggeler, Clingempeel, Brondino, & Pickrel, 2002	MST vs. standard community-based services; 4 year follow-up	n = 80 substance abusing or dependent juvenile delinquents and their families	Alcohol and marijuana use Criminal Behavior Illicit Drug Use Psychiatric Symptoms Arrest/incarceration/ recidivism
Schoenwald, Halliday-Boykins, & Henggeler, 2003	Multi-site comparison of MST	n = 233 families n = 66 therapists (16 teams in 9 organizations)	Adherence Criminal offenses Substance abuse Arrests/recidivism School suspensions Caregiver/therapist ethnic match Economic disadvantage
Strengthening Families Program			
Kumpfer, Molgaard, and Spoth, 1996	Quasi-Experimental with 5 year follow-up	n = 421 parents and 703 high risk youth (6-13 yrs.)	Family conflict/ communication Parenting behavior Child emotional status
Aktan, Kumpfer, & Turner, 1996	Quasi-Experimental with matched comparison	n = 88 Inner City African-American youth (age 6-12) and families with substance-using parent n = 56 comparison group	Parenting efficacy Parental substance use Retention/completion in treatment
Kamoeoka, 1996	Quasi-Experimental	n = 136 Asian and Pacific-Island youth and families	Substance use Retention in treatment Parenting skills Depression Children behaviors
Spoth, Redmond, & Shin, 1998	"Preparing for the drug free years" program vs. SFP vs. minimal contact control	n = 523 families of students in 33 rural Midwestern schools	Parenting methods Retention in treatment Child academic status

Reference	Design	Sample	Outcome Variables
Multi-Systemic Therapy			
Spoth, Reyes, & Redmond, 1999	"Preparing for the drug free years" program vs. SFP vs. control follow-up	n = 329 10th grade adolescents	Current and past use of Alcohol/tobacco/ marijuana Parenting methods Retention in treatment Child academic status
Spoth, Redmond, & Lepper, 1999	Longitudinal, efficacy study	n = 446 adolescents and families	Alcohol initiation behaviors Parenting methods Retention in treatment Child academic status
Spoth, Redmond, & Shin, 2001; Spoth, Guyll, & Day, 2002	"Preparing for the drug free years" program vs. SFP vs. control	n = 667 6th graders and their families in 33 public schools Random assignment	Cost of treatment Current and past use of Alcohol/tobacco/ marijuana Parenting methods Retention in treatment Child academic status
Kumpfer, Alvarado, & Tait, 2002	"I Can Problem Solve" program vs. "I Can Problem Solve" program combined with SFP vs. SFP only	n = 655 1st graders from 12 rural schools Random assignment	Social competency Self-regulations Family relationships Parenting School bonding Parenting skills
Spoth, Guyll, & Chao, 2003	Exploratory with wait list control	n = 85 African-American families with youth 10-14 years of age from general population Random selection	Retention rates Treatment adherence Child behaviors Child participation in family meetings Child and family living skills
Brief Strategic Family Therapy			
Szapocznik, Santisteban, Rio, Perez-Vidal, & Kurtines, 1986	BSFT vs. Bicultural Effectiveness Training	n = 41 Cuban American adolescents with a behavior problem and families Random assignment	Adolescent problem behaviors Family functioning
Szapocznik, Santisteban, Rio, Perez-Vidal, Kurtines, & Hervis, 1986	Family Effectiveness Training vs. Minimum Contact Control	n = 79 Hispanic 6- to 11-year-old children with emotional and behavior problems and families Random assignment	Structural family functioning Child behavior problems Child self-concept
Szapocznik, 1986	Conjoint family therapy with entire family versus One-person family therapy	n = 35 Hispanic-American families with drug-using adolescents	Individual and family Functioning Behavioral acculturation

TABLE 1 (continued)

Reference	Design	Sample	Outcome Variables
Multi-Systemic Therapy			
Szapocznik, Kurtines, Foote, Perez-Vidal, & Hervis, 1983, 1986	Conjoint family therapy with entire family vs. One-person family therapy	n = 72 Hispanic drug abusing 12- to 17-year-old adolescent and families Random assignment	Youth drug use Behavior problems Family functioning
Sazpocznik et al., 1988	Engagement as Usual vs. Strategic Structural Systems Engagement	n = 108 Cuban Hispanic families and adolescents suspected of/observed using drugs by their parents or school counselors Random assignment	Engagement in treatment Retention to treatment Family functioning
Szapocznik, Rio, Murray et al., 1989	BSFT vs Psychodynamic Child Therapy vs. Recreational Control Condition	n = 69 Hispanic boys with emotional and behavioral problems (aged 6 to 12) Random Assignment	Emotional and behavioral problems Retention in treatment Child functioning Family integrity
Santisteban et al., 1996	BSFT plus Strategic Structural Systems Engagement vs. BSFT plus Engagement as usual vs. group counseling plus Engagement as usual	n = 193 Hispanic families Random Assignment	Engagement in treatment Retention to treatment Hispanic cultural/ethnic identity
Coatsworth, Santisteban, & McBride, 2001	BSFT vs. standard community services	n = 104 African American or Hispanic families and adolescents with behavioral, emotional, academic and substance use problems Random Assignment	Engagement to treatment Retention to treatment Conduct problems Anxiety Disruptive behaviors
Santisteban, Coatsworth, & Perez-Vidal, 2003	BSFT vs. Group treatment control	n = 126 Hispanic families and adolescents with behavioral problems and drug-use Random assignment	Conduct problems Delinquency Substance use Family functioning
Multi-Dimensional Family Therapy			
Liddle et al., 2001	MDFT vs. adolescent group therapy and multifamily educational intervention	n = 182 clinically referred marijuana and alcohol-abusing 13-18-yr.-olds and families Random Assignment	Substance use Acting out GPA Family competence

Reference	Design	Sample	Outcome Variables
Multi-Systemic Therapy			
Liddle, in press	MDFT vs. Cognitive-Behavioral Therapy	n = 224 African-American males from low-income families Random Assignment	Substance use Conduct problems Anxiety/depression Family functioning
Dennis et al., in press	MDFT vs. Motivational Enhancement Therapy (MET) vs. Cognitive Behavioral Therapy (CBT) vs. Family Support Network (FSN), vs. Adolescent Community Reinforcement Approach (ACRA) vs. Multidimensional Family Therapy (MDFT)	n = 600 adolescents between 12- 18 years of age, used marijuana in the past 90 days, and met one or more criteria of abuse or dependence Random assignment	Substance use Cost and cost/benefit ratio Substance use Conduct problems Anxiety/depression Family functioning Academic behaviors
Hogue, Liddle, Becker, & Johnson-Leckrone, 2002	MDFT vs. control condition	n = 124 inner-city African-American youths (11-14 yrs.) Random assignment	Drug use Self-competence Family functioning School involvement Peer associations Global self-worth Family cohesion
Integrated Behavioral Family Therapy			
Waldron, Slesnick, & Brody, 2001	IBFT vs. individual cognitive behavioral therapy vs. combination	n = 114 substance-abusing adolescents Random assignment	Substance use
Latimer, Winters, & D'Zurilla, 2003	IBFT vs. "Drug's Harm" psycho-educational curriculum	n = 43 adolescents meeting diagnostic criteria for substance use disorder	Alcohol and marijuana use Rational problem solving Learning strategy skills Problem avoidance skills

The effects of MST on drug use have been examined in trials using juvenile offenders as participants (Henggeler et al., 1991; Henggeler, Melton, & Smith, 1992; Borduin, Mann, Cone et al., 1995). In these trials, MST significantly reduced self-reported drug use, criminal activity, violence, incarceration (Henggeler, et al., 1992), incarceration recidivism, aggression with peers, family cohesion (Henggeler, Melton, Smith et al., 1993), and drug-related and other arrests (Borduin et al., 1995).

An experimentally designed study compared home-based MST with usual community services for 118 substance using juvenile delinquents. MST showed higher rates of client completion of the full course of the treatment, which averaged 130 days (Henggeler, Pickrel, Brondino, & Crouch, 1996). The MST group showed significantly decreased self-reported alcohol and marijuana use, although urine screen results did not confirm the youth self-reports and the positive outcomes were not maintained at 6 months post-treatment (Henggeler, Pickrel, & Brondino, 1999). However, the MST group showed increased school attendance and these treatment gains were maintained at 6-month follow-up (Brown, Henggeler, & Schoenwald, 1999). Additionally, it was found that the cost of MST was mitigated by the reduced incarceration costs (Schoenwald, Ward, & Henggeler, 1996).

Based on the negative results related to urine screening for substance use, several enhancements were made to the MST treatment protocol to thoroughly address adolescent substance use. These enhancements were based on the Community Reinforcement Approach (CRA), an approach specifically geared toward substance use (Randall & Cunningham, 2003; Randall, Henggeler, & Cunningham, 2001). In a recent follow-up study, MST was compared with usual community services among substance abusing juvenile offenders four years following participation. Significantly less aggressive criminal activity was found. While findings for illicit drug use were mixed, significantly higher rates of marijuana abstinence was found among MST participants (Henggeler, Clingempeel, Brondino, & Pickrel, 2002).

In terms of adherence to MST, a recent study of 233 families indicated that adherence ratings were lower for youths referred for both criminal offenses and substance abuse, but not for either referral individually. Adherence ratings were negatively associated with pretreatment arrests and school suspensions, and positively associated with education disadvantage and caregiver-therapist ethnic match. They were also marginally associated with economic disadvantage (Schoenwald, Halliday-Boykins, & Henggeler, 2003).

STRENGTHENING FAMILIES PROGRAM

The Strengthening Families Program (SFP) provides a family-based intervention for families with substance abusing parents aimed at developing drug resistance skills in their children. Framed within the social ecological model of adolescent substance abuse (Kumpfer & Turner,

1990-1991), the SFP holds that the family climate is responsible for child substance abuse. Based on this model, the family influences school bonding and self-efficacy, which in turn determines the amount of peer influence and later alcohol and drug use (Kumpfer, Molgaard, & Spoth, 1996; Kumpfer & Turner, 1990-1991; Oetting, 1992; Newcomb, 1992). The SFP program focuses on strengthening the family in order to mediate peer influence related to drug and alcohol use in adolescents.

The highly structured SFP program consists of a 14-week curriculum involving parent training, child skills training, and family skills training (Kumpfer et al., 1996). The approach is highly detailed in terms of manuals and training (Kumpfer et al., 1989). In fact, versions of SFP have been culturally-adapted for African-Americans, Hispanic-Americans, Asian/Pacific Islanders, and American-Indian families. The culturally adapted versions can increase retention, but may reduce positive outcomes (Kumpfer, Alvarado, & Smith, 2002).

SFP references empirical research that focuses on risk and protective factors in order to examine the family's influence on child's substance use. It is believed that a child's risk of substance use increases as the number of risk factors increases relative to protective factors (Kumpfer et al., 1996). This is especially true when the level of risk is elevated above one or two risk factors (Bry & Krinsley, 1992; Newcomb & Bentler, 1989).

Research suggests that SFP has been effective with substance-abusing parents and parents from racial and ethnic minority groups (Kumpfer et al., 1996; Kumpfer & Alvarado, 1995, Kumpfer, Alverado, & Tait, 2002; Aktan, Kumpfer, & Turner, 1996; Kamoeoka, 1996; Kumpfer, Wamberg, & Martinez, 1996). In a recent study, 56 rigorous evaluations of interventions for alcohol misuse were reviewed and summarized. It was noted that SFP showed promise as an effective prevention intervention (Foxcroft, Ireland, & Lister-Sharp, 2003)

The program's effectiveness was originally established with school-aged children of drug abusers (Kumpfer et al., 1989). Three groups (parent training program only, parent training with a children's training program, and parent and child training with a family skills training and relationship enhancement program) were compared. The study concluded that the combined intervention including all three components caused the most improvement on: (1) children's problem behaviors, emotional status, and prosocial skills, (2) parents' parenting skills, and (3) family environment and family functioning. Each program component was effective in reducing risk factors targeted by that component.

Subsequent studies have found consistent support for SFP with parent and child behaviors and drug use (Aktan, 1995; Aktan et al., 1996), especially for high-risk families (Kumpfer et al., 1996). SFP has also been found effective with modifications for African-American, Hawaiian, Hispanic, rural, and multi-ethnic families (Spoth, Guyll, & Chao, 2003). For example, a five-year follow-up of high risk, ethnic minority families demonstrated that family management skills were still in use many years following participation in SFP (Kumpfer et al., 1996).

Using a substance initiation index, Spoth and colleagues have consistently found evidence suggesting the potential of SFP to delay the onset of substance use and the possibility of avoiding substantial costs to society with relatively small intervention costs (Spoth, Guyll, & Day, 2002; Spoth, Redmond, & Trudeau, 2002; Spoth, Reyes, & Redmond, 1999; Spoth, Redmond, & Lepper, 1999; Spoth, Redmond, & Shin, 1998; Spoth, Redmond, & Shin, 2001; Spoth, Redmond, & Trudeau, 2002). A seven-session version of SFP, developed for early adolescence and based on resilience principles, showed positive results during a 5-year randomized clinical trial with rural sixth-grade students (Kumpfer, 1998). Spoth (1998) also found positive results in terms of tobacco and alcohol rates with this program.

In a recent study (Kumpfer, Alvarado, & Tait, 2002), 655 first graders from 12 rural schools were randomly assigned to either the "I Can Problem Solve" program alone, in combination with SFP, or parent training only. Results suggested that there were significant improvements on school bonding, parenting skills, family relationships, social competency, and behavioral self-regulation for the group receiving the combined intervention. Adding the parenting skills program only, social competency and self-regulation were more improved, but family relationships were negatively impacted. Alternatively, adding SFP improved family relationships, parenting, and school bonding.

BRIEF STRATEGIC FAMILY THERAPY

Brief Strategic Family Therapy (BSFT) was developed through the integration of theory, research, and practice of structural and strategic methods (Szapocznik & Williams, 2000). BSFT is especially appropriate for treatment of substance use that co-occurs with other behavior problems, including conduct disorders, oppositional behavior, delinquency, associating with antisocial peers, aggressive and violent behavior, and risky sexual behavior (Szapocznik, Rio, & Murray, 1989; Santisteban, Szapocznik, Perez-Vidal et al., 2000; Newcomb and Bentler, 1989; Perrino, Gonzalez-Soldevilla, Pantin & Szapocznik, 2000). BSFT is a family-based intervention specifically created to address conduct problems and drug abuse among Hispanic (Szapocznik & Williams, 2000; Robbins, Szapocznik, & Santisteban, 2003; Robbins, Mitrani, & Zarate, 2002) and African American youths (Szapocznik & Williams, 2000), and has been proposed for use with other populations as well, such as Chinese Americans (Soo-Hoo, 1999).

Three basic principles typify BSFT: The family as a system, structure/patterns of interactions, and strategy (Szapocznik & Kurtines, 1989). The concept of family systems reflects the understanding that family members are interdependent and that individual behaviors affect others in the family. The structure/patterns of interactions indicate that the behaviors of family members are habitual and repeat over time. This structure contributes to behavior problems, such as substance abuse and BSFT targets these interactions. The third principle relates to the notion that intervention must be practical and deliberate, and linked directly to problem behaviors (Szapocznik & Williams, 2000).

BSFT is built into the youth's daily family life and can be implemented in eight to twenty-four sessions. The therapy is manualized (Szapocznik, Hervis, & Schwartz, 2001), with training programs available. BSFT is a flexible approach that appeals to cultures that emphasize family and interpersonal relationships. BSFT has been well established in the treatment of adolescents with problems ranging from substance use to conduct problems, associations with antisocial peers, and impaired family functioning (Szapocznik, Perez-Vidal, Hervis et al., 1989).

Engagement and retention issues have also been examined, with encouraging results. Structural Strategic Systems Engagement was developed specifically in relation to family therapy, with the belief that resistance to treatment can be understood in terms of family interactions (Szapocznik & Kurtines, 1989; Szapocznik et al. 1989). Studies have shown positive results in engaging and retaining clients in BSFT (Coatsworth, Santisteban, & McBride, 2001), and in Structural Strategic Systems Engagement specifically (Santisteban, Szapocznik, Perez-Vidal et al., 1996; Szapocznik, Perez-Vidal, Brickman et al., 1988).

In clinical trials, BSFT has been compared with other therapies. Individual psychodynamic child therapy and a recreational control condition were compared with BSFT in a randomized study with sixty-nine Hispanic boys with emotional and behavioral problems, aged six to eleven. Findings indicated that the control condition was significantly less effective in retaining cases, the two treatment conditions were equally effective in reducing emotional and behavior problems, and the BSFT group alone reported continued significant improvement of family functioning at the one-year follow-up (Szapocznik, Rio, & Murray, 1989; Szapocznik, Santisteban, Rio et al., 1986).

Other studies have compared BSFT in conjunction with other methods. For example, BSFT was compared to a Bicultural Effectiveness Training; however, no significant differences were found (Szapocznik et al., 1986). Following these results, the researchers compared a combination of BSFT and Bicultural Effectiveness Training (Family Effectiveness Training) and group controls. The Family Effectiveness Training condition showed significantly greater improvement than control families on structural family functioning, child behavior problems, and child self-concept (Szapocznik, Santisteban, Rio et al., 1986).

Two types of BSFT have also been compared: conjoint family therapy (including the entire family) with one-person family therapy. In a study with 35 Hispanic-American families (Szapocznik, Kurtines, Foote, Perez-Vidal, & Hervis, 1983), it was found that one-person family therapy was as effective as conjoint family therapy in reducing youth drug use and behavior problems, as well as improving individual and family functioning. Additionally, one-person family therapy was more effective in sustaining improved family functioning at follow-up (Szapocznik, Kurtines, Foote, Perez-Vidal, & Hervis, 1986).

BSFT has been shown to be effective with adolescent behavior problems. One study (Santisteban et al., 2000) reviewed the ability of BSFT to reduce behavior problems in twelve to eighteen year old Hispanic adolescents and their families. In this study, BSFT was compared to a group control condition. Adolescents in the BSFT condition showed significantly decreased levels of conduct disorder and socialized aggression from pre- to post-treatment, while the control condition showed no change. Another recent study compared BSFT to a group treatment control (Santisteban, Coatsworth, & Perez-Vidal, 2003). One hundred twenty-six Hispanic families were randomly assigned to one of the two conditions. BSFT families showed significant improvement in conduct problems and delinquency, as well as marijuana use and family functioning.

MULTIDIMENSIONAL FAMILY THERAPY (MDFT)

Multidimensional Family Therapy (MDFT) focuses on changing systemic influences that establish and maintain problem behaviors in adolescents. MDFT was first introduced as a weekly, clinic-based intervention (Liddle & Hogue, 2000). A newer version provides a home-based, intensive intervention that incorporates alterations for severely impaired co-morbid substance abusing youth. MDFT is based on the integration of existing therapeutic work in areas such as case management, school interventions, drug counseling methods, use of multimedia, and HIV/AIDS prevention (Rowe, Liddle, & McClintic, 2002).

MDFT is manualized and treatment duration and intensity has been tested for 16 sessions over five months, as well as a variable number of sessions over six months. Generally, an average of 2-3 sessions with various combinations of family members is held weekly, averaging 1-2 hours each. Phone contacts should be frequent and provide opportunities for "mini-sessions." MDFT assesses and intervenes in five domains: Interventions with the adolescent, parent, parent-adolescent relationship, other family members, and systems external to the family (Liddle & Dakof, 1995). MDFT encompasses a collaborative, individualized approach that requires a high degree of engagement by families. Strategies for engagement is employed to capture the interest of the family and assess risk and protective factors within the specific ecological context of the family in order to create a working agenda for preventive intervention (Becker, Hogue, & Liddle, 2002).

MDFT has been empirically supported as a therapy for substance abusing teens. Its efficacy has been supported by studies comparing MDFT with alternate therapies in four controlled trials (Dennis, Titus, Diaond et al., in press; Hogue, Liddle, Becker, & Johnson-Leckrone, 2002; Liddle et al., 2001). Specifically, three randomized clinical trials have explored the use of MDFT with adolescent substance use cessation. The first study split 182 substance-using adolescents of varying ethnicities into three groups: MDFT, Adolescent Group Therapy, and Multifamily Education Intervention (Liddle et al., 2001). The results showed overall improvement for all three groups, but the greatest improvement for the MDFT group. Only the MDFT group reported significant improvement in family competence and academic grades. The MDFT group also maintained the improvement at 3-month and 12-month follow-ups.

The second study compared MDFT to Cognitive-Behavioral Therapy (Liddle, Dakof, Turner, & Tejeda, in press). The clients were primarily African-American males from low-income families. It was found that both treatments were somewhat efficacious from intake to termination. However, clients who participated in MDFT maintained gains after termination. The third study focused on issues of cost and suggested that MDFT compared favorably in terms of cost (less than the median). MDFT was also found to have an impact that was maintained at three-month follow-up (Dennis et al., in press).

A prevention study with Multidimensional Family Prevention (MDFP) (Hogue & Liddle, 1999; Liddle & Hogue, 2000) showed greater gains when compared to controls on mediators of substance use. Domains studied included self-competence, family functioning, school involvement, and peer associations. Preliminary evidence of short-term efficacy indicated strengthened family cohesion, school bonding, and reduced peer delinquency compared to controls (Hogue et al., 2002).

INTEGRATED BEHAVIORAL FAMILY THERAPY

There is some evidence for the effectiveness of IBFT, especially in terms of long-term maintenance of results. The therapy combines two common and well-established family treatment approaches for adolescent substance abuse: family systems therapy and individual cognitive-behavioral therapy. IFBT has been manualized and typically includes weekly or bi-weekly meetings with the adolescent and the parents. The duration of the intervention usually ranges from a few months to a year, depending on the need for the intensity of the treatment. Booster sessions have been used following termination of treatment, and are recommended beginning at three months after treatment termination, as this is a typical time for recurrences in substance abuse (Whisman, 1990). The use of IFBT with minority clients has also been explored (Moncher, Holden, & Schinke, 1990).

IBFT (also known as Targeted Family Intervention) involves assessment and intervention based on assessment. During the assessment phase, the therapist elicits statements regarding desired outcomes, assesses past attempts to address the problem, collects information about current reinforcement of the problem, and elicits maladaptive explanatory statements from the family. The intervention goal is to help families establish environments that will promote desired behaviors. This is accomplished by taking one complaint at a time, modeling and coaching non-aversive communication behaviors, modeling and guiding members through sequential verbal problem-solving, focusing on consistent consequences for undesired behavior, and suggesting evidence for more adaptive explanatory statements about undesired outcomes (Bry & Krinsley, 1992).

In a randomized trial comparing IBFT, individual cognitive-behavioral therapy, and IBFT combined with individual cognitive-behavioral therapy, each intervention demonstrated a level of efficacy (Waldron, Slesnick, & Brody, 2001). However, the IBFT alone and in combination with individual therapy showed a significant decrease in days of substance use. In order to explore ways to lengthen the effects of IBFT and other family therapies, the long-term effects of IBFT on substance abuse have been examined. In a small group of subjects receiving IBFT (n = 1 control, 3 experimental), maintenance of decreased substance use was seen after six months in youth that received booster sessions (Bry & Krinsley, 1992).

In another recent study (Latimer, Winters, & D'Zurilla, 2003), IBFT was compared with a psychoeducational curriculum. Forty-three substance abusing youth participated in the study. During the 6-month post-treatment period, the IBFT group showed significantly lower rates of alcohol and marijuana use, and problem avoidance; significantly higher levels of rational problem-solving and learning strategy skills was also found.

OTHER FAMILY THERAPIES

Other family therapies have been developed and are currently being examined; however, limited empirical support exists. Some of the leading therapies in this category will be discussed briefly and include: Purdue Brief Family Therapy, Project STAR, the Seattle Social Development Project, and the Community Reinforcement Approach and Family Training.

Purdue Brief Family Therapy (PBFT) integrates structural, strategic, functional, and behavioral family therapies. Goals include reduction of resistance to change, restraint of immediate change, reestablishment of parental control, assessment, and interruption of dysfunctional patterns, provision of adolescent assertion skills training and positive therapeutic changes (Trepper, Piercy, & Lewis, 1993). In a study of 84 adolescents and their families (Lewis, Piercy, & Sprenkle, 1990), the Purdue Brief Family Therapy model was compared to a parenting skills program. Both programs were found to significantly reduce drug use, but a greater percentage of the PBFT group showed decreased drug use.

Project STAR has gained recognition focusing on prevention with preschool children. The program includes a classroom-based curriculum and also parent training and home visits. In a longitudinal study (Kaminski, Stormshak, Good, & Goodman, 2002), Head Start classrooms were randomly assigned to experimental and control groups. An increase in positive parenting and parent-school involvement over the first year of intervention and positive parenting and social competence through kindergarten suggests the possible usefulness of this program in preventing substance abuse.

The Seattle Social Development Project (SSDP) is based on the social development model, which incorporates empirical predictive and protective factors related to antisocial behavior in adolescents. The social development model is based on control theory, social learning theory, and differential association theory (Catalano & Hawkins, 1996). One study (Lonczak, 2000) found encouraging results for risky sexual abuse in adolescents. Additionally, it has been tested for use with adolescent substance use and findings indicate that the model's factors are potential targets for the prevention or reduction of adolescent alcohol use (Lonczak, Huang, & Catalano, 2001; Catalano, Kosterman, & Hawkins, 1996). Positive effects of the program have been found for students' attitudes, achievement, and behavior (Hawkins, Catalano, & Morrison, 1992).

CONCLUSIONS

From this review of the literature it is evident that most studies indicated the effectiveness of family-based interventions in reducing youth substance use behaviors. Although the findings are somewhat inconclusive concerning the lasting effects, the evidence clearly indicates that these interventions are helpful in reducing youth substance use and other high-risk behaviors. Various studies demonstrated that the short-term effectiveness of these interventions appear comparable to the effectiveness of individually based interventions; however, long-term effects of family-based interventions appear more promising than adolescent therapy alone. Also encouraging is the fact that these treatments are manualized, making future replication possible.

However, many of the studies reviewed used quasi-experimental or exploratory methods with a small sample sizes. Very few studies meet the criteria for strong validity in experimental design and sensitivity (Spoth, 1998). Additionally, the validity of some studies is questionable, as self-report measures of substance use and other highly sensitive issues were employed. Some studies measured potential substance use based on indirect measures, such as drug-related arrests or family functioning measures. Clearly, the issue of social desirability in self-report findings may affect the validity of the results; thus, future studies on family-based interventions must utilize multi-method, multi-informant measurement procedures.

Although adaptation of existing successful family-based models to address substance use among youth is needed, few studies of family-based interventions addressed the serious problem of engagement and retention in the treatment process. Research has shown that time in treatment (retention) is the single best predictor of positive outcomes (Simpson, 2001) and higher levels of engagement early in treatment lead to extended retention rates (Joe, Simpson, & Broome, 1998; Simpson, Joe, Rowan-Szal, & Greener, 1995). Engagement is typically defined across general dimensions of therapeutic involvement and session participation (Joe et al., 1998) and involves rapport, treatment confidence, and commitment (De Leon, 1996; Simpson, Joe, & Brown, 1997). Thus, a client who is 'engaged' is more likely to bond with counselors, endorse treatment goals, and participate to a greater degree (Broome, Joe, & Simpson, 2001). In addition, a high degree of treatment readiness is considered an important predictor of client participation and positive outcomes (Broome, Knight, Hiller, & Simpson, 1997; Gainey, Wells, Hawkins, & Catalano, 1993). Treatment retention is highly associated with engagement and, like engagement, is considered an important criterion for judging the effectiveness of an intervention (Szapocznik & Kurtines, 1990). These studies point to the need for further development and research of strategies to improve engagement and retention, especially for difficult to recruit and retain populations.

In light of these findings, more studies are needed to explore the use of family-based interventions for this population. These findings should be replicated in experimental studies with larger sample sizes and more rigorous methodologies. Additionally, the treatments should be studied across diverse ethnic groups, and developed with cultural sensitivity. Given the encouraging results related to the long-term effects of family-based interventions on adolescent substance use, factors related to these positive findings should be explored in more depth.

REFERENCES

Aktan, G. (1995). Organizational framework for a substance use prevention program. *International Journal of Addition, 30,* 185-201.

Aktan, G., Kumpfer, K.L., & Turner, C. (1996). Effectiveness of a family skills training program for substance abuse prevention with inner-city African-American families. *International Journal of Addition, 31,* 158-175.

Becker, D., Hogue, A., & Liddle, H.A. (2002). Methods of engagement in family-based preventive intervention. *Child & Adolescent Social Work Journal, 19(2),* 163-179.

Borduin, C.M., Mann, B.J., Cone, L.T., Henggeler, S.W., Fucci, B.R., Blaske, D.M., & Williams, R.A. (1995). Multisystemic treatment of serious juvenile offenders: Long-term prevention of criminality and violence. *Journal of Consulting & Clinical Psychology, 63,* 569-578.

Broome, K.M., Joe, G.W., & Simpson, D.D. (2001). Engagement Models for Adolescents in DATOS-A. *Journal of Adolescent Research, 16(6),* 608-610.

Broome, K.M., Knight, D.K., Knight, K., Hiller, M.L., & Simpson, D.D. (1997). Peer, family, and motivational influences on drug treatment process and recidivism for probationers. *Journal of Clinical Psychology, 53*(4), 387-397.

Brown, T.L., Henggeler, S.W., & Schoenwald, S.K. (1999). Multisystemic treatment of substance abusing and dependent juvenile delinquents: Effects on school attendance at posttreatment and 6-month follow-up. *Children's Services: Social Policy, Research, and Practice, 2(2),* 81-93.

Bry, B.H., & Krinsley, K.E. (1992). Booster sessions and long-term effects of behavioral family therapy on adolescent substance use and school performance. *Journal of Behavior Therapy & Experimental Psychiatry, 23(3),* 183-189.

Burns, B.J., & Weisz, J. (2000). *Implementing child services and interventions: At the crossroads.* Rockville, MD: Discussion and Plenary Session, NIMH Challenges for the 21st Century: Mental Health Services Research.

Catalano, R.F., & Hawkins, J.D. (1996). The social development model: A theory of antisocial behavior. In J.D. Hawkins (Ed.), *Delinquency and crime: Current theories.* New York: Cambridge University Press.

Catalano, R.F., Kosterman, R., & Hawkins, J.D. (1996). Modeling the etiology of adolescent substance use: A test of the social development model. *Journal of Drug Issues, 26(2),* 429-455.

Cauce, A.M., Reid, M., Landesman, S., & Gonzales, N.A. (1990). Social support in young children: Measurement, structure, and behavioral impact. In Sarason, B.R., Sarason, I.G., & Pierce, G.R. (Eds.), *Social support: An interactional view* (pp. 64-94). New York: Wiley.

Coatsworth, J.D., Santisteban, D.A., & McBride, C.K. (2001). Brief strategic family therapy versus community control: Engagement, retention, and an exploration of the moderating role of adolescent symptom severity. *Family Process, 40(3),* 313-332.

DeLeon, G. (1996). Integrative recovery: A state paradigm. *Substance Abuse, 17,* 51-63.

Dennis, M., Titus, J., Diamond, G., Babor, T., Donaldson, J., Godley, S.H., Tims, F., Webb, C., Liddle, H.A., & Scott, C. (in press). The Cannabis Youth Treatment (CYT) experiment: A multi-site study of five approaches to outpatient treatment for adolescents. *Addiction.*

Formoso, D., Gonzales, N.A., & Aiken, L.S. (2000). Family conflict and children's internalizing and externalizing behavior: Protective factors. *American Journal of Community Psychology, 28*(2), 175-199.

Foxcroft, D.R., Ireland, D., & Lister-Sharp, D.J. (2003). Longer-term primary prevention for alcohol misuse in young people: A systematic review. *Addiction, 98(4),* 397-411.

Gainey, R.R., Wells, E.A., Hawkins, J.D., & Catalano, R.F. (1993). Predicting treatment retention among cocaine users. *International Journal of the Addictions, 28(6)*, 487-505.

Haley, J. (1973). Strategic therapy when a child is presented as the problem. *Journal of the American Academy of Child Psychiatry, 12(4)*, 641-659.

Hawkins, J., Catalano, R.F., & Miller, J.Y. (1992). Risk and protective factors for alcohol and other drug problems in adolescence and early adulthood: Implications for substance abuse prevention. *Psychological Bulletin, 112*(1), 64-105.

Hawkins, J. D., Catalano, R.F., & Morrison, D. M. (1992). The Seattle Social Development Project: Effects of the first four years on protective factors and problem behaviors. In McCord, J., & Tremblay, R. (Eds.), *Preventing antisocial behavior: Interventions from birth through adolescence*. New York, NY, US: The Guilford Press (pp. 139-161).

Henggeler, S.W. (1986). Multisystemic treatment of juvenile offenders: Effects on adolescent behavior and family interaction. *Developmental Psychology, 22(1)*, 132-141.

Henggeler, S.W., Borduin, C.M., Melton, G.B., Mann, B.J., Smith, L., Hall, J.A., Cone, L., & Fucci, B.R. (1991). Effects of multisystemic therapy on drug use and abuse in serious juvenile offenders: A progress report from two outcome studies. *Family Dynamics of Addiction Quarterly, 1*, 40-51.

Henggeler, S.W., Clingempeel, W.G., Brondino, M.J., & Pickrel, S.G. (2002). Four year follow-up of multisystemic therapy with substance abusing and dependent juvenile offenders. *Journal of the American Academy of Child & Adolescent Psychiatry, 41*, 868-874.

Henggeler, S.W., Melton, G.B., & Smith, L.A. (1992). Family preservation using multisystemic therapy: An effective alternative to incarcerating serious juvenile offenders. *Journal of Consulting & Clinical Psychology, 60*, 953-961.

Henggeler, S.W., Melton, G.B., Smith, L.A., Schoenwald, S.K., & Hanley, J.H. (1993). Family preservation using multisystemic treatment: Long-term follow-up to a clinical trial with serious juvenile offenders. *Journal of Child & Family Studies, 2*, 283-293.

Henggler, S.W., Pickrel, S.G., Brondino, M.J., & Crouch, J.L. (1996). Eliminating (almost) treatment dropout of substance abusing or dependent delinquents through home-based multisystemic therapy. *American Journal of Psychiatry, 153*, 427-428.

Henggeler, S.W., Pickrel, S.G., & Brondino, M.J. (1999). Multisystemic treatment of substance abusing and dependent delinquents: Outcomes, treatment fidelity, and transportability. *Mental Health Services Research, 1*, 171-184.

Henggeler, S.W., Schoenwald, S.K., Borduin, C.M., Rowland, M.D., & Cunningham, P.B. (1998). *Multisystemic Treatment of Antisocial Behavior in Children and Adolescents*. New York, NY: The Guildford Press.

Hogue, A., & Liddle, H.A. (1999). Family-based preventive intervention: An approach to preventing substance use and antisocial behavior. *American Journal of Orthopsychiatry, 69(3)*, 278-293.

Hogue, A.T., Liddle, H.A., Becker, D. and Johnson-Leckrone, J., (2002). Family-based prevention counseling for high risk young adolescents: Immediate outcomes. *Journal of Community Psychology* 30(1), 1-22.

Huizinga, D., Loeber, R., & Thornberry, T.P. (1994). *Urban delinquency and substance abuse: Initial findings.* Washington, DC: U.S. Government Printing Office.

Joe, G.W., Simpson, D.D., & Broome, K.M. (1998). Effects of readiness for drug abuse treatment on client retention and assessment of process. *Addiction, 93*(8), 1177-1190.

Johnston, L.D., O'Malley, P.M., & Bachman, J.G. (2002). Demographic subgroup trends for various licit and illicit drugs, 1975-2001. (Monitoring the Future Occasional Paper No. 57). Ann Arbor, MI: Institute for Social Research. Available: http://monitoringthefuture.org.

Kaminski, R.A., Stormshak, E.A., Good, R.H.., & Goodman, M.R. (2002). Prevention of Substance Abuse With Rural Head Start Children and Families: Results of Project STAR. *Psychology of Addictive Behaviors, 16 (Suppl4),* S11-S26.

Kamoeoka, V.A. (1996). *The effects of a family-focused intervention on reducing risk for substance abuse among Asian and Pacific-Island youths and families: Evaluation of the Strengthening Hawaii's Families Project.* Honolulu: University of Hawaii, Social Welfare Evaluation and Research Unit.

Kumpfer, K.L. (1998). Selective prevention approaches for drug use prevention: Overview of outcome results from multi-ethnic replications of the Strengthening Families Program. In: Ashery, R., Kumpfer, K.L., and Robertson, E. (Eds.), *Drug Abuse Prevention Through Family Interventions.* National Institute on Drug Abuse Research Monograph 177. U.S. Department of Health and Human Services, National Institutes of Health, National Institute on Drug Abuse.

Kumpfer, K.L., Alexander, L.B., McDonald, L., & Olds, D.L. (1998). *Family-focused substance abuse prevention: What has been learned from other fields* (No. Monograph 177). Rockville, MD: National Institute of Drug Abuse.

Kumpfer, K.L., & Alvarado, R. (1995). Strengthening families to prevent drug use in multi-ethnic youth. In G. Botvin, S. Schinke, & M. Orlandi (Eds.), *Drug abuse prevention with multi-ethnic youth* (pp. 253-292). Newbury Park, CA: Sage.

Kumpfer, K.L., Alvarado, R., & Smith, P. (2002). Cultural sensitivity and adaptation in family-based prevention interventions. *Prevention Science, 3(3),* 241-246.

Kumpfer, K.L., Alvarado, R., & Tait, C. (2002). Effectiveness of school-based family and children's skills training for substance prevention among 6-8-year-old rural children. P*sychology of Addictive Behaviors, 16*(Suppl4), S65-S71.

Kumpfer, K.L., DeMarsh, J.P., & Child, W. (1989). *Strengthening Families Program: Children's Skills Training Curriculum Manual, Parent Training Manual, Children's Skill Training Manual, and Family Skills Training Manual* (Prevention Services to Children of Substance-Abusing Parents). Salt Lake City: Social Research Institute, Graduate School of Social Work, University of Utah.

Kumpfer, K.L., Molgaard, V., & Spoth, R. (1996). The Strengthening Families Program for prevention of delinquency and drug use in special populations. In R. DeV Peters, & R.J. McMahon (Eds.), *Childhood disorders, substance abuse, and delinquency: Prevention and early intervention approaches.* Newbury Park, CA: Sage.

Kumpfer, K.L., & Turner, C.W. (1990-1991). The social ecology model of adolescent substance abuse: Implications for prevention. *Internal Journal of the Addictions, 25(4-A),* 435-463.

Kumpfer, K.L., Wamberg, K., & Martinez, D. (1996). *Strengthening Hispanic Families Program*. Paper presented at the Center for Substance Abuse Prevention, High Risk Youth Conference, Washington, DC.

Latimer, W.W., Winters, K.C., & D'Zurilla, T. (2003). Integrated Family and Cognitive-Behavioral Therapy for adolescent substance abusers: A Stage I efficacy study. *Drug & Alcohol Dependence, 71(3)*, 303-317.

Letourneau, E.J., Cunningham, P.B., & Henggeler, S.W. (2002) Multisystemic treatment of antisocial behavior in adolescents. In Hofmann, S.G., & Tompson, M.C. (Eds.), *Treating chronic and severe mental disorders: A handbook of empirically supported interventions*. (pp. 364-381). New York, NY, U.S.: The Guilford Press.

Lewis, R.A., Piercy, F.P., & Sprenkle, D.H. (1990). Family-based interventions for helping drug-abusing adolescents. *Journal of Adolescent Research, 5(1)*, 82-95.

Liddle, H.A., & Dakof, G.A. (1995). Efficacy of family therapy for drug abuse: Promising but not definitive. *Journal of Marital & Family Therapy, 21(4)*, 511-539.

Liddle, H.A., Dakof, G.A., Parker, K., Diamond, G.S., Barrett, K., & Tejeda, M. (2001). Multidimensional family therapy for adolescent drug abuse: Results of a randomized clinical trial. *American Journal of Drug & Alcohol Abuse, 27*(4), 651-688.

Liddle, H.A., Dakof, G.A., Turner, R.M., & Tejeda, M. (in press). Treating adolescent substance abuse: a comparison of individual and family therapy interventions. *NIDA Monograph on the 2001 CPDD Conference* (paper presented at Adolescent Drug Abuse Treatment Research Symposium [A. Morral, & M. Dennis, Chairs], CPDD, June, 2001).

Liddle, H.A., & Hogue, A. (2000). A family-based, developmental-ecological preventive intervention for high-risk adolescents. *Journal of Marital & Family Therapy, 26(3)*, 265-279.

Lonczak, H.S. (2000). An examination of the long-term effects of the Seattle Social Development Project on sexual behavior and related outcomes, and of the consequences of adolescent motherhood. (Washington, early intervention). *Dissertation Abstracts International Section A: Humanities & Social Sciences, Vol 60(7-A)*, 2371.

Lonczak, H.S., Huang, B., & Catalano, R.F. (2001). The social predictors of adolescent alcohol misuse: A test of the Social Development Model. *Journal of Studies on Alcohol, 62(2)*, 179-189.

Lundahl, L.H., Davis, T.M., Adesso, V.J., & Lukas, S.E. (1997). Alcohol expectancies: effects of gender, age, and family history of alcoholism. *Addictive Behaviors, 22(1)*, 115-125.

Minuchin, S. (1974). *Families & family therapy*. Oxford, England: Harvard University Press, pp. 268.

Moncher, M.S., Holden, G.W., & Schinke, S.P. (1990). Behavioral family treatment of the substance abusing Hispanic adolescent. In Feindler, E.L., & Kalfus, G.R. (Eds.), *Adolescent behavior therapy handbook*. New York, NY: Springer Publishing Co., 329-349.

Newcomb, M.D. (1992). Understanding the multidimensional nature of drug use and abuse: The role of consumption, risk factors, and protective factors. In Glantz, M.D., & Pickens, R.W. (Eds.), *Vulnerability to drug abuse*. Washington, DC: American Psychological Association.

Newcomb, M.D., & Bentler, P.M. (1989). Substance use and abuse among children and teenagers. *American Psychologist* 44, 242-248.

Nichols, M.P., & Schwartz, R.C. (1995). Family Therapy: Concepts and Methods. Needham Heights, MA: Allyn and Bacon.

Oetting, E.R. (1992). Planning programs for prevention of deviant behavior: A psychosocial model. *Drugs & Society, 6(3-4)*, 313-344.

Paradise, M., Cauce, A.M., Ginzler, J., Wert, S., Wruck, K., & Brooker, M. (2001). The role of relationships in developmental trajectories of homeless and runaway youth. In Sarason, B.R., & Duck, S. (Eds.), *Personal relationships: Implications for clinical and community psychology*. New York: John Wiley & Sons.

Perrino, T., Gonzalez-Soldevilla, A., Pantin, H., & Szapocznik, J. (2000). The role of families in adolescent HIV prevention: A review. *Clinical Child and Family Psychology Review*, 3(2), 81-96.

Rahdert, E., & Czechowicz, D. (Eds.). (1995). *Adolescent drug abuse: Clinical assessment and therapeutic interventions*. Washington, DC: NIDA Research Monograph 156. U.S. Government Printing Office.

Randall, J., & Cunningham, P.B. (2003). Multisystemic therapy: A treatment for violent substance-abusing and substance-dependent juvenile offenders. *Addictive Behaviors, 28(9)*, 1731-1739.

Randall, J., Henggeler, S.W., & Cunningham, P.B. (2001). Adapting multisystemic therapy to treat adolescent substance abuse more effectively. *Cognitive & Behavioral Practice, 8(4)*, 359-366.

Robbins, M.S., Mitrani, V.B., & Zarate, M. (2002). Change processes in family therapy with Hispanic adolescents. *Hispanic Journal of Behavioral Sciences, 24(4)*, 505-519.

Robbins, M.S., Szapocznik, J., & Santisteban, D.A. (2003). Brief strategic family therapy for Hispanic youth. In Kazdin, A.E. (Ed.), *Yale University School of Medicine, Child Study Center. Evidence-based psychotherapies for children and adolescents*. New York, NY: The Guilford Press, 407-424.

Rowe, C., Liddle, H.A., & McClintic, K. (2002). Integrative treatment development: Multidimensional family therapy for adolescent substance abuse. In: Kaslow, F.W. (Ed.), *Comprehensive handbook of psychotherapy: Integrative/eclectic*. New York, NY: John Wiley & Sons, Inc. 133-161.

Santisteban, D.A., Coatsworth, J.D., & Perez-Vidal, A. (2003). Efficacy of brief strategic family therapy in modifying Hispanic adolescent behavior problems and substance use. *Journal of Family Psychology, 17(1)*, 121-133.

Santisteban, D.A., Szapocznik, J., Perez-Vidal, A., Kurtines, W.M., Coatsworth, J.D., & LaPerriere, A. (2000). *The efficacy of brief strategic/structural family therapy in modifying behavior problems and an exploration of the role that family functioning plays in behavior change*. Manuscript in preparation, University of Miami, Center for Family Studies.

Santisteban, D.A., Szapocznik, J., Perez-Vidal, A., Kurtines, W.M., Murray, E.J., & LaPerriere, A. (1996). Efficacy of intervention for engaging youth and families into treatment and some variables that may contribute to differential effectiveness. *Journal of Family Psychology, 10*, 35-44.

Schoenwald, S.K., Halliday-Boykins, C.A., & Henggeler, S.W. (2003). Client-level predictors of adherence to MST in community service settings. *Family Process, 42(3)*, 345-359.

Schoenwald, S.K., Ward, D.M., & Henggeler, S.W. (1996). Multisystemic therapy treatment of substance abusing or dependent adolescent offenders: Costs of reducing incarceration, inpatient, and residential placement. *Journal of Child & Family Studies, 5(4)*, 431-444.

Sheidow, A.J., & Woodford, M.S. (2003). Multisystemic therapy: An empirically supported, home-based family therapy approach. *Family Journal-Counseling & Therapy for Couples & Families, 11(3)*, 257-263.

Simpson, D.D. (2001). Modeling treatment process and outcomes. *Addiction, 96(2)*, 207-211.

Simpson, D.D., Joe, G.W., & Brown, B.S. (1997). Treatment retention and follow-up outcomes in the Drug Abuse Treatment Outcome Study (DATOS). *Psychology of Addictive Behaviors, 11(4)*, 294-307.

Simpson, D.D., Joe, G.W., Rowan-Szal, G., & Greener, J. (1995). Client engagement and change during drug abuse treatment. *Journal of Substance Abuse, 7(1)*, 117-134.

Soo-Hoo, T. (1999). Brief strategic family therapy with Chinese Americans. *American Journal of Family Therapy, 27(2)*, 163-179.

Spoth, R. (1998). *Results From Iowa Strengthening Families Program for Drug Use.* Paper presented to the Society for Prevention Research Annual Conference, Baltimore, MD.

Spoth, R., Guyll, M., & Chao, W. (2003). Exploratory Study of a Preventive Intervention with General Population African American Families. *Journal of Early Adolescence, 23(4)*, 435-468.

Spoth, R.L., Guyll, M., & Day, S.X. (2002). Universal family-focused interventions in alcohol-use disorder prevention: Cost-effectiveness and cost-benefit analyses of two interventions. *Journal of Studies on Alcohol, 63(2)*, 219-228.

Spoth, R., Redmond, C., & Lepper, H. (1999). Alcohol initiation outcomes of universal family-focused preventive interventions: One-and two-year follow-ups of a controlled study. *Journal of Studies on Alcohol, supp 13*, 103-111.

Spoth, R., Redmond, C., & Shin, C. (1998). Direct and indirect latent-variable parenting outcomes of two universal family-focused preventive interventions: Extending a public health-oriented research base. *Journal of Consulting & Clinical Psychology, 66(2)*, 385-399.

Spoth, R.L., Redmond, C., & Shin, C. (2001). Randomized trial of brief family interventions for general populations: Adolescent substance use outcomes 4 years following baseline. *Journal of Consulting & Clinical Psychology, 69(4)*, 627-642.

Spoth, R.L., Redmond, C., & Trudeau, L. (2002). Longitudinal substance initiation outcomes for a universal preventive intervention combining family and school programs. *Psychology of Addictive Behaviors, 16(2)*, 129-134.

Spoth, R., Reyes, M.L., & Redmond, C. (1999). Assessing a public health approach to delay onset and progression of adolescent substance use: Latent transition and log-linear analyses of longitudinal family preventive intervention outcomes. *Journal of Consulting & Clinical Psychology, 67(5)*, 619-630.

Stanton, M.D., & Shadish, W.R. (1997). Outcomes, attrition, and family-couple treatment for drug abuse: A meta-analysis and review of the controlled, comparative studies. *Psychological Bulletin, 122*, 170-191.

Szapocznik, J., Hervis, O., & Schwartz, S. (2001). *Brief Strategic Family Therapy Manual [NIDA Treatment Manual Series]*. Rockvill, MD: National Institute on Drug Abuse.

Szapocznik, J., & Kurtines, W.M. (1989). *Breakthroughs in family therapy with drug abusing problem youth*. New York: Springer.

Szapocznik, J., & Kurtines, W. (1990). Interplay of advances between theory, research, and application in treatment interventions aimed at behavior problem children and adolescents. *Journal of Consulting & Clinical Psychology, 58(6)*, 696-703.

Szapocznik, J., Kurtines, W.M., Foote, F., Perez-Vidal, A., & Hervis, O.E. (1983). Conjoint versus one-person family therapy: Some evidence for the effectiveness of conducting family therapy through one person with drug-abusing adolescents. *Journal of Consulting & Clinical Psychology, 51*, 889-899.

Szapocznik, J., Kurtines, W.M., Foote, F., Perez-Vidal, A., & Hervis, O.E. (1986). Conjoint versus one-person family therapy: Further evidence for the effectiveness of conducting family therapy through one person with drug-abusing adolescents. *Journal of Consulting & Clinical Psychology, 54(3)*, 395-397.

Szapocznik, J., Perez-Vidal, A., Brickman, A., Foote, F.H., Santisteban, D., Hervis, O.E., & Kurtines, W.M. (1988). Engaging adolescent drug abusers and their families into treatment: A strategic structural systems approach. *Journal of Consulting & Clinical Psychology, 56*, 552-557.

Szapocznik, J., Perez-Vidal, A., Hervis, O.E., Brickman, A.E., & Kurtines, W.M. (1989). Innovations in family therapy: Strategies for overcoming resistance to treatment. In R.A. Wells & V.J. Giannetti (Eds.), *Handbook of brief psychotherapies*. (pp. 93-114). New York: Plenum Press.

Szapocznik, J., Rio, A., & Murray, E. (1989). Structural family versus psychodynamic child therapy for problematic Hispanic boys. *Journal of Consulting & Clinical Psychology, 57(5)*, 571-578.

Szapocznik, J., Santisteban, D., Rio, A., Perez Vidal, A., & Kurtines, W.M. (1986). Family effectiveness training for Hispanic families: Strategic structural systems intervention for the prevention of drug abuse. In H.P. Lefley, & P.B. Pedersen (Eds.), *Cross cultural training for mental health professionals*. (pp. 245-261). Springfield, IL: Charles C Thomas.

Szapocznik, J., Santisteban, D., Rio, A., Perez Vidal, A., Kurtines, W.M., & Hervis, O.E. (1986). Bicultural effectiveness training (BET): An intervention modality for families experiencing intergenerational/intercultural conflict. *Hispanic Journal of Behavioral Sciences, 6*, 303-330.

Szapocznik, J., & Williams, R.A. (2000). Brief Strategic Family Therapy: Twenty-five years of interplay among theory, research and practice in adolescent behavior problems and drug abuse. *Clinical Child & Family Psychological Review, 3(2)*, 117-134.

Trepper, T.S., Piercy, F.P., & Lewis, R.A. (1993). Family therapy for adolescent alcohol abuse. In O'Farrell, T. J. (Ed.), *Treating alcohol problems: Marital and family interventions*. New York, NY, US: Guilford Press. pp. 261-278.

Waldron, H.B., Slesnick, N., & Brody, J.L. (2001). Treatment outcomes for adolescent substance abuse at 4-and 7-month assessments. *Journal of Consulting & Clinical Psychology, 69(5)*, 802-813.

Whisman, M.A. (1990). The efficacy of booster maintenance sessions in behavior therapy: Review and methodological critique. *Clinical Psychology Review, 10*, 155-170.

Wills, T.A.V., & D McNamara, G. (1992). The role of life events, family support, and competence in adolescent substance use: A test of vulnerability and protective factors. *American Journal of Community Psychology, 20(3)*, 349-374.

Winters, K.C. (1999). *Treatment of adolescents with substance use disorders.* (SMA 99-3283). Rockville MD: Center for Substance Abuse Treatment.

Behavioral Couples Therapy for Alcoholism and Drug Abuse: Rationale, Methods, Findings, and Future Directions

Keith Klostermann, PhD
William Fals-Stewart, PhD
Christie Gorman, MA
Cheryl Kennedy, CSW
Cynthia Stappenbeck, MA

SUMMARY. Behavioral Couples Therapy (BCT) is an evidence-based family treatment for alcoholism and drug abuse. The results of multiple

---

Keith Klostermann, William Fals-Stewart, Christie Gorman, Cheryl Kennedy, and Cynthia Stappenbeck are affiliated with the Research Institute on Addictions, University at Buffalo, The State University of New York.

Address correspondence to: William Fals-Stewart, Research Institute on Addictions (www.addictionandfamily.org), 1021 Main Street, Buffalo, NY 14203-1016 (E-mail: wstewart@ria.buffalo.edu).

This project was supported, in part, by grants from the National Institute on Drug Abuse (R01DA12189, R01DA014402, R01DA014402-SUPL, R01DA015937, R01DA016236), the National Institute on Alcohol Abuse and Alcoholism (R21AA013690), and the Alpha Foundation.

[Haworth co-indexing entry note]: "Behavioral Couples Therapy for Alcoholism and Drug Abuse: Rationale, Methods, Findings, and Future Directions." Klostermann et al. Co-published simultaneously in *Journal of Evidence-Based Social Work* (The Haworth Social Work Practice Press, an imprint of The Haworth Press, Inc.) Vol. 2, No. 1/2, 2005, pp. 235-255; and: *Addiction, Assessment, and Treatment with Adolescents, Adults, and Families* (ed: Carolyn Hilarski) The Haworth Social Work Practice Press, an imprint of The Haworth Press, Inc., 2005, pp. 235-255. Single or multiple copies of this article are available for a fee from The Haworth Document Delivery Service [1-800-HAWORTH, 9:00 a.m. - 5:00 p.m. (EST). E-mail address: docdelivery@haworthpress.com].

http://www.haworthpress.com/web/JEBSW
Digital Object Identifier: 10.1300/J394v02n01_13

studies conducted during the last 3 decades indicate that participation in BCT by married or cohabiting substance-abusing patients, compared to more traditional individual-based interventions, results in greater reductions in substance use, higher levels of relationship satisfaction, greater reductions in partner violence, and more favorable cost-benefit and cost-effectiveness. This review examines the rationale for using BCT, the empirical literature supporting its use, methods used as part of this intervention, and future research directions. *[Article copies available for a fee from The Haworth Document Delivery Service: 1-800-HAWORTH. E-mail address: <docdelivery@haworthpress.com> Website: <http://www.HaworthPress. com> © 2005 by The Haworth Press, Inc. All rights reserved.]*

KEYWORDS. Family, treatment, adolescents, substance use, risky behaviors

The critical role of the family in the development and maintenance of substance abuse is now widely acknowledged by researchers and practitioners alike. As a result, more and more service providers are intervening with the family as a way to reduce or eliminate abusive drinking or drug use by one or more of its members. During the last 3 decades, the effectiveness of family-based treatment approaches for substance abuse has been demonstrated consistently in multiple empirical clinical studies. Recent meta-analytic reviews of randomized clinical trials have concluded that family-involved treatments result in higher levels of abstinence compared to individual-based interventions that focus exclusively on the substance-abusing client (e.g., Stanton & Shadish, 1997).

Behavioral Couples Therapy (BCT) is a partner-involved family intervention with strong empirical support for its effectiveness (O'Farrell & Fals-Stewart, 2003). In this review of BCT for alcoholism and drug abuse, we discuss the following: (a) the theoretical rationale for the use and effectiveness of BCT, (b) typical treatment methods used as part of the BCT intervention, and (c) research findings supporting the effectiveness of BCT in multiple domains of functioning. In addition, we also note some of the existing gaps in the BCT literature and the future directions of this programmatic line of research.

BCT FOR ALCOHOLISM AND DRUG ABUSE: RATIONALE AND METHODS

Theoretical Rationale for Use of Couples Therapy to Treat Substance Use Disorders

The dynamic interplay between substance use and relationship functioning is quite complex and appear to interact reciprocally. For example, couples in which one of the partners abuses substances usually have extensive relationship problems; these couples often experience high levels of relationship dissatisfaction, instability (i.e., partners making significant steps toward relationship dissolution), and a desire for substantial change in multiple facets of the relationship (e.g., Fals-Stewart, Birchler, & O'Farrell, 1999). In addition, spouses' chronic substance use is often correlated with reduced marital satisfaction (e.g., Dunn, Jacob, Hummon, & Seilhamer, 1987). Consequently, relationship distress is associated with increased problematic substance use and is related to relapse among alcoholics and drug abusers after treatment (e.g., Fals-Stewart & Birchler, 1994; Maisto et al., 1988). Thus, as shown in Figure 1, the relationship between substance use and marital problems forms a mutually causal "vicious cycle."

Given the strong interrelationship between substance use and family interaction, it seems that interventions that focus largely or exclusively on the individual substance-abusing client may not be optimally effective. Yet, the standard format for substance abuse treatment is individual-based therapy. In contrast, BCT (and most other family-based treatment models for alcoholism and drug abuse) has two primary objectives that evolve from the conceptualization of the interrelationship between substance use and family interaction described above: (1) reduce or eliminate substance use and utilize the family to positively support the clients' efforts to change and (2) alter dyadic and family interaction patterns to promote a family environment that is more conducive to long-term stable abstinence.

Primary BCT Treatment Elements

In the early stages of treatment, therapists delivering BCT concentrate on shifting the focus from negative feelings and interactions about past and possible future drinking or drug use to positive behavioral exchanges between partners. In later sessions, emphasis is placed on com-

FIGURE 1. The Vicious Cycle of Substance Abuse and Relationship Distress

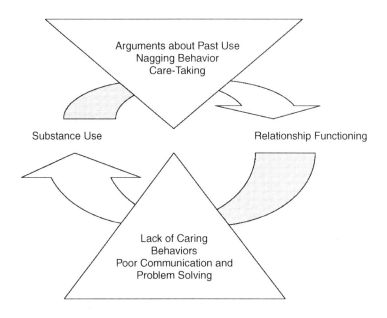

munication skills training, problem-solving strategies, negotiating behavior change agreements, and continuing recovery strategies.

BCT methods used to address substance use. A BCT therapist works to build support from within the dyadic system for abstinence by treating the substance-abusing client with his or her intimate partner. Together, the therapist and couple develop a Recovery Contract in which the partners agree to engage in a daily *Abstinence Trust Discussion.* In this brief verbal exchange, the substance-abusing partner states his or her intent not to drink or use drugs that day (in the tradition of "one day at a time" from Alcoholics Anonymous). In turn, the nonsubstance-abusing partner verbally expresses positive support for the client's efforts to remain abstinent. In addition to participating in the daily Abstinence Trust Discussion, the nonsubstance-abusing partner may witness and verbally reinforce the daily ingestion of abstinence-related medications (e.g., naltrexone, disulfiram) for a substance-abusing client who is medically cleared to do so and willing. The nonsubstance-abusing partner tracks the performance of the Abstinence Trust Discussion (and consumption of medication, if applicable) on a daily Recovery Calendar, which is provided by the therapist.

A central tenant of the Recovery Contract is the agreement between partners to not discuss past drinking or drug use or fears of future substance use when at home (i.e., between scheduled BCT sessions), and to save such discussions for therapy sessions. This agreement is designed to reduce the likelihood of substance-related conflicts occurring between therapy sessions, which can trigger relapses. Instead, partners are asked to only discuss these issues during BCT therapy sessions, which can be monitored by the therapist. In addition, many contracts require partners' regular attendance at self-help meetings (e.g., Alcoholics Anonymous, Nar-Anon, Al-Anon), which are also marked on the provided calendar during the course of treatment.

In the beginning of each BCT session, the therapist reviews the Recovery Calendar to determine overall compliance with the contract. The calendar not only provides a daily record of progress (which is rewarded verbally by the therapist at each session), but it also provides a visual (and temporal) record of any problems with adherence which can be addressed in couples' sessions. Typically, the partners are asked to perform behaviors that are components of their Recovery Contract (e.g., Abstinence Trust Discussion, consumption of abstinence-supporting medication) in each scheduled BCT session. The purpose of this in-session practice is to highlight the importance of the Recovery Contract and to allow the therapist to observe the partners' behaviors providing corrective feedback as needed.

BCT methods used to enhance relationship functioning. BCT seeks to increase positive feelings, shared activities, and constructive communication through the use of standard couple-based behavioral assignments. These relationship factors are viewed as conducive to supporting and maintaining abstinence. For example, *Catch Your Partner Doing Something Nice* asks each partner to notice and acknowledge one pleasing behavior performed by their mate each day. In the *Caring Day* assignment, each partner chooses a day to surprise his or her significant other with a special activity to demonstrate how much he or she cares. In *Shared Rewarding Activities*, the partners plan and engage in mutually agreed upon activities. This assignment is especially important because many substance abusers' families have ceased engaging in shared pleasing activities. In fact, participating in such activities has been associated with positive recovery outcomes (Moos et al., 1990). By learning *Communication Skills* (e.g., paraphrasing, empathizing, validating), the substance-abusing client and his or her partner are better prepared to handle any stressors that arise, and thus, reduce the risk of relapse.

Couples-based relapse prevention and planning. Relapse prevention occurs during the final stages of BCT. At the end of each session, the partners develop a written plan (i.e., *Continuing Recovery Plan*) designed to promote stable abstinence (e.g., continuation of a daily Abstinence Trust Discussion, attending self-help support meetings) and list contingency plans should a relapse occur (e.g., re-contacting the therapist, re-engaging in self-help support meetings, contacting a sponsor). A key element in creating the Continuing Recovery Plan for many couples is the negotiation of the posttreatment duration of the agreed-to activities. Couples often have difficulty agreeing upon the duration of the contract activities; the substance-abusing partner typically wants a life that does not involve the structured exercises and homework that are part of BCT whereas the nonsubstance-abusing partner is often apprehensive about progress made in treatment (i.e., relationship improvement, abstinence) and thus advocates for continued involvement with certain activities (e.g., self-help meeting attendance, Abstinence Trust Discussions). For example, those couples in which the substance-abusing partner is taking medication to assist with abstinence maintenance (e.g., Antabuse) may express a desire to eventually forgo the daily Abstinence Trust Discussion with the observation of medication taking. In this situation, partners develop a mutually agreed-to, long-term gradual reduction of the frequency of the activity until it is eliminated (e.g., for the first month, daily Abstinence Trust Discussion with observed medication-taking, as was done during active treatment; for the second month, the Abstinence Trust Discussion is performed three times per week with observed medication taking; for the third month, the Abstinence Trust Discussion is performed once per week with observed medication taking, and so forth). If problems arise with any of the planned transitions, partners are encouraged to contact their BCT counselor.

Session structure and treatment duration. BCT sessions tend to be moderately-to-highly structured. Typically, the therapist sets a specific agenda for the session from the outset of each meeting. For example, a typical BCT session begins with an update on any drinking or drug use that has occurred since the last session. Compliance with different aspects of the Recovery Contract is reviewed and any difficulties with compliance are discussed and addressed. The session then transitions to a review of any homework from the previous session. Relationship or other difficulties that may have arisen during the last week are then addressed during the session, with the goal being problem resolution. Next, new material (e.g., instruction in and rehearsal of skills to be practiced at home during the week) is introduced. At the end of each session, partners are given specific homework assignments to complete before the next scheduled session.

Typically, the substance-abusing client and his or her partner are seen together for approximately 15-20 outpatient couple sessions over 5-6 months. However, a briefer (i.e., six-session) variant of BCT has recently been developed (Fals-Stewart, Birchler, & O'Farrell, 2001) and is currently being evaluated. Moreover, BCT can be delivered as a stand-alone intervention or as an adjunct to treatment-as-usual substance abuse counseling procedures. Appropriate candidates for BCT are (a) couples in which partners are married or cohabiting for at least one year; (b) couples in which neither partner has a co-occurring psychiatric condition that may significantly interfere with participation in BCT (e.g., schizophrenia, psychosis); and (c) dyads in which only one member of the couple has a current problem with alcoholism or drug abuse.

RESEARCH FINDINGS ON BCT

Primary Outcomes:
Effects on Substance Use and Relationship Adjustment

Numerous studies over the past 30 years have compared drinking and relationship outcomes for alcoholic clients and their partners treated with BCT to various forms of individual-based therapy. Outcomes were measured at 6-months posttreatment in earlier studies and at 18-24 months after treatment in more recent investigations. The results of these investigations have consistently demonstrated BCTs clinical superiority. More specifically, these results reveal a pattern of less frequent drinking, fewer alcohol-related problems, happier relationships, and lower risk of marital separation for alcoholic clients who receive BCT than for clients who receive only individual-based treatment (Azrin, Sisson, Meyers, & Godley, 1982; Bowers & Al-Rehda, 1990; Hedberg & Campbell, 1974; McCrady et al., 1991).

Traditionally, BCT research has been focused on the effects of BCT for alcoholism. More recently, investigators have started examining the effects of BCT for married or cohabiting clients who abuse substances other than alcohol (e.g., Winters, Fals-Stewart, O'Farrell, Birchler, & Kelley, 2002). The first randomized study of BCT with married or cohabiting drug-abusing clients compared BCT plus individual treatment to an equally intensive individual-based treatment for married or cohabiting male clients entering outpatient treatment (Fals-Stewart, Birchler, & O'Farrell, 1996). Compared to clients who participated in individual-based treatment, those who received BCT had fewer days of drug use, fewer drug-related arrests and hospitalizations, and a longer time to relapse after treatment completion. Along these lines, couples who received BCT also reported more positive relationship adjustment and fewer days separated due to relationship discord than couples whose partners received individual-based treatment only. Moreover, very similar results favoring BCT over individual-based counseling were observed in another randomized clinical trial in which married or cohabiting male clients were in a methadone maintenance program (Fals-Stewart, O'Farrell, & Birchler, 2001a).

Fals-Stewart and O'Farrell (2003) examined behavioral family counseling and naltrexone for male opioid-dependent clients. These clients were randomly assigned to one of two equally intensive 24-week treatments: (a) Behavioral Family Counseling (BFC) plus individual treatment (clients had both individual and family sessions and took naltrexone daily in the presence of a family member) or (b) Individual-Based Treatment only (IBT; clients were prescribed naltrexone and were asked in counseling sessions about their compliance but there was no family involvement or compliance contract). BFC clients, compared with their IBT counterparts, ingested more doses of naltrexone, attended more scheduled treatment sessions, remained continuously abstinent longer, and had significantly more days abstinent from opiate-based and other illicit drugs during treatment and during the year after treatment. Consequently, BFC clients also had significantly fewer drug-related, legal, and family problems at 1-year follow-up.

Although the BCT studies with alcoholic and drug-abusing clients have recruited samples that consisted largely or exclusively of married or cohabiting male clients and their nonsubstance-abusing female partners, Winters and colleagues (2002) recently conducted the first BCT study that focused exclusively on female drug-abusing clients. Results indicated female clients who received BCT had significantly fewer days of substance use, longer periods of continuous abstinence, and higher levels of relationship satisfaction. The results of this study were very similar to those found with male substance-abusing clients, indicating BCT may work equally well with both types of couples.

Secondary Outcomes: Effects on Other Areas

Historically, BCT research has focused primarily on substance use and relationship outcomes. BCT for substance abuse is designed primarily to have a direct effect on substance use and relationship outcomes. However, it is plausible that effective reductions in drinking and improvements in the relationship could result in improvements in other problematic areas as well (e.g., secondary outcomes). Consequently, during the last decade, investigators have started to examine the effect of BCT on areas such as intimate partner violence (IPV), cost outcomes, the emotional and behavioral adjustment of children living in homes with substance-abusing parents, and HIV risk behaviors.

IPV. Recently, several studies have examined the effect of BCT on the occurrence of IPV. The results of multiple studies suggest that IPV is a highly prevalent problem among substance-abusing clients and their partners. Roughly two-thirds of the married or cohabiting men entering treatment for alcoholism, or their partners, report at least one episode of male-to-female physical aggression in the year prior to program entry, which is four times higher than IPV prevalence estimates from nationally representative surveys (e.g., O'Farrell, Fals-Stewart, Murphy, & Murphy, 2003). Fals-Stewart (2003) found that the likelihood of male-to-female physical aggression was nearly eight times higher on days of drinking than on days of no drinking for married or cohabiting men entering alcoholism treatment.

In a recent study, O'Farrell and colleagues (2003) examined partner violence before and after BCT. In the year before BCT, 60% of alcoholic clients had been violent toward their female partners, five times the comparison sample rate of 12%. In the year after BCT, violence decreased significantly to 24% among the alcoholic sample but remained higher than the comparison group. Among remitted alcoholics after BCT, violence prevalence of 12% was identical to the comparison sample and less than half the rate among relapsed clients (30%). Results for the second year after BCT yielded similar findings to those found for the first year outcomes. Thus, partner violence decreased after BCT, and clinically significant violence reductions occurred for clients who ceased drinking after BCT.

Fals-Stewart, Kashdan, O'Farrell, and Birchler (2002) examined changes in IPV among married or cohabiting drug-abusing clients and their partners. Although nearly half of the couples in each condition reported male-to-female physical aggression during the year before treatment, the number reporting violence in the year after treatment was significantly lower for BCT (17%) than for individual treatment (42%). Results indicated BCT reduced violence better than individual treatment because BCT reduced drug use, drinking, and relationship problems to a greater extent than individual treatment.

Cost Outcomes. In the current era of limited resources, the control of costs has become an increasingly important concern. As pressure for cost containment intensifies, not only are clinicians, administrators and investigators more frequently asked to answer the question, "Does this treatment work?" but also "What does it cost and is it really worth it?" (e.g., McGuire, 1989). Thus, several authors have maintained that researchers must conduct economic evaluations (i.e., cost-benefit and cost-effectiveness analyses) as part of any comprehensive examination of clinical interventions (e.g., Yates, 1994). Cost-benefit analysis compares the resources used to deliver a given service to the benefits of the intervention, with both costs and benefits expressed in monetary units. Cost-effectiveness analysis compares different interventions on the cost per unit of clinical effect (e.g., cost of a day of abstinence from drugs and alcohol during the year after substance abuse treatment completion).

O'Farrell and colleagues (1996b) presented cost outcomes comparing equally intensive, manualized treatments: (a) BCT plus individual counseling, (b) interactional couples therapy plus individual counseling, and (c) individual counseling only. The cost-benefit analysis of BCT plus individual alcoholism counseling showed: (a) average costs per case for alcohol-related hospital treatments and jail stays decreased from about $7,800 in the year before to about $1,100 in the two years after BCT with cost savings averaging about $6,700 per case; and (b) a benefit-to-cost ratio of $8.64 in cost savings for every dollar spent to deliver BCT. None of the positive cost-benefit results observed for BCT were true for subjects given interactional couples therapy plus individual alcoholism counseling for which posttreatment utilization costs increased. Participants in the interactional therapy condition had fewer days abstinent during treatment than those in BCT, and interactional cases that failed to stay abstinent during treatment incurred substantial hospital and jail costs during follow-up. Thus, adding BCT to individual alcoholism counseling produced a positive cost-benefit effect while the addition of interactional couples therapy did not. Individual counseling alone had a significantly more positive benefit-to-cost ratio than BCT plus individual counseling. More specifically, the cost of delivering individual counseling was about half the cost of delivering BCT plus individual counseling. Cost-effectiveness analyses indicated that the addition of BCT to individual counseling was less cost-effective than individual counseling only and modestly more cost-effective than interactional therapy in producing abstinence from drinking. Regarding marital adjustment outcomes, the three treatments were equally cost-effective except during the active treatment phase when BCT was more cost-effective than interactional couples therapy.

O'Farrell and colleagues (1996a) presented cost outcomes for a second study in which manualized BCT with added couples relapse prevention (RP) sessions was compared with manualized BCT alone. Costs of treatment delivery and health and legal service utilization were measured for 12 months before and 12 months after BCT. Cost-benefit analysis results for both standard BCT and for the longer and more costly form of BCT with additional RP sessions showed decreases in health care and legal costs after treatment as compared to before treatment with average cost savings per case of $5,053 for BCT only and $3,365 for BCT-plus-RP. The benefit-to-cost ratios showed $5.97 for BCT only and $1.89 for BCT-plus-RP in cost savings for every dollar spent to deliver the respective treatment. Despite the fact that adding RP to BCT led to less drinking and better relationship adjustment, it did not lead to greater cost savings (e.g., decrease in health and legal service utilization) or a more favorable benefit-to-cost ratio than BCT-only. Adding RP to BCT nearly doubled the cost of delivering the basic BCT program. The results of cost-effectiveness analyses indicated that BCT only was more cost effective than BCT plus RP in producing abstinence from drinking, however, the two treatments were equally cost-effective when marital adjustment outcomes were considered. Since BCT only was less effective clinically than BCT plus RP in producing abstinent days, it was the lower cost of BCT only that produced its greater cost-effectiveness in relation to abstinence.

In addition, cost-benefit analyses of participants in this study also favor BCT over cognitive-behavioral individual treatment for substance abuse (Fals-Stewart, O'Farrell, & Birchler, 1997). Social costs (i.e., drug abuse-related health care, criminal justice system use, income from illegal sources, and public assistance) in the year before treatment averaged about $11,000 per case for clients in both treatment groups. In the year after treatment, social costs for the BCT group decreased significantly, to about $4,900 per case, with an average cost savings of about $6,600 per client. Similarly, results of cost-effectiveness analyses also favored the BCT group, producing significantly greater clinical improvements (e.g., fewer days of substance use) per dollar spent to deliver BCT than did individual treatment.

Children's emotional and behavioral adjustment. Over the last century, an extensive literature has evolved examining the functioning of Children of Alcoholics (COAs; for a review, see Windle and Searles, 1990). In general, these investigations have concluded COAs are more likely to experience psychosocial problems than children of nonsubstance-abusing parents. For example, COAs experience increased somatic complaints, internalizing (e.g., anxiety, depression) and externalizing behavior problems (e.g., conduct disorder, alcohol use), lower academic achievement, and lower verbal ability (e.g., Moos & Billings, 1982; Sher, 1991). Along these lines, available research also suggests that children of parents who abuse illicit drugs (i.e., Children of Substance Abusers; COSAs) display significant emotional and behavioral problems (for a review, see Johnson and Leff, 1999). In fact, preliminary studies indicate the psychosocial functioning of COSAs may be significantly worse than that of demographically matched COAs (e.g., Fals-Stewart, Kelley, Cooke, & Golden, 2003c).

Despite the emotional and behavioral problems observed among COAs, surveys of clients entering substance abuse treatment who also have custodial children suggest that these parents are very reluctant to allow their children to engage in any type of mental health treatment (Fals-Stewart et al., 2003c). Thus, the most readily available approach to improve the psychosocial functioning of these children may be by successfully treating their parents. The successful treatment of parental substance abuse (e.g., reduced substance use, improved communication, reduced conflict) may lead to secondary improvements in the lives of their children.

Kelley and Fals-Stewart (2002) completed two studies that involved a parallel replication of the same study design with alcoholic and drug-dependent male clients. In this investigation, participants were randomly assigned to one of three equally intensive outpatient treatments: (a) BCT, (b) Individual-Based Treatment (IBT), or (c) couples-based Psychoeducational Attention Control Treatment (PACT). Results in the year after treatment indicated that for both alcohol-and drug-abusing fathers, BCT improved children's functioning more than did individual-based or couple psychoeducation. Of these 3 treatments, only BCT showed reductions in the number of children with clinically significant psychosocial impairment.

HIV risk behaviors. In a recently completed investigation, Fals-Stewart and colleagues (2003a) found that roughly 40% of married or cohabiting drug-abusing men engaged in some behavior that placed them at high risk for HIV exposure (e.g., risky needle practices, unprotected sexual intercourse with a partner other than their spouse). Unfortunately, in this study, more than 70% of the wives of these men were unaware of their husbands' high risk behaviors *and* were also having unprotected sexual intercourse with their husbands. Thus, these wives were unknowingly placed at high indirect risk of exposure for HIV by their husbands. HIV risk behavior is a significant problem for both partners in these couples.

In a preliminary study, Hoebbel and Fals-Stewart (2003) found that participation in BCT significantly reduced the proportion of male partners ($N = 270$) who engaged in high risk behaviors during the year after treatment compared to an equally intensive individual-based manualized 12-step facilitation treatment (Crits-Christoph et al., 1997) or a couples-based psychoeducational attention control condition. Although roughly 40% of the male partners in each of the conditions reported engaging in one or more high-risk behaviors during the year before entering treatment, significant differences between the groups emerged during the year after treatment. Among male partners who received BCT with their wives, 19% reported they had engaged in one or more high risk behaviors during the year after treatment, compared to 33% of the male partners in both the individual counseling condition and 34% of the male partners in the attention control treatment. Mediation analyses indicated that differential improvements in dyadic adjustment and reductions in substance use (both favoring BCT over individual-based treatment and the attention control) partially explained these posttreatment group differences.

FUTURE DIRECTIONS

Important gaps in the BCT research, some of which have been recognized for many years while others have only recently been identified, are only now ready to be addressed. Investigations in the following four areas seem most pressing: (a) dissemination of BCT to community-based treatment programs; (b) exploration of the effects of BCT with dual drug-abusing couples (i.e., dyads in which both partners have current drug and/or alcohol problems) and couples in which only female partners abuse alcohol or other drugs; (c) examination of mechanisms of action underlying the effects of BCT; and (d) addition of other intervention components to standard BCT specifically targeted to enhance important secondary outcomes, particularly decreases in IPV, reductions in HIV risk behaviors, economic evaluations, and improvements in children's psychosocial adjustment.

Dissemination. Despite strong empirical support and clinical efficacy, BCT has yet to be widely adopted in community-based alcoholism and drug abuse treatment settings. Fals-Stewart and Birchler (2001) conducted a national survey of 398 randomly selected U.S. substance abuse treatment programs that treated adults to determine the proportion of settings that use different family- and couples-based therapies. Based on responses from program administrators, 27% of the facilities provided some type of service that included couples treatment, which was mostly confined to assessment. Less than 5% of the agencies used behaviorally oriented couples therapy and none used BCT specifically.

In this survey, program administrators were also queried about significant barriers to the implementation of BCT. Two primary concerns were raised: (1) BCT was viewed as too costly to deliver, requiring too many sessions in its standard form; and (2) most BCT studies used master's-level therapists as treatment providers, while most community-based treatment programs employ counselors with less formal education or clinical training. Thus, the concern was that counselors who typically work in substance abuse treatment programs could not effectively deliver BCT.

Two recently completed studies addressed each of these concerns. First, Fals-Stewart and colleagues (2001a) evaluated the effectiveness of a briefer version of BCT. Couples ($N = 80$) were randomly assigned for a 12-week period to either (a) Brief BCT (12 sessions-6 couples sessions alternating with 6 individual sessions); (b) standard BCT (24 sessions-12 BCT sessions alternating with 12 individual counseling sessions); (c) Individual-Based Treatment (IBT; 12 individual sessions); or (d) Psychoeducational Attention Control Treatment (PACT; 12 sessions-6 individual sessions alternating with 6 educational sessions for the couple). Group comparisons indicated Brief BCT and standard BCT were significantly more effective than IBT or PACT in terms of male partners' percentage of days abstinent and other outcome indicators during the year after treatment. Furthermore, Brief BCT and standard BCT produced equivalent post-treatment outcomes. A second parallel study with male drug-abusing clients produced similar findings as with the alcohol clients (Fals-Stewart et al., 2001b).

Fals-Stewart and Birchler (2002) examined the effectiveness of BCT as a function of counselors' educational background, comparing outcomes of couples randomly assigned to be treated by either bachelor's- or master's-level BCT counselors. Results for 48 alcoholic men and their female partners showed that, in comparison to master's-level counselors, bachelor's-level counselors were equivalent in terms of adherence ratings to a BCT treatment manual, but were rated lower in terms of quality of treatment delivery. However, couples who received BCT from the bachelor's-level or the master's-level counselors reported equivalent levels of (a) satisfaction with treatment, (b) relationship happiness during treatment, (c) relationship adjustment, and (d) the alcoholic clients' percentage of days abstinent at posttreatment, 3, 6, 9, and 12-month follow-ups. Along these lines, the bachelor's-level counselors reported that BCT was very easy to learn, the concepts were not difficult to understand, and that the structured therapy format provided a very clear set of guidelines for working with couples (which was a generally unfamiliar clinical subpopulation for these counselors).

The findings of these investigations suggest the primary identified barriers to BCT implementation in community-based settings (i.e., concerns about counselors with limited educational backgrounds and that BCT required too many sessions) either were not found when tested (i.e., no differential effectiveness of BCT based on counselors' educational background) or could be effectively overcome (i.e., use of an abbreviated version of BCT). Thus, the results of these studies suggest BCT could potentially be delivered effectively in the context of community-based substance abuse treatment programs.

BCT for dual substance-abusing couples. Historically, couples in which both partners have a diagnosis of an alcohol or other substance use disorder have typically been excluded from BCT clinical trials. A primary tenant of BCT as a treatment for substance abuse is that there is support within the dyadic and family systems for abstinence, particularly from the nonsubstance-abusing partner. In general, couples in which both partners abuse drugs or alcohol are almost always not supportive of abstinence.

Therefore, the problem faced by BCT investigators is that a significant proportion of married or cohabiting clients who enter substance abuse treatment are co-habitating with individuals who also have current problems with drugs or alcohol. This appears to be particularly true of women seeking treatment for substance abuse. For instance, in the Winters and colleagues (2002) study examining the effects of BCT on drug-abusing women and their nonsubstance-abusing male partners, nearly 70% of married or cohabiting substance-abusing women entering treatment at the recruitment site were excluded from the investigation because their male partners met criteria for a substance use disorder.

Although there is a paucity of research on these couples, our clinical experience with partners in these couples suggests they have fairly poor outcomes. Oftentimes, one partner's success in eliminating his or her substance use results in the dissolution of the relationship. In most instances, however, the treatment-seeking partner fails to stop drinking or using drugs and the relationship survives. The lack of support for abstinence within dual substance-abusing couples has resulted in BCT being largely ineffective with these couples.

Among these couples, the family system is strongly intertwined with the substance use behavior, with many of these couples forming drinking or drug use partnerships. In fact, for some couples, substance use often becomes the central shared recreational activity, despite its negative consequences. Barring separation or dyadic dissolution (which, in our experience, is infrequent), treatments are needed to address the family and the substance use together. A variant of BCT may be a strong candidate as an approach to address these issues among such couples. However, some modification to the standard BCT approach is clearly necessary since there is typically a lack of support for abstinence within the dyad. At present, contingency management approaches (i.e., providing voucher incentives for attendance and abstinence by both partners) are being used with these couples. Although the initial findings are encouraging, this research effort is in its infancy and more data is necessary before more definitive conclusions can be drawn.

Mediators and Moderators of Effect. Although the results of multiple randomized clinical trials demonstrate the effectiveness of BCT, no studies to date have empirically established *how* it works. More precisely, the mechanisms of action that produce the observed outcomes have not been empirically tested. As described earlier, the general theoretical rationale for the effects of BCT on substance abuse has been that certain dyadic interactions reinforce continued substance use or relapse and that relationship distress, in general, is a trigger for substance use. In turn, the BCT intervention package that has evolved from this rationale involves (a) teaching and promoting methods to reinforce abstinence from within the dyad (e.g., engaging in the Recovery Contract); (b) improving communication skills to address problems and conflict appropriately when it arises; and (c) encouraging participation in relationship enhancement exercises (e.g., Shared Rewarding Activities) to increase dyadic adjustment.

However, it is not clear which, if any, of these aspects of the BCT intervention results in the observed improvements. For example, although most BCT studies have found that participation in BCT results in improvements in relationship adjustment and reductions in substance use, none have conducted a formal test of mediation to determine if changes in relationship adjustment (i.e., either during treatment or after treatment completion) partially or fully mediate the relationship between type of treatment received (e.g., BCT, individual counseling, an attention control condition) and substance use outcomes. Indeed, it is important to highlight that most studies have generally failed to find strong relationships between theoretical mechanisms of action and subsequent outcomes, both in general psychotherapy (e.g., Orlinski, Grawe, &

Parks, 1994; Stiles & Shapiro, 1994), and in substance abuse treatment (e.g., Longabaugh & Wirtz, 2001). Thus, it is important for future studies to formally test the theoretical mechanisms thought to underlie the observed BCT effects.

Additionally, there is very little understanding of characteristics of those for whom BCT may, or may not, be effective. For example, is BCT differentially effective with male alcoholic patients versus female alcoholic patients? To date, BCT have not used a sufficient number of male and female alcoholic patients to examine these potential effects with sufficient statistical power. Moreover, much of the BCT research has been conducted with white male alcoholics; it is not clear if race or ethnicity may moderate the effects observed. Far more research is needed to examine these and other potential moderating factors.

Additions to standard BCT targeted to enhance secondary outcomes. Future research needs to examine if the effects of BCT can be enhanced by modifying the intervention to specifically target secondary outcome domains (in addition to reducing substance use and increasing relationship satisfaction). Preliminary research is currently being conducted to examine the effect of adding such circumscribed interventions to the standard BCT intervention package.

For example, Fals-Stewart, Fincham, Vendetti, and Kelley (2003b) recently completed a study exploring the impact of adding parent skills training to BCT to ascertain the effects on school-aged children living with participating parents. In this study, 72 couples, in which the male partners abused drugs and who were raising a school-aged child, were randomly assigned to one of four conditions: (a) a 24-session manualized BCT condition, consisting of 12 sessions of BCT plus 12 sessions of 12-step group drug counseling (Daley, Mercer, & Carpenter, 1998); (b) a 24-session manualized Parent Skills training plus BCT (PSBCT) condition, consisting of 6 sessions of BCT, 6 sessions of parent skills training, and 12 sessions of 12-step group drug counseling; (c) a manualized 24-session Parent Skills Training (PS) condition, consisting of 12 sessions of parent skills training and 12 sessions of group drug counseling; or (d) a manualized 24-session group drug counseling condition for the male partner only. Results indicate that the positive effects of standard BCT on children's emotional and behavioral adjustment can be enhanced with the addition of parent skills training. In addition, the results of the study have implications for similarly designed investigations exploring the effects of adding other components to standard BCT to enhance secondary outcomes of interest. Pilot studies are also underway to determine if components added to BCT designed to reduce HIV risk behaviors and IPV will also enhance the effects of standard BCT on these secondary outcomes.

CONCLUSION

From the initial small-scale pilot studies conducted in the early 1970s to the large, well-funded randomized clinical trials that are ongoing, research on BCT for substance abuse continues to evolve. What the next 30 years of BCT research holds is unclear; many of the future directions for BCT research described in this review were only identified during the last several years as the findings of new and ongoing studies were reported and illuminated new avenues to explore. Thus, based on the findings from current BCT investigations and results from studies in other disciplines, as well as changing public health priorities, the direction of BCT can and will most likely change from what has been outlined here. However, the overarching objectives of this programmatic line of research will remain unchanged, as they have been for the last quarter century. First, from a research perspective, BCT investigators will continue to modify, refine, and re-evaluate the intervention to make what is already a very effective intervention even more so. Second, from a clinical vantage point, a fundamental goal continues to be a transfer of this well-established treatment technology to standard substance abuse treatment providers to, in turn, make BCT more available to drug-and alcohol-abusing couples who are likely to benefit from participating in the program.

REFERENCES

Azrin, N. H., Sisson, R. W., Meyers, R., & Godley, M. (1982). Alcoholism treatment by disulfiram and community reinforcement therapy. *Journal of Behavior Therapy & Experimental Psychiatry, 13*, 105-112.

Bowers, T. G., & Al-Rehda, M. R. (1990). A comparison of outcome with group/marital and standard/individual therapies with alcoholics. *Journal of Studies on Alcohol, 51*, 301-309.

Crits-Christoph, P., Siqueland, L., Blaine, J., Frank, A., Luborsky, L., Onken, L. S., Muenz, L., Thase, M., Weiss, R. D., Gastfriend, D. R., Woody, G., Barber, J. P., Butler, S. F., Daley, D., Bishop, S., Najavits, L. M., Lis, J., Mercer, D., Griffin, M. L., Moras, K., & Beck, A. T. (1997). The NIDA Collaborative Cocaine Treatment Study: Rationale and Methods. *Archives of General Psychiatry, 54*, 721-726.

Daley, D., Mercer, D., & Carpenter, G. (1998). *Group drug counseling manual*. Holmes Beach, FL: Learning Publications, Inc.

Dunn, N. J., Jacob, T., Hummon, N., & Seilhamer, R. A. (1987). Marital stability in alcoholic-spouse relationships as a function of drinking pattern and location. *Journal of Abnormal Psychology, 96*, 99-107.

Fals-Stewart, W. (2003). The occurrence of interpartner violence on days of alcohol consumption: A longitudinal diary study. *Journal of Consulting & Clinical Psychology, 71*, 41-52.

Fals-Stewart, W., & Birchler, G. R. (1994). *Marital functioning among substance-abusing patients in outpatient treatment*. Poster presented at the Annual Meeting of the Association for Advancement of Behavior Therapy, San Diego, CA.

Fals-Stewart, W., & Birchler, G. R. (2001). A national survey of the use of couples therapy in substance abuse treatment. *Journal of Substance Abuse Treatment, 20*, 277-283.

Fals-Stewart, W., & Birchler, G. R. (2002). Behavioral couples therapy for alcoholic men and their intimate partners: The comparative effectiveness of master's-and bachelor's-level counselors. *Behavior Therapy, 33*, 123-147.

Fals-Stewart, W., Birchler, G. R., Hoebbel, C., Kashdan, T. B., Golden, J., & Parks, K. (2003a). An examination of the indirect risk of exposure to HIV among wives of substance-abusing men. *Drug and Alcohol Dependence, 70* (1), 65-76.

Fals-Stewart, W., Birchler, G. R., & O'Farrell, T. J. (1996). Behavioral couples therapy for male substance-abusing patients: Effects on relationship adjustment and drug-using behavior. *Journal of Consulting & Clinical Psychology, 64*, 959-972.

Fals-Stewart, W., Birchler, G. R., & O'Farrell, T. J. (1999). Drug-abusing patients and their intimate partners: Dyadic adjustment, relationship stability, and substance use. *Journal of Abnormal Psychology, 108*(1), 11-23.

Fals-Stewart, W., Birchler, G. R., & O'Farrell, T. J. (2001). Use of abbreviated couples therapy in substance abuse treatment. In J.V. Cordova (Chair), *Approaches to Brief Couples Therapy: Application and efficacy*. Symposium conducted at the World Congress of Behavioral and Cognitive Therapies, Vancouver, CA.

Fals-Stewart, W., Fincham, F., Vendetti, K., & Kelley, M. L. (2003b). *The effect of adding parent skills training to behavioral couples therapy*. Poster presented at the 110th Annual Convention of the American Psychological Association, Toronto, Ontario, CA.

Fals-Stewart, W., Kashdan, T. B., O'Farrell, T. J., & Birchler, G. R. (2002). Behavioral couples therapy for drug-abusing patients: Effects on partner violence. *Journal of Substance Abuse Treatment, 21*, 1-10.

Fals-Stewart, W., Kelley, M. L., Cooke, C. G., & Golden, J. (2003c). Predictors of the psychosocial adjustment of children living in households in which fathers abuse drugs: The effects of postnatal social exposure. *Addictive Behaviors, 28* (6), 1013-1031.

Fals-Stewart, W., O'Farrell, T.J., & Birchler, G. R. (1997). Behavioral couples therapy for male substance abusing patients: A cost outcomes analysis. *Journal of Consulting & Clinical Psychology, 65*, 789-802.

Fals-Stewart, W., O'Farrell, T. J., & Birchler, G. R. (2001a). Behavioral couples therapy for male methadone maintenance patients: Effects on drug-using behavior and relationship adjustment. *Behavior Therapy, 32*, 391-411.

Fals-Stewart, W., O'Farrell, T. J., & Birchler, G. R. (2001b). Both brief and extended behavioral couples therapy produce better outcomes than individual treatment for alcoholic patients. In T. J. O'Farrell (Chair), *Behavioral Couples Therapy for alcohol and drug problems: Recent advances.* Symposium conducted at the 24th Annual Scientific Meeting of the Research Society on Alcoholism, Montreal, CA.

Fals-Stewart, W., & O'Farrell, T. J. (2003). Behavioral family counseling and naltrexone for male opioid-dependent patients. *Journal of Consulting & Clinical Psychology, 7* (3), 432-442.

Hedberg, A. G., & Campbell, L. (1974). A comparison of four behavioral treatments of alcoholism. *Journal of Behavior Therapy & Experimental Psychiatry, 5,* 251-256.

Hoebbel, C., & Fals-Stewart, W. (2003, June). *Changes in HIV risk behaviors of husbands who participate in behavioral couples therapy.* Poster presented at the College on Problems of Drug Dependence, Boca Raton, FL

Johnson, J. L., & Leff, M. (1999). Children of substance abusers: Overview of research findings. *American Academy of Pediatrics, 103,* 1085-1099.

Kelley, M. L., & Fals-Stewart, W. (2002). Couples-versus individual-based therapy for alcoholism and drug abuse: Effects on children's psychosocial functioning. *Journal of Consulting & Clinical Psychology, 70,* 417-427.

Longabaugh, R., & Wirtz, P. W. (2001). *Project MATCH hypotheses: Results and causal chain analyses.* Project MATCH Monograph Series, Vol. 8. Bethesda, MD: National Institute on Alcohol Abuse and Alcoholism.

Maisto, S. A., O'Farrell, T. J., McKay, J., Connors, G. J., & Pelcovitz, M. A. (1988). Alcoholics' attributions of factors affecting their relapse to drinking and reasons for terminating relapse events. *Addictive Behaviors, 13,* 79-82.

McCrady, B., Stout, R., Noel, N., Abrams, D., & Nelson, H. (1991). Comparative effectiveness of three types of spouse involved alcohol treatment: Outcomes 18 months after treatment. *British Journal of Addiction, 86,* 1415-1424.

McGuire, T. (1989). Outpatient benefits for mental health services in Medicare: Alignment with the private sector? *American Psychologist, 44,* 818-824.

Moos, R. H., & Billings, A. G. (1982). Children of alcoholics during the recovery phase. Alcoholic and matched control families. *Addictive Behavior, 7,* 155-163.

Moos, R. J., Finney, J. W., & Cronkite, R. C. (1990). *Alcoholism treatment: Context, process and outcome.* New York: Oxford University Press.

O'Farrell, T. J., Choquette, K. A., Cutter, H. S. G., Brown, E. D., Bayog, R., McCourt, W., Lowe, J., Chan, A., & Deneault, P. (1996a). Cost-benefit and cost-effectiveness analyses of behavioral marital therapy with and without relapse prevention sessions for alcoholics and their spouses. *Behavior Therapy, 27,* 7-24.

O'Farrell, T. J., Choquette, K. A., Cutter, H. S. G., Floyd, F. J., Bayog, R. D., Brown, E. D., Lowe, J., Chan, A., & Deneault, P. (1996b). Cost-benefit and cost-effectiveness analyses of behavioral marital therapy as an addition to outpatient alcoholism treatment. *Journal of Substance Abuse, 8,* 145-166.

O'Farrell, T. J., & Fals-Stewart, W. (2003). Alcohol abuse. *Journal of Marital & Family Therapy, 29,* 97-120.

O'Farrell, T. J., Fals-Stewart, W., Murphy, M., & Murphy, C. M. (2003). Partner violence before and after individually-based alcoholism treatment for male alcoholic patients. *Journal of Consulting & Clinical Psychology, 71,* 92-102.

Orlinski, D. E., Grawe, K., & Parks, B. K. (1994). Process and outcome in psychotherapy-Noch einmal. In A. E. Bergin, & S. L. Garfield (Eds.), *Handbook of psychotherapy and behavior change* (pp. 270-283). New York: Wiley.

Sher, K. J. (1991). *Children of alcoholics.* Chicago: University of Chicago Press.

Stanton, M. D., and Shadish, W. R. (1997). Outcome, attrition, and family-couple treatment for drug abuse: A meta-analysis and review of the controlled, comparative studies. *Psychological Bulletin, 122* (2), 170-191.

Stiles, W. B., & Shapiro, D. A. (1994). Disabuse of the drug metaphor: Psychotherapy process-outcome correlation. *Journal of Consulting & Clinical Psychology, 62,* 942-948.

Windle, M., & Searles, J. S. (1990). *Children of alcoholics: Critical perspectives.* New York: The Guildford Press.

Winters, J., Fals-Stewart, W., O'Farrell, T. J., Birchler, G. R., & Kelley, M. L. (2002). Behavioral couples therapy for female substance-abusing patients: Effects on substance use and relationship adjustment. *Journal of Consulting & Clinical Psychology, 70,* 344-355.

Yates, B. T. (1994). Toward the incorporation of costs, cost-effectiveness analysis, and cost-benefit analysis into clinical research. *Journal of Consulting & Clinical Psychology, 62,* 729-736.

Index

Numbers followed by "t" indicate tabular material.

AA. *See* Alcoholics Anonymous (AA)
Abstinence, 97,104,201
    as sole indicator of treatment
        success, 194
    substance abuse prevention
        programs and, 92,93
Abstinence Trust Discussion, 238-239
Abstinence violation effect, 193-194
Adapted Motivational Interviewing
    (AMI), 58-59. *See also*
    Motivational interviewing
    (MI)
Addiction Severity Index, 117
Adolescents. *See also* Juvenile
    offenders
    alcohol and, 176
    attachment and alcohol and drug
        use by, 178-179
    with conduct disorder, 80-82
    development of self-concept for,
        94-95
    group therapy for, 80
    substance abuse and,
        92-93,156,176,208-209
Advice, in articles on motivational
    interviewing, 67-68
Alcoholics Anonymous (AA), 20. *See*
    also Alcohol treatment;
    Twelve-Step Program of
    Alcoholics Anonymous
    effectiveness of, 197
    faith-related service settings of,
        27-28

    spiritual and religious aspects of,
        21-24
Alcoholism. *See also* Children of
    Alcoholics (COAs)
    disease attributions of, 22
    drinking goals and, 196
    harm reduction approaches to, 26
    holistic models for treating, 22-23
    individual variation and, 194-196
    Rational Recovery approach to, 26
    as relapsing condition, 193-194
Alcohol Skills Training Program
    (ASTP), 100-101
Alcohol treatment. *See also* Relapse
    approaches to, 197-200
    non-confrontational, client-focused
        approaches to, 197
    relapse prevention for, 197-198
    resistance and, 192
    spending on, 192
Alcohol Use Disorders Identification
    Test (AUDIT),
        139,141,148-149,150,153-
        154
AMI. *See* Adapted Motivational
    Interviewing (AMI)
Antisocial behavior, 83-84
Assessment instruments. *See* Rapid
    assessment instruments
ASTP (Alcohol Skills Training
    Program), 100-101
Attachment theory, 177-178
    adolescent alcohol and drug use,
        178-179

    257

BOOK ORDER FORM!

Order a copy of this book with this form or online at:
http://www.haworthpress.com/store/product.asp?sku=5584

Addiction, Assessment, and Treatment
with Adolescents, Adults, and Families

____ in softbound at $34.95 ISBN-13: 978-0-7890-2887-7. / ISBN-10: 0-7890-2887-5.
____ in hardbound at $59.95 ISBN-13: 978-0-7890-2886-0. / ISBN-10: 0-7890-2886-7.

COST OF BOOKS _____

POSTAGE & HANDLING _____
US: $4.00 for first book & $1.50
for each additional book
Outside US: $5.00 for first book
& $2.00 for each additional book.

SUBTOTAL _____

In Canada: add 7% GST. _____

STATE TAX _____
CA, IL, IN, MN, NJ, NY, OH, PA & SD residents
please add appropriate local sales tax.

FINAL TOTAL _____
If paying in Canadian funds, convert
using the current exchange rate,
UNESCO coupons welcome.

❑ BILL ME LATER:
Bill-me option is good on US/Canada/
Mexico orders only; not good to jobbers,
wholesalers, or subscription agencies.

❑ Signature _____

❑ Payment Enclosed: $ _____

❑ PLEASE CHARGE TO MY CREDIT CARD:

❑ Visa ❑ MasterCard ❑ AmEx ❑ Discover
❑ Diner's Club ❑ Eurocard ❑ JCB

Account # _____

Exp Date _____

Signature _____
(Prices in US dollars and subject to change without notice.)

PLEASE PRINT ALL INFORMATION OR ATTACH YOUR BUSINESS CARD

Name

Address

City   State/Province   Zip/Postal Code

Country

Tel   Fax

E-Mail

May we use your e-mail address for confirmations and other types of information? ❑ Yes ❑ No We appreciate receiving
your e-mail address. Haworth would like to e-mail special discount offers to you, as a preferred customer.
We will never share, rent, or exchange your e-mail address. We regard such actions as an invasion of your privacy.

Order from your **local bookstore** or directly from
The Haworth Press, Inc. 10 Alice Street, Binghamton, New York 13904-1580 • USA
Call our toll-free number (1-800-429-6784) / Outside US/Canada: (607) 722-5857
Fax: 1-800-895-0582 / Outside US/Canada: (607) 771-0012
E-mail your order to us: orders@haworthpress.com

For orders outside US and Canada, you may wish to order through your local
sales representative, distributor, or bookseller.
For information, see http://haworthpress.com/distributors

(Discounts are available for individual orders in US and Canada only, not booksellers/distributors.)

Please photocopy this form for your personal use.
www.HaworthPress.com